Substance Use and Addiction Medicine

Editors

JEFFREY H. SAMET
PATRICK G. O'CONNOR
MICHAEL D. STEIN

MEDICAL CLINICS
OF NORTH AMERICA

www.medical.theclinics.com

Consulting Editor
BIMAL H. ASHAR

July 2018 • Volume 102 • Number 4

ELSEVIER

1600 John F. Kennedy Boulevard ● Suite 1800 ● Philadelphia, Pennsylvania, 19103-2899

http://www.theclinics.com

MEDICAL CLINICS OF NORTH AMERICA Volume 102, Number 4
July 2018 ISSN 0025-7125, ISBN-13: 978-0-323-61066-7

Editor: Jessica McCool
Developmental Editor: Kristen Helm

Medical Clinics of North America (ISSN 0025-7125) is published bimonthly by Elsevier Inc., 360 Park Avenue South, New York, NY 10010-1710. Months of publication are January, March, May, July, September, and November. Business and editorial offices: 1600 John F. Kennedy Boulevard, Suite 1800, Philadelphia, PA 19103-2899. Periodicals postage paid at New York, NY, and additional mailing offices. Subscription prices are USD $273.00 per year (US individuals), $574.00 per year (US institutions), $100.00 per year (US Students), $336.00 per year (Canadian individuals), $746.00 per year (Canadian institutions), $200.00 per year (Canadian and foreign students), $402.00 per year (foreign individuals), and $746.00 per year (foreign institutions). To receive student/resident rate, orders must be accompanied by name of affiliated institution, date of term, and the signature of program/residency coordinator on institution letterhead. Orders will be billed at individual rate until proof of status is received. Foreign air speed delivery is included in all Clinics' subscription prices. All prices are subject to change without notice. **POSTMASTER:** Send address changes to *Medical Clinics of North America*, Elsevier Health Sciences Division, Subscription Customer Service, 3251 Riverport Lane, Maryland Heights, MO 63043. **Customer Service: Telephone: 1-800-654-2452** (U.S. and Canada); **1-314-447-8871** (outside U.S. and Canada). **Fax: 314-447-8029. E-mail: journalscustomerserviceusa@elsevier.com** (for print support); **journalsonlinesupport-usa@elsevier.com** (for online support).

Reprints. For copies of 100 or more of articles in this publication, please contact the Commercial Reprints Department, Elsevier Inc., 360 Park Avenue South, New York, NY 10010-1710. Tel.: 212-633-3874; Fax: 212-633-3820; E-mail: reprints@elsevier.com.

Medical Clinics of North America is also published in Spanish by McGraw-Hill Interamericana Editores S. A., P.O. Box 5-237, 06500 Mexico, D.F., Mexico.

Medical Clinics of North America is covered in *MEDLINE/PubMed (Index Medicus), Current Contents, ASCA, Excerpta Medica, Science Citation Index,* and *ISI/BIOMED.*

and is not intended to promote off-label use of these medications. If you have any questions, contact the medical affairs department of the manufacturer for the most recent prescribing information.

TO ENROLL
To enroll in the *Medical Clinics of North America* Continuing Medical Education program, call customer service at 1-800-654-2452 or sign up online at http://www.theclinics.com/home/cme. The CME program is available to subscribers for an additional annual fee of USD $300.90.

METHOD OF PARTICIPATION
In order to claim credit, participants must complete the following:
1. Complete enrolment as indicated above.
2. Read the activity.
3. Complete the CME Test and Evaluation. Participants must achieve a score of 70% on the test. All CME Tests and Evaluations must be completed online.

CME INQUIRIES/SPECIAL NEEDS
For all CME inquiries or special needs, please contact elsevierCME@elsevier.com.

Contributors

CONSULTING EDITOR

BIMAL H. ASHAR, MD, MBA, FACP
Associate Professor of Medicine, Division of General Internal Medicine, Johns Hopkins University School of Medicine, Baltimore, Maryland, USA

EDITORS

JEFFREY H. SAMET, MD, MA, MPH
Chief, General Internal Medicine, John Noble MD Professor in General Internal Medicine and Professor of Public Health, Clinical Addiction Research and Education Unit, Section of General Internal Medicine, Department of Medicine, Boston University School of Medicine, Boston Medical Center, Department of Community Health Sciences, Boston University School of Public Health, Boston, Massachusetts, USA

PATRICK G. O'CONNOR, MD
Dan Adams and Amanda Adams Professor of General Medicine, Chief, General Internal Medicine, Yale University School of Medicine, Yale-New Haven Hospital, Yale University, New Haven, Connecticut, USA

MICHAEL D. STEIN, MD
Professor and Chair, Department of Health Law, Policy, and Management, Boston University School of Public Health, Boston, Massachusetts, USA

AUTHORS

ANA ABRANTES, PhD
Butler Hospital, Behavioral Medicine and Addictions Research, Butler, Pennsylvania, USA; Department of Psychiatry and Human Behavior, The Warren Alpert Medical School of Brown University, Providence, Rhode Island, USA

SARAH M. BAGLEY, MD, MSc
Division of General Pediatrics, Department of Pediatrics, Section of General Internal Medicine, Department of Medicine, Boston University School of Medicine, Departments of Pediatrics and Medicine, Boston Medical Center, Grayken Center for Addiction, Boston, Massachusetts

WILLIAM C. BECKER, MD
Core Investigator, Opioid Reassessment Clinic, VA Connecticut Healthcare System, Pain Research, Informatics, Multimorbidities and Education (PRIME) Center, West Haven, Connecticut, USA; Assistant Professor, Department of Medicine, Yale School of Medicine, New Haven, Connecticut, USA

INGRID A. BINSWANGER, MD, MPH, MS
Senior Investigator, Institute for Health Research, Kaiser Permanente Colorado,
Associate Professor, Department of Medicine, Division of General Internal Medicine,
University of Colorado, Aurora, Colorado, USA

MEGAN E. BURESH, MD
Division of Chemical Dependence, Johns Hopkins University School of Medicine,
Baltimore, Maryland, USA

DEEPA R. CAMENGA, MD, MHS
Assistant Professor of Emergency Medicine, Yale School of Medicine, New Haven,
Connecticut, USA

NICHOLAS CHADI, MD
Adolescent Substance Use and Addiction Program, Division of Developmental
Medicine, Department of Pediatrics, Boston Children's Hospital, Harvard Medical School,
Boston, Massachusetts

SUBHAJIT CHAKRAVORTY, MD
Assistant Professor of Psychiatry, Perelman School of Medicine, Corporal Michael J.
Crescenz VA Medical Center, Philadelphia, Pennsylvania, USA

KAREN J. DEREFINKO, PhD
Assistant Professor, The University of Tennessee Health Science Center, Memphis,
Tennessee, USA

E. JENNIFER EDELMAN, MD, MHS
Yale University School of Medicine and Public Health, New Haven, Connecticut, USA

NADIA FAIRBAIRN, MD
British Columbia Centre on Substance Use, St. Paul's Hospital, Department of Medicine,
University of British Columbia, Vancouver, British Columbia, Canada

CHRISTOPHER FAIRGRIEVE, MD
Department of Family Medicine, University of British Columbia, St. Paul's
Hospital, British Columbia Centre on Substance Use, Vancouver, British Columbia,
Canada

RYAN GRADDY, MD
Division of Chemical Dependence, Johns Hopkins University School of Medicine,
Baltimore, Maryland, USA

SCOTT E. HADLAND, MD, MPH, MS
Division of General Pediatrics, Department of Pediatrics, Section of General Internal
Medicine, Department of Medicine, Boston University School of Medicine, Boston,
Massachusetts

SEAN HE, BS
Student, Post-baccalaureate Studies Program, College of Liberal Arts and Professional
Studies, University of Pennsylvania, Corporal Michael J. Crescenz VA Medical Center,
Philadelphia, Pennsylvania, USA

STEPHEN R. HOLT, MD, MS, FACP
Assistant Professor of Medicine, Department of Internal Medicine, Yale University School
of Medicine, New Haven, Connecticut, USA

ANNIE LÉVESQUE, MD, MSc
Assistant Professor, Icahn School of Medicine at Mount Sinai, Department of Psychiatry, Mount Sinai West Hospital, New York, New York, USA

BERNARD LE FOLL, MD, PhD
Head, Translational Addiction Research Laboratory, Medical Head of Addiction Medicine Service, Addiction Division, Centre for Addiction and Mental Health (CAMH), Professor, Departments of Pharmacology and Toxicology, Psychiatry, Family and Community Medicine, Institute of Medical Sciences, University of Toronto, Toronto, Ontario, Canada

AJAY MANHAPRA, MD
Research Scientist, Veteran Affairs New England Mental Illness Research, Education and Clinical Center (MIRECC), West Haven, Connecticut, USA; Lead Physician, Advanced PACT Pain Clinic, VA Hampton Medical Center, Hampton, Virginia, USA; Lecturer, Department of Psychiatry, Yale School of Medicine, New Haven, Connecticut, USA

SEONAID NOLAN, MD
Clinician Researcher, British Columbia Centre on Substance Use, St. Paul's Hospital, Clinical Assistant Professor, Department of Medicine, University of British Columbia, Vancouver, British Columbia, Canada

BENJAMIN J. OLDFIELD, MD
National Clinician Scholars Program, Yale University School of Medicine, New Haven, Connecticut, USA

CHRISTINE A. PACE, MD, MSc
Assistant Professor of Medicine, Section of General Internal Medicine, Boston University School of Medicine, Boston Medical Center, Boston, Massachusetts, USA

STEPHANIE LEE PEGLOW, DO, MPH
Assistant Professor, Department of Psychiatry and Behavioral Sciences, Norfolk, Virginia, USA

DARIUS A. RASTEGAR, MD
Division of Chemical Dependence, Johns Hopkins University School of Medicine, Baltimore, Maryland, USA

FRANCISCO I. SALGADO GARCÍA, PhD
The University of Tennessee Health Science Center, Memphis, Tennessee, USA

JEFFREY H. SAMET, MD, MA, MPH
Chief, General Internal Medicine, John Noble MD Professor in General Internal Medicine and Professor of Public Health, Clinical Addiction Research and Education Unit, Section of General Internal Medicine, Department of Medicine, Boston University School of Medicine, Boston Medical Center, Department of Community Health Sciences, Boston University School of Public Health, Boston, Massachusetts, USA

MICHAEL D. STEIN, MD
Professor and Chair, Department of Health Law, Policy, and Management, Boston University School of Public Health, Boston, Massachusetts, USA

DANIEL D. SUMROK, MD, FAAFP, DABAM, DFASAM
Assistant Professor, The University of Tennessee Health Science Center, Memphis, Tennessee, USA

JEANETTE M. TETRAULT, MD
Department of Internal Medicine, Yale University School of Medicine, New Haven, Connecticut, USA

HILARY A. TINDLE, MD, MPH
Associate Professor of Medicine, Vanderbilt University Medical Center, Nashville, Tennessee, USA

DANIEL G. TOBIN, MD, FACP
Associate Professor of Medicine, Department of Internal Medicine, Yale University School of Medicine, New Haven, Connecticut, USA

BABAK TOFIGHI, MD, MSc
Assistant Professor, Department of Population Health, Division of General Internal Medicine, New York University School of Medicine, New York, New York, USA

LISA A. UEBELACKER, PhD
Associate Professor (Research), Departments of Psychiatry and Human Behavior, and Family Medicine, The Warren Alpert Medical School of Brown University, Providence, Rhode Island, USA; Assistant Director, Psychosocial Research, Butler Hospital, Butler, Pennsylvania, USA

RYAN G. VANDREY, PhD
Associate Professor of Psychiatry and Behavioral Sciences, Behavioral Pharmacology Research Unit, Johns Hopkins University School of Medicine, Baltimore, Maryland, USA

SARAH E. WAKEMAN, MD
Assistant Professor, Department of Medicine, Harvard Medical School, Massachusetts General Hospital, Boston, Massachusetts, USA

ZOE M. WEINSTEIN, MD, MS
Assistant Professor, Department of Medicine, Boston University School of Medicine, Boston Medical Center, Boston, Massachusetts, USA

Contents

> Unhealthy substance use is common in primary care populations and is a major contributor to morbidity and mortality. Two key strategies to address unhealthy substance use in primary care are the process of screening, brief intervention, and referral to treatment (SBIRT) and integration of treatment for substance use disorders into primary care. Implementation of SBIRT requires buy-in from practice leaders, careful planning, and staff and primary care provider training. Primary care–based treatment of opioid and alcohol use disorders can be effective; more data are needed to better understand the benefits of these models and identify means of treating other substance use disorders in primary care.

> Substance use disorders are highly prevalent and are a large driver of costly inpatient medical care; however, historically the substance use disorder has gone unaddressed during an inpatient stay. Inpatient addiction consult services are an important intervention to use the reachable moment of hospitalization to engage patients and initiate addiction treatment. Addiction consultation involves taking an addiction-specific history, motivational interviewing, withdrawal symptom management, and initiation of long-term pharmacotherapy. Addiction consult services have the potential to decrease readmissions and utilization costs for medical systems and improve substance-related outcomes for patients.

> Adolescents and young adults (AYAs) have unique needs and important biopsychosocial differences when compared with older adults who use substances. As their brains continue to develop, youth are especially susceptible to the reinforcing effects of substances in the context of a still-developing capacity for executive control and decision making. In this article, the authors highlight key differences in the neurobiologic, epidemiologic, and relational aspects of substance use found in AYA. They also discuss how best to engage with youth who use substances and how

prevention and intervention can be adapted for optimal effectiveness for this distinct and high-risk population.

Drawing from existing opioid prescribing guidelines, this article describes how medical providers can reduce the risk of overdose. Through primary prevention, providers can prevent initial exposure and associated risks by educating patients, using risk stratification, minimizing opioid dose and duration, and avoiding coprescribing with sedatives. Secondary prevention efforts include monitoring patients with urine toxicology and prescription monitoring programs and screening for opioid use disorders. Tertiary prevention includes treating opioid use disorders and providing naloxone to prevent overdose death. Specific preventive strategies may be required for those with psychiatric disorders or substance use disorders, adolescents, the elderly, and pregnant women.

Primary care is an important setting for delivering evidence-based treatment to address substance use disorders. To date, effective approaches to treat, care largely incorporate pharmacotherapy with counseling-based interventions and rely on multidisciplinary teams. There is strong support for primary care–based approaches to address alcohol and opioid use disorder, with growing data focused on people living with human immunodeficiency virus and those experiencing incarceration. Future work should focus on the implementation of these effective approaches to decrease health disparities among people with substance use and to identify optimal approaches to address substance use in primary care and specialty settings.

Alcohol use disorder is a common, destructive, and undertreated disease. As understanding of alcohol use disorder has evolved, so has our ability to manage patients with pharmacotherapeutic agents in addition to nondrug therapy, including various counseling strategies. Providers now have a myriad of medications, both approved and not approved by the US Food and Drug Administration, to choose from and can personalize care based on treatment goals, comorbidities, drug interactions, and drug availability. This article explores these treatment options and offers the prescriber practical advice regarding when each option may or may not be appropriate for a specific patient.

Cannabis (marijuana) is a drug product derived from the plant *Cannabis sativa*. Cannabinoid is a general term for all chemical constituents of the cannabis plant. Legalization of marijuana in numerous US states, the availability of cannabis of higher potency, and the emergence of synthetic cannabinoids may have contributed to the increased demand for related medical services. The most effective available treatments for cannabis use disorder are psychosocial approaches. There is no pharmacotherapy-approved treatment. This article reviews the current state of knowledge regarding effective treatments for cannabis use disorder.

Despite the availability of effective medications and psychosocial interventions for the management of a substance use disorder, some individuals repeatedly fail the most aggressive treatment regimens. For such individuals, alternative treatment options exist seeking to mitigate the negative consequences of the use of harmful substances. Participation in a managed alcohol program, the use of sustained-release oral morphine or injectable opioid agonist treatment, or the creation of safe injecting facilities are examples of such nonstandard approaches. This article reviews the available evidence of these treatment modalities.

Several novel psychoactive substances have emerged in recent years. Users are typically young men who use other substances. In the category of stimulants, cathinones ("bath salts") have predominated and can lead to agitation, psychosis, hyperthermia, and death. Synthetic cannabinoids ("spice") are more potent than marijuana and can lead to agitation, psychosis, seizures, and death. There are no rapid tests to identify these substances, and general treatment includes benzodiazepines for agitation and supportive therapy. Many synthetic opioids are potent analogues of fentanyl and carry a high risk of overdose. In addition, there are several designer benzodiazepines that have emerged.

The burden of alcohol and drug use disorders (substance use disorders [SUDs]) has intensified efforts to expand access to cost-effective psychosocial interventions and pharmacotherapies. This article provides an overview of technology-based interventions (eg, computer-based and Web-based interventions, text messaging, interactive voice recognition, smartphone apps, and emerging technologies) that are extending the reach of effective addiction treatments both in substance use treatment and primary care settings. It discusses the efficacy of existing technology-based interventions for SUDs, prospects for emerging technologies, and special considerations when integrating technologies in primary care (eg, privacy and regulatory protocols) to enhance the management of SUDs.

> Sleep and substance use disorders commonly co-occur. Insomnia is commonly associated with the use of and withdrawal from substances. Circadian rhythm abnormalities are being increasingly linked with psychoactive substance use. Other sleep disorders, such as sleep-related breathing disorder, should be considered in the differential diagnosis of insomnia, especially in those with opioid use or alcohol use disorder. Insomnia that is brief or occurs in the context of active substance use is best treated by promoting abstinence. A referral to a sleep medicine clinic should be considered for those with chronic insomnia or when another intrinsic sleep disorder is suspected.

> The current opioid crisis highlights an urgent need for better paradigms for prevention and treatment of chronic pain and addiction. Although many approach this complex clinical condition with the question "Is this pain or is this addiction?" it is more than the sum of its parts. Chronic pain among those with dependence and addiction often evolves into a complex disabling condition with pain at multiple sites, psychosocial dysfunctions, medical and psychiatric disorders, polypharmacy, and polysubstance use, all interacting with each other in complex ways (multimorbidity). The authors offer an integrative therapeutic approach to manage this complex clinical scenario.

> This article reviews the current evidence on electronic cigarette (e-cigarette) safety and efficacy for smoking cessation, with a focus on smokers with cardiovascular disease, pulmonary disease, or serious mental illness. In the United States, adult smokers use e-cigarettes primarily to quit or reduce cigarette smoking. An understanding of the potential risks and benefits of e-cigarette use may help clinicians counsel smokers about the potential impact of e-cigarettes on health.

> This article summarizes the literature regarding the similar biopsychosocial mechanisms of tobacco use and alcohol and substance use disorders and the evidence for and against the provision of tobacco cessation for those in treatment for alcohol and substance use disorders. The practicality of treatment, focusing on methods, timing, and breadth of intervention strategies, is also presented. Common methodologies that may be used across tobacco use and alcohol and substance use disorder to prevent lapse and relapse are discussed. Physicians can and should adhere to the policy that tobacco use is a common and dangerous comorbid condition that demands concomitant treatment.

MEDICAL CLINICS OF NORTH AMERICA

Foreword

More than "Just Say No"

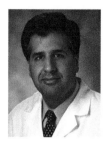

Bimal H. Ashar, MD, MBA, FACP
Consulting Editor

In 2001, the Joint Commission on the Accreditation of Healthcare Organizations issued standards for hospitals designed to draw attention to the underassessment and undertreatment of pain. Many organizations reacted by adopting the "5th vital sign" of pain assessment. The Wong-Baker FACES Pain Rating scale was used widely by practices to identify the pain status in all patients. Narcotic prescriptions, which had already been rising, increased even further as providers were "educated" by pharmaceutical companies as to the safety of opioids. Physicians welcomed having something "safe and effective" in their armamentarium to help relieve their patients' suffering. It took more than a decade to realize the harms from chronic opioid use. The Centers for Disease Control and Prevention estimates that in 2016 more than 2 million Americans suffered from substance use disorders related to prescription opioid pain relievers and more than 60,000 people in the United States died of an opioid overdose. In October of 2017, President Trump directed the Department of Health and Human Services to declare the opioid crisis a "public health emergency." He went on to say that the government would initiate "really tough, really big, really great advertising" aimed at persuading Americans not to start taking drugs. "This was an idea that I had, where if we can teach young people not to take drugs," the President said, "it's really, really easy not to take them."

Despite the recent focus on narcotic use and abuse, other substances continue to negatively impact health. It is estimated that 80% of the more than 21 million Americans suffering from a substance abuse disorder have an alcohol use disorder. Providers are often uncomfortable dealing with such disorders and/or feel limited in their ability to address the psychosocial issues surrounding the abuse. Physicians appear to be more comfortable assessing and addressing tobacco use. Despite this, tobacco use continues to be the leading cause of preventable death in the United States.

Although it would be great if the entire population "just said no" to abusing substances, it seems unrealistic. Physicians need to know how to assist patients in dealing

Med Clin N Am 102 (2018) xv–xvi
https://doi.org/10.1016/j.mcna.2018.04.002
0025-7125/18/© 2018 Published by Elsevier Inc.

medical.theclinics.com

with their addiction. In this issue of the *Medical Clinics of North America*, Drs Samet, O'Connor, and Stein enlisted experts to assist clinicians in identifying, assessing, and treating substance abuse disorders. In addition to focusing on tobacco, alcohol, and opioids, the authors have also addressed issues relating to newer popular potential agents for abuse, including novel drugs and e-cigarettes.

Bimal H. Ashar, MD, MBA, FACP
Division of General Internal Medicine
Johns Hopkins University School of Medicine
601 North Caroline Street
#7143
Baltimore, MD 21287, USA

E-mail address:
Bashar1@jhmi.edu

Preface

The Internist's Challenge: Addressing Our Patients' Unhealthy Substance Use

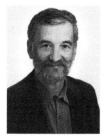 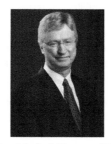 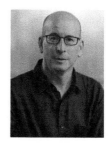

Jeffrey H. Samet, MD, MA, MPH   Patrick G. O'Connor, MD   Michael D. Stein, MD

Editors

The first two decades of the twenty-first century will be remembered as the time when the harm of illicit drug use, longstanding cause of substantial morbidity and mortality, gained the undivided attention of North Americans due to a devastating opioid crisis. Remarkably, the adverse consequences of opioids and other drugs are an almost-daily feature in the media as deaths from overdoses mount. At the same time, legal substances, alcohol and tobacco, continue to quietly but dreadfully leave even greater overall health consequences in their wake. Other substances without clear medication treatments increasingly produce negative health effects (eg, cannabinoids, stimulants, and designer drugs).

To address the harm caused by these substances, new opportunities have emerged to identify and engage individuals at risk, prevent substance use-related consequences, and optimize treatment for those seeking help for problems caused by substance use. To highlight these efforts, articles in this issue of *Medical Clinics of North America* describe medical innovations and models of treatment to advance substance use care in the following domains: engaging patients when they are hospitalized; providing addiction treatment within primary care clinics and other general medical settings; increasing clinicians' awareness of the scope of addiction-related problems, such as sleep disruption; considering novel approaches for those who have failed traditional treatments, including adolescents and young adults as a group with special needs; and using new technologies to achieve addiction treatment goals.

In 2016 the American Board of Medical Specialties established Addiction Medicine as a new subspecialty. Soon after, the accreditation council for graduate medical education approved fellowship training in addition. Since then, over 50 Addiction Medicine Fellowship programs have taken shape. Addiction Medicine subspecialty-trained

Med Clin N Am 102 (2018) xvii–xviii
https://doi.org/10.1016/j.mcna.2018.04.001
0025-7125/18/© 2018 Published by Elsevier Inc.

physicians can assist general internists, family physicians, psychiatrists, and physicians from all medical specialties in the treatment of complicated patients who are suffering from addiction and its consequences. The expansion and dispersion of an addiction-trained workforce, often integrated into general treatment settings, offer new hope for millions of North Americans and substance users worldwide.

This is an incredibly exciting time in medicine. Medications to address addictive disorders are now available and have been tested in clinical trials. Physicians are working in new teams and configurations with greater attention to the breadth of addiction's effects. Health system administrators are becoming aware of the health and cost benefits of assisting substance-using patients at every contact point. The notion that Addiction Medicine addresses mainstream medical problems that demand the attention of all generalist physicians is becoming the norm. This timely issue of *Medical Clinics of North America*, Substance Use and Addiction Medicine, will serve as a resource to all who want to provide medical care around these important issues in a well-informed and effective manner.

We very much appreciate the support of Katherine Calver, PhD, who worked with the editors and authors to produce the high quality articles in this volume of Medical Clinics of North America.

Jeffrey H. Samet, MD, MA, MPH
General Internal Medicine
Boston University Schools of
Medicine & Public Health
Boston Medical Center
801 Massachusetts Avenue, 2nd Floor
Boston, MA 02118, USA

Patrick G. O'Connor, MD
General Internal Medicine
Yale University School of Medicine
Yale-New Haven Hospital
Yale University
PO Box 208056
333 Cedar Street
New Haven, CT 06520-8056, USA

Michael D. Stein, MD
Health Law, Policy & Management
Boston University School of Public Health
715 Albany Street
Boston, MA 02118, USA

E-mail addresses:
jsamet@bu.edu (J.H. Samet)
patrick.oconnor@yale.edu (P.G. O'Connor)
mdstein@bu.edu (M.D. Stein)

Addressing Unhealthy Substance Use in Primary Care

Christine A. Pace, MD, MSc[a,*], Lisa A. Uebelacker, PhD[b,c,d]

KEYWORDS

- Screening and brief intervention • Collaborative care • Behavioral health integration
- Medication-assisted treatment

KEY POINTS

- Unhealthy substance use is a major contributor to morbidity, mortality, and health care costs, and is common in primary care populations.
- Many barriers have prevented primary care providers from adequately identifying and responding to it.
- Screening, brief intervention, and referral to treatment in primary care can reduce unhealthy alcohol use.
- Primary care–based treatment of opioid and alcohol use disorders can be effective, with collaborative care models showing particular promise; more data are needed to better understand the benefits of these models and to identify means of treating other substance use disorders in primary care.

INTRODUCTION

Unhealthy substance use is defined as a level of substance use that can incur health consequences, and includes both risky use that does not meet substance use disorder (SUD) criteria, as well as use that reflects an SUD (**Fig. 1**). Unhealthy substance use is among the most common preventable causes of death, contributes to significant morbidity,[1] is a driver of health care–related and societal costs,[1] and is prevalent among patients seen in primary care settings.[2,3] SUDs have much in common with the

Disclosure: Dr C. Pace has no relationship with a commercial company that has a direct financial interest in the subject matter or materials discussed in this article or with a company making a competing product. Dr L. Uebelacker's spouse is employed by Abbvie Pharmaceuticals. Dr C. Pace receives support from a Health Resources and Services Administration award (K02HP30814).
[a] Section of General Internal Medicine, Boston University School of Medicine, Boston Medical Center, 801 Massachusetts Avenue, 2nd Floor, Boston, MA 02118, USA; [b] Department of Psychiatry and Human Behavior, Warren Alpert School of Medicine, Brown University, Box G-BH, 700 Butler Drive, Providence, RI 02906, USA; [c] Department of Family Medicine, Brown University, Memorial Hospital of RI, 111 Brewster Street, Pawtucket, RI 02860, USA; [d] Psychosocial Research, Butler Hospital, 345 Blackstone Boulevard Providence, RI 02906, USA
* Corresponding author.
E-mail address: Christine.Pace@bmc.org

https://doi.org/10.1016/j.mcna.2018.02.004
0025-7125/18/© 2018 Elsevier Inc. All rights reserved.
medical.theclinics.com

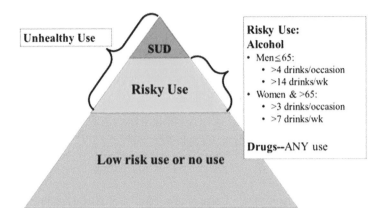

Fig. 1. Unhealthy substance use. (*Adapted from* Pace CA, Samet JH. In the clinic. Substance use disorders. Ann Intern Med 2016;164(7):ITC49-ITC64 Copyright © 2016; American College of Physicians. All Rights Reserved. Reprinted with the permission of American College of Physicians, Inc.)

chronic conditions, such as diabetes, hypertension, and asthma, that primary care providers (PCPs) routinely manage. SUDs have a biological basis in that genetics contribute to SUD risk and use of substances may result in persistent brain changes.[4] SUDs can require lifelong management, often including medication such as buprenorphine, and self-management and behavior change is essential in recovery.[5]

Despite the prevalence and chronicity of unhealthy substance use and SUDs, PCPs do not consistently embrace identification, evaluation, and management of these conditions. Reasons may include the historical separation between general medical and addiction services[6]; concerns about confidentiality and federal law[7]; barriers to reimbursement for substance use treatment[8]; PCPs' perception of a lack of adequate clinic staff to support work with patients with SUDs[9]; limited SUD resources in the community[10]; lack of PCP education about unhealthy substance use[8]; and persistent stigma on the part of health care providers[11] as well as patients, who may be reluctant to disclose use to their medical providers. Although many of these barriers apply to mental health care as well, overall primary care has more readily embraced integration of mental health services than substance use services.[10]

There is increasing interest in overcoming these barriers. The opioid epidemic in particular has shed light on the paucity of easily accessed substance use treatment, and on the role for medication treatment of opioid use disorders in primary care and other ambulatory settings.[12] Concurrently, alternative health care payment models have drawn increased attention to the cost-savings potential of addressing unhealthy substance use in primary care.[13]

What evidence justifies the resources and culture change needed to advance primary care's engagement with unhealthy substance use, and how can such resources be deployed? This article reviews the evidence base for key strategies through which unhealthy substance use can be identified and addressed in the primary care setting, and identifies key steps in implementation. It focuses on screening, brief intervention and referral to treatment (SBIRT) and the integration of SUD treatment into primary care through models such as collaborative care.

DEFINITION AND PREVALENCE OF UNHEALTHY SUBSTANCE USE IN PRIMARY CARE

Alcohol is the most widely consumed drug of unhealthy use in the United States. Like all unhealthy substance use, unhealthy alcohol use encompasses a spectrum from risky use alone (ie, without symptoms or impairment sufficient to meet Diagnostic and Statistical Manual of Mental Disorders, Fifth revision (DSM-V) criteria for alcohol use disorder[5]) to an alcohol use disorder (see **Fig. 1**). As defined in the United States, for men 65 years of age and younger, unhealthy use means more than 4 drinks per occasion or more than 14 drinks per week; for women and for men more than 65 years old, unhealthy use is defined as more than 3 drinks per occasion or more than 7 drinks per week.[14] Nearly 30% of Americans 18 years of age and older drink more than the recommended limits for alcohol use.[15] Most of these drinkers are in the risky category. A substantial minority drink in a way that constitutes an alcohol use disorder: 12-month prevalence of alcohol use disorder among adults in the United States is 14%.[2] The health consequences of unhealthy alcohol use are significant; alcohol is the fourth leading cause of death in the United States.[1] Because patients with risky use do not meet criteria for an SUD (which is the focus of the substance use treatment system), and these patients may not identify that there is a problem, primary care is the ideal context for identifying and addressing risky levels of use.

Unhealthy drug use beyond alcohol is also widespread. Because of the diverse risks associated with any use of an illicit drug or misuse of a prescription drug (ie, taken differently or for a purpose other than prescribed, or taking another person's prescription),[16] even a single episode of such use is considered unhealthy use. As with alcohol, only some patients with unhealthy drug use meet criteria for an SUD. Although prevalence likely varies by site of care, recent data from multiple primary care sites found that 28% of adult patients reported use of an illicit drug or misuse of a prescription drug (not including alcohol or tobacco) in the past 12 months.[3] Marijuana was included in this category and was the most common drug used, with a prevalence of 21%.[3] Approximately 7% of the sample misused prescription medicines (such as benzodiazepines or opioid analgesics) in the past year, and similar proportions used cocaine.[3] Fourteen percent of the entire sample of patients met criteria for a 12-month SUD (not including alcohol or tobacco as the target substance).[3] More than half of those with a SUD are likely also to meet criteria for SUD with a second substance.[17]

Both risky substance use and SUDs are associated with physical and mental health comorbidities. For example, unhealthy alcohol consumption is associated with liver disease, cardiovascular disease, pancreatitis, gastritis, esophagitis, bone marrow suppression, peripheral neuropathy, chronic infectious diseases, pneumonia, and several cancers.[18] Many people with SUDs have difficulties with sleep[19] and chronic pain.[20,21] Further, more than 40% of persons with an SUD have a mood disorder and about a third have an anxiety disorder.[22]

INTEGRATING SCREENING AND BRIEF INTERVENTION FOR UNHEALTHY SUBSTANCE USE INTO PRIMARY CARE

Despite its prevalence, unhealthy substance use often goes unidentified in primary care settings. For example, in 2011, only 1 in 6 adults in the United States reported ever talking about alcohol with their primary care providers.[23] Screening alone is likely insufficient for changing substance use behavior. Research studies have thus primarily evaluated the health effects of screening not as a stand-alone service but as part of a series of clinical steps called SBIRT.[24] As described later, SBIRT has shown efficacy in reducing unhealthy alcohol use, and may have other benefits for drug use. The United States Preventive Services Task Force (USPSTF) has made universal screening coupled with brief intervention for unhealthy alcohol use a grade B recommendation (meaning there is high certainty that the net benefit is moderate or there is moderate certainty that the net benefit is moderate to substantial).[25,26] In contrast, the USPSTF has determined that there is insufficient evidence to determine whether screening for unhealthy drug use would be useful in primary care practices.[27] Screening instruments, the evidence base for SBIRT, and key steps in implementation are reviewed here.

Specific Screening Instruments

Although the health effects of substance use screening on its own have not been examined, studies have tested the validity of several brief screening instruments against the in-depth clinical assessments that are impractical in primary care. In general, a widely accepted and pragmatic strategy for screening for unhealthy alcohol and drug use is to use a brief screening tool first and then, for patients who screen positive, a longer instrument intended to distinguish risky use from use that meets criteria for an SUD.

For alcohol screening, the briefest validated tool is the single-item alcohol question. This question asks how many times the patient has consumed alcohol in excess of recommended limits (ie, 3 drinks per occasion for women and for men more than 65 years of age, and 4 drinks per occasion for men 65 years of age and younger) in the past year. A response of 1 or more is 82% sensitive and 79% specific for unhealthy alcohol use.[28] An alternative to the single-item alcohol test, the Alcohol Use Disorders Identification Test (AUDIT)-C is a 3-item tool assessing frequency of alcohol intake, amount of intake, and frequency of binges (6 or more drinks on 1 day).[29] The 3 multiple choice questions are, "How often do you have a drink containing alcohol?", "How many standard drinks containing alcohol do you have on a typical day?", and "How often do you have 6 or more drinks on 1 occasion?" A response of 1 or more on the single-item alcohol question or a score of 3 or more (for women) or 4 or more (for men) on the AUDIT-C should be followed by further assessment to determine whether the patient has risky use or an alcohol use disorder. The full 10-item AUDIT[30] or the modified Alcohol, Smoking, and Substance Involvement Screening Test (ASSIST) can help with this determination.[31]

For drug use, screening options are similar. A single-item drug question is, "How many times in the past year have you used an illegal drug or used a prescription medication for nonmedical reasons?" where nonmedical use is defined as "for reasons or in doses other than prescribed."[31–33] With a cutoff of 1 episode or more being positive for unhealthy use, this question is 85% sensitive and 96% specific for past-year drug use that is detectable either by self-report or via urine drug testing, and 100% sensitive and 73% specific for an SUD. Any positive response prompts further assessment, including identification of drugs used. The National Institute on Drug Abuse (NIDA) recommends the modified ASSIST as follow-up[34] and provides online support for its use. Other secondary screening questionnaires that have been validated in primary care and can follow the single-item drug screen[35] include the Drug Abuse Screening Test (DAST),[36] and the unmodified ASSIST.[37]

An additional option for assessment of both drug and alcohol use is the recently developed Tobacco, Alcohol, Prescription Medication, and other Substance Use (TAPS) tool.[38] The tool can be self-administered using a tablet computer, or a staff member can ask the questions of the patient. This multistep tool includes an initial brief screen (TAPS-1), which is similar to the single-item alcohol and drug screens. Patients scoring more than a certain threshold on the TAPS-1 then receive the TAPS-2, which includes more detailed questions for relevant substances. Initial studies show the TAPS to be highly sensitive and specific for certain substances but to be insensitive for prescription drug use disorder.[38] Later studies showed that the TAPS-1 may even be used on its own to detect SUDs.[39]

Evidence for Screening, Brief Intervention, and Referral to Treatment

In primary care, as well as other medical settings, screening for unhealthy alcohol use, followed by a form of brief counseling known as a brief intervention, can reduce self-reported alcohol consumption. A 2012 meta-analysis found that brief interventions for primary care patients with risky alcohol use led to reductions in self-reported consumption of 3.6 drinks (on average) per week from baseline, with some evidence for reduced hospital days among patients receiving brief interventions as well.[25] Greater effects seem to be achieved with interventions that were brief (up to 15 minutes) but involved multiple patient contacts (2 or more), compared with single contact or very brief interventions.[25] Most of the multicontact studies involved brief intervention by PCPs, sometimes assisted by a nurse. For example, in the Trial for Early Alcohol Treatment (TrEAT) study, PCPs conducted 2 brief interventions 1 month apart, and nurses made follow-up calls.[40] However, interventions by nonphysician providers also seem to have some effectiveness.[41] Notably, technologically assisted brief interventions (eg, a Web site or app on which patients complete screening instruments and receive instantaneous personalized feedback and suggestions for next steps) could reduce workload for primary care clinicians and staff. A meta-analysis found that there is a small but statistically significant effect of these interventions for reducing alcohol use.[42]

Studies suggest some important limitations to screening and brief intervention for unhealthy alcohol use. Brief interventions have been shown to reduce self-reported alcohol use for those with risky alcohol use but not for those who have an alcohol use disorder.[25] In theory, those with alcohol use disorders should receive specialty treatment, which could range from outpatient counseling to detoxification services depending on the patient's needs and readiness for change. However, evidence suggests that brief interventions do not improve the use of specialty treatment when referrals are made.[43,44] Further, studies of SBIRT have failed to consistently show an impact on biological markers of alcohol use, leading to skepticism among some experts about the intervention's effectiveness on more than self-reported use.[43] These experts have suggested that current guidelines for alcohol SBIRT may exceed the scope of the evidence,[43] and they suggested that randomized controlled trials using outcomes that are most relevant to PCPs and patients are needed.[43]

SBIRT for drug use is even more controversial. Several research groups have tested the efficacy of SBIRT interventions in primary care patients with varying levels of risky drug use. Two large-scale, well-designed studies have failed to show that SBIRT, compared with treatment as usual, results in decreased drug use or other improved outcomes, such as substance use treatment engagement, decreased emergency department visits or inpatient hospitalizations, or decreased legal involvement.[45–47] Both studies included patients who screened positive for risky drug use (including possible SUDs) in primary care clinics, with most participants using marijuana. Both studies tested a 30-minute to 45-minute motivational interviewing intervention by non-PCP clinicians or health educators, followed by a telephone booster a few weeks later. Not only were there no benefits to the treatment group, in 1 study the intervention group was less likely than the control group to receive addiction treatment within the 6 months after the index visit.[47] In contrast, 2 other large studies did find that SBIRT in primary care had a significant impact on drug use. There were some key differences between positive and negative studies. Bernstein[48] only enrolled people with risky opiate or cocaine use and found increased abstinence over time for both substances. In Project QUIT (Quit Using

Drugs Intervention Trial), researchers tested SBIRT versus treatment as usual in primary care (n = 334). In the intervention group, the primary care provider provided 5 minutes of scripted brief advice to quit or reduce drug use. Participants then received 2 calls of 20 to 30 minutes from a drug-health educator that included motivational interviewing and referrals. This intervention was successful in reducing number of days of drug use 3 to 4 months after the index visit.[49] Thus, a key difference between this study and the negative studies include the involvement of the primary care provider in the intervention.

In summary, SBIRT for alcohol use is modestly effective in reducing at least self-reported drinking among those patients with risky alcohol use (a large proportion of those with unhealthy use), although not clearly effective for patients with alcohol use disorder. Although SBIRT for alcohol remains controversial among some experts, it is generally embraced by guidelines. SBIRT for drug use has a more conflicted evidence base and is not yet widely recommended. Regardless of whether SBIRT for unhealthy substance use reduces use, systematic screening and consequent identification of patients with unhealthy substance use might have other benefits. It can alert PCPs that a patient may be at increased risk for substance-related health problems, ranging from increased blood pressure or fatty liver disease from risky alcohol use, to the cognitive or pulmonary risks of marijuana use, to the cardiovascular risks of cocaine use, to the infectious complications of injection drug use. Knowledge of unhealthy substance use can help PCPs make safer choices about medications for such conditions as hypertension, depression, and pain. Moreover, PCPs may use a positive screen to pursue additional preventive care measures, such as human immunodeficiency virus (HIV) or hepatitis C testing, pneumonia vaccination (recommended in patients with alcohol use disorder), or hepatitis B vaccination (recommended in persons who inject drugs).

Implementation of Screening, Brief Intervention, and Referral to Treatment

In a primary care practice, the SBIRT work flow involves first screening for unhealthy substance use, using the process described earlier. When patients screen positive, the primary care provider, an on-site behavioral health clinician, or practice staff can conduct a brief intervention, to give feedback about the patient's level of alcohol use, offer advice, and elicit goals and next steps from the patient. Steps in a specific type of brief intervention inspired by motivational interviewing principles, called the brief negotiated interview,[50] are outlined in **Table 1**. If there is concern that a patient not only has risky use but may meet criteria for an SUD, the patient should be referred for further treatment.

Implementation of SBIRT in a clinical practice is a multistep process that requires the following:

- Identification of a team to lead change. This team should include a PCP "champion", who can enthusiastically promote SBIRT and help other clinicians to change their practice behaviors,[51] as well as a person with an administrative role (such as a practice manager or project manager) who can execute a work plan and address logistical challenges. In order to increase buy-in from all staff, the team should also include representation from any other disciplines who will be involved in SBIRT.
- Buy-in from practice leadership. This step is key because of the number of personnel who must be involved in successful SBIRT, as well as the potential need for changes in the electronic medical record (EMR). In many cases, implementation of SBIRT may already be a priority for leaders, because of quality

Table 1 Approach to brief intervention in primary care	
Task	**Suggested Communication Strategy**
Explore pros and cons	• Begin by asking permission: "Is it OK if we talk about your use of [substance]?" • Then: "What do you like about using [substance]? What do you like less about using [substance]?"
Review health risks of use	• Preface feedback by asking, "What do you know about how [substance] affects your health?" or, "How do you see your use of [substance]?" • Then: "Is it ok if I share other risks with you?" • Point out any links between use of substance and current health conditions. • For alcohol, review NIAAA guidelines regarding alcohol use
Summarize and key question	• "So, on the one hand you've said [pros]… and on the other hand you've said [cons and risks]…Where does that leave you with your [substance] use?"
Explore readiness	• "Given what we've been discussing, on a scale of 0–10, how ready are you to change your use of [substance]?" • Then: "Why didn't you choose a lower number?"
Negotiate goals	• "What type of changes might you make?" • Support realistic and concrete change. • If needed: "Can I give you my best advice based on what you have told me?" • This advice may be: (1) for risky substance use only, to cut back to lower risk amounts; (2) for a screening test suggestive of an SUD and/or symptoms suggestive of SUD, such as use despite negative consequences, referral to addiction treatment
Explore confidence	• "On a scale of 0–10, how confident are you that you can change your use of [substance]?" • "What challenges can you imagine?" • "How can you overcome these challenges?" • "Can I suggest strategies that have helped other patients?"

A brief intervention is a brief, nonconfrontational, directive conversation, using motivational interviewing (MI) principles and strategies to enhance motivation to change use of alcohol (and other drugs). Key MI principles include that ambivalence is normal to any change process; the patient is the active decision maker; and advocating for change evokes resistance to change.

Abbreviation: NIAAA, National Institute on Alcohol Abuse and Alcoholism.

Adapted from Alford DP, Ellenberg L. Boston University evidence-based SBIRT student training project. 2017. Available at: http://www.masbirt.org/besst. Accessed September 12, 2017.

metrics related to screening, and the fact that screening for unhealthy alcohol use is a USPSTF recommendation.[25]

• Combatting stigma. Stigma and lack of understanding about SUDs may be major barriers in obtaining buy-in from leaders as well as PCPs and office staff.[11] Describing case studies of institutions that have provided substance use treatment and achieved outcomes that are meaningful to the organization (not only substance use outcomes but also reduced health care costs, for example[52]) may be helpful in persuading leaders, as may visits to nearby institutions that have made these changes. For clinical staff, the problem of stigma can be difficult to solve, although educational interventions, including ones that involve patients[53,54] or are administered online,[55] may be useful.

- Determine screening strategy. Specific questions to answer include:
  - Will the practice screen all patients or only certain groups? How often?
  - Will the practice screen for alcohol use only, or include illicit drugs and misuse of prescription drugs as well?
  - Which instruments will be used for screening?
  - Who will do the screening: front desk staff, medical assistants, PCPs, nurses, patients working on tablets in the waiting areas, or some combination? The resources available for screening also affect the selection of a tool; for example, the TAPS requires either staff with time to do face-to-face screening or tablet computers, because it does not have a paper-and-pencil option.
  - Can the instrument be linked to another screening instrument (eg, for depression) that is already in use?
  - How will staff members create time for screening?
  - Will the practice maintain a registry to track patients who screen positive? If so, what will be the strategy for follow-up for these patients?
- EMR integration. After the practice has selected tools and developed the screening workflow, it will ideally integrate these into the available EMR to facilitate documentation and tracking. The EMR should ideally allow for rapid result entry so that the team member responsible for brief interventions for patients who screen positive can become aware of the patient's result in real time. Having patients enter their own results using a tablet computer in the waiting room is efficient, when feasible. Ideally, practices should also be able to devise means to track when a brief intervention or referral takes place. These data also allow for population estimates of unhealthy substance use across practice providers.
- Process for brief interventions. The clinic must decide which team members will conduct brief interventions for patients who screen positive for unhealthy alcohol/drug use. Some data suggest a brief intervention by the PCP may be particularly effective.[25] However, PCP visits are typically brief, and PCPs may struggle to incorporate even a 5-minute brief intervention into their encounters, limiting their enthusiasm for the process as well as the benefits for the patient. If staff such as medical assistants conduct brief interventions, they need training. Behavioral health clinicians usually have training in motivational interviewing, and, if they do a brief intervention, they can arrange for follow-up in their own schedule if indicated. However, they may not have the capacity to accommodate all patients with risky use in their schedules. Further, even some mental health professionals may have insufficient training in working with people with risky substance use.
- Referral resources. How can the primary care practice increase the likelihood that patients with SUDs are connected to appropriate treatment? Referrals to outside programs can be challenging to patients, staff, and PCPs because of the complexity of referral options and levels of care in addiction treatment. However, this step in SBIRT must be emphasized and allocated appropriate resources. It may be useful to designate and train a small group of staff who can become experts in local treatment options, develop relationships with external sites, help patients set up intake appointments, address barriers to attendance, and follow up with patients and providers.
- Training. Training of all team members on the rationale for SBIRT, their new roles, and referral options is fundamental to successful implementation. In our experience, the concepts of unhealthy and risky substance use in particular are new for PCPs and require explanation with as many concrete, case-based examples as possible. As discussed earlier, training should likely address the problem of

stigma against people with SUDs. Training in brief interventions should also include opportunities for skills practice. Booster sessions and ongoing supervision help to maintain quality.

- Reimbursement. The practice must also consider whether to facilitate billing for brief interventions. Medicare reimburses for SBIRT conducted by a range of health care professionals as long as certain documentation criteria are met. For example, brief intervention must be at least 15 minutes long for billing purposes.[56] Some state Medicaid programs and commercial payers also reimburse.
- Performance management. As SBIRT is implemented, use of formal quality improvement processes can help practices set performance goals, monitor performance and share results with staff, rapidly identify barriers to implementation, and test solutions. Ideally, practices track screening rates and the numbers of patients who screen positive, who receive brief intervention, and who receive referrals.

INTEGRATED APPROACHES TO TREATMENT OF SUBSTANCE USE DISORDERS INTO PRIMARY CARE

Patients with SUDs need more than screening and brief intervention but rarely receive it; in 2015, only 11% of Americans with SUDs received treatment.[57] Offering not only referral to treatment but treatment itself within primary care has the potential to expand access, particularly to medication treatment of opioid use disorder, for which the number of current providers falls far short of demand.[58] Moreover, patients with an SUD report being more willing to enter substance use treatment in a primary care setting than in a specialty care setting.[59] In the case of medication treatment, which some patients choose to take for several years or more, PCPs may be ideally positioned to effectively prescribe because of their familiarity with patients' medical histories, comorbidities, and other medications, as well as their long-term engagement with patients.

Evidence-Based Treatment Modalities for Substance Use Disorders

This article first briefly reviews evidence-based treatment of SUDs irrespective of setting. Nonpharmacologic treatment of SUDs typically takes the form of individual or group counseling, or 12-step facilitation such as Alcoholics Anonymous or Narcotics Anonymous. Effective counseling techniques include motivational interviewing and varieties of cognitive behavior therapy.[60] Cognitive behavior therapy typically involves helping patients to understand antecedents and consequences of substance use behavior and to develop coping skills that help them cope with stress or specific antecedents to substance use.[61]

For some SUDs, medication maintenance is effective either in addition to or instead of counseling. US Food and Drug Administration (FDA)–approved medications for alcohol use disorders include naltrexone, acamprosate, and disulfiram. Naltrexone, an opioid antagonist, may reduce the pleasurable effects of alcohol intake and modestly reduced alcohol use in clinical trials of heavy drinkers when administered either as a daily tablet or a monthly intramuscular injection.[62,63] Acamprosate reduces symptoms associated with abstinence, but its efficacy is debatable.[64] In addition, disulfiram discourages alcohol use by causing uncomfortable physical symptoms when alcohol is consumed; however, rates of noncompliance are high.[65,66]

For opioid use disorders, methadone, buprenorphine (with or without naloxone), and naltrexone are all FDA approved. Methadone, a full opioid agonist, must be dispensed by licensed clinics in the United States; ample data support its efficacy in reducing opioid use as well as in reduction of HIV and hepatitis C transmission.[67] Buprenorphine is a partial opioid agonist that is usually formulated with naloxone for nonpregnant adults to deter injection; it too is highly effective in reducing opioid use,[68] including in primary care clinics.[69,70] Physicians, physician assistants, and nurse practitioners in the United States must receive specialized training in order to receive a waiver to prescribe the medication, and they must have the capacity to provide counseling, either in their own practices or through referrals to community services.[71] Naltrexone is a newer option, with efficacy in reducing opioid use when used monthly as an intramuscular injection.[72]

Evidence for Models of Substance Use Treatment Integrated into Primary Care

Numerous studies have shown that substance use treatment, particularly for opioid use disorders, can be effectively delivered in primary care settings.[73,74] However, the heterogeneity of studies and programs makes it challenging to determine which programmatic features drive effectiveness and to make decisions about resource allocation accordingly.

Given this difficulty, a framework for overall integration of behavioral health services into primary care can help categorize and interpret studies of SUD treatment in primary care. The Substance Abuse and Mental Health Services Administration (SAMHSA) provides one such framework, as shown in **Table 2**. Behavioral health integration is conceptualized as a continuum, from no integration to fully integrated care. Less intensive strategies (occupying level 2) might include a practice having a referral relationship with community providers, in which PCPs and staff can contact the community provider with information about the referral to better coordinate care, and in some cases may be able to secure expedited access to treatment. Intermediate models (occupying levels 3 and 4) could mean having specially trained providers of medication and/or psychosocial treatment colocated in the primary care setting without formal integration of workflows or avenues for collaboration.

Integrated behavioral health models (levels 5 and 6) that can address unhealthy substance use include the chronic care model and collaborative care. The philosophy of these integrated models is that the primary care practice is responsible for the physical and behavioral health of a population of people (ie, population-based care). To accomplish this, care must be evidence based and measurement based.[75] Fully integrated care includes the following elements: reorganization of the health care system, including its reward structure to promote quality; changes in the way care is delivered so that roles are redefined and appropriate members of the care team work together and communicate effectively with patients; integration of evidence-based guidelines, provider education, and specialist expertise into the workflow; use of clinical information systems to provide tools for registries, reminders, measurement of outcomes, feedback, and care coordination; explicit and structured ways of supporting patient self-management; and systematic ways to link patients to community resources.[4]

In collaborative care for unhealthy substance use, the clinic has systems and staff in place not only for screening and brief intervention but also for treatment, although some patients still require referrals to specialty settings such as inpatient detoxification or intensive outpatient treatment. A multidisciplinary team is involved. Medical assistants might screen patients, PCPs might conduct brief intervention for unhealthy use and medication management for SUDs, and an on-site behavioral health consultant (eg, social worker, addiction counselor, or psychologist) might provide SUD counseling. Specialty behavioral health providers such as psychiatrists may provide medication consultation, either as on-site direct patient care or via case reviews with PCPs. A care manager might use a registry to track relevant patients, provide outreach,

Table 2
Levels of behavioral health and primary care integration

Type of Care	Specific Level	Description
Coordinated care	Level 1: minimal collaboration	• Behavioral health and primary care in separate locations with separate medical records, billing systems, and other systems • Minimal communication between behavioral health and primary care
	Level 2: basic collaboration at a distance	• Behavioral health and primary care in separate locations with separate medical records, billing systems, and other systems • Periodic communication between behavioral health and primary care about shared patients
Colocated care	Level 3: basic collaboration on site	• Behavioral health and primary care occurs in the same facility, and sometimes in the same practice space • EMR and billing systems are separate from each other • Periodic communication between behavioral health and primary care about shared patients • Behavioral health and primary care function fairly independently
	Level 4: close collaboration with some system integration	• Behavioral health and primary care occur in the same practice space, often by placing a behavioral health provider in primary care space • Behavioral health and primary care may share an electronic health record (EHR), front desk staff, and billing staff • Consultation about challenging patients occurs as needed
Integrated care	Level 5: close collaboration approaching an integrated practice	• Behavioral and primary care functions as team and communicates frequently • Providers start to change the way care is provided and the structure of the system • May still be some barriers to full integration, such as lack of a shared EMR
	Level 6: full collaboration in a transformed/ merged practice	• Behavioral health and primary care operate as a single system with full collaboration between providers, who view their mission as the treatment of the whole person for their entire patient population • Example: primary care staff, as a group, would routinely screen for SUDs and, when these are detected, all members of the staff, including but not limited to behavioral health specialists, work together and with the patient to address the problem

Adapted from Heath B, Wise Romero P, Reynolds K. A review and proposed standard framework for levels of integrated healthcare. Washington, DC: SAMHSA-HRSA Center for Integrated Health Solutions; 2013; with permission.

encourage patient self-management, and assist with linkages to community resources including self-help groups and various levels of specialty addiction treatment. Decision supports could include validated screening instruments, clinical practice guidelines, and guidance for implementing brief behavioral interventions.[4] Ideally, the team would have regular meetings to discuss how best to provide care to patients.

A systematic review of studies evaluating medication treatment of opioid use disorders in primary care applied a framework that has some overlap with SAMHSA's, classifying 41 studies according to their models of care.[73] Thirty-two of the models were coordinated care models, defined as at least 2 different types of health care professionals actively communicating and working together to share care responsibilities. For example, nurse case managers or pharmacists could serve functions such as supporting buprenorphine induction, coordinating appointments, supporting medication adherence, and often offering some behavioral counseling, in collaboration with physician prescribers. Notably, these models were diverse and did not always include all the aspects of true collaborative care (eg, only 3 included a registry). Notably, in the few studies that compared specialty care with primary care treatment, outcomes were either similar across settings or better in primary care. However, many of the buprenorphine studies were observational, without any comparison group, whereas others compared only specific aspects of a model (such as induction strategies or the presence of counseling services) across groups, rather than comparing different overall models of care. Moreover, the heterogeneity of studies and outcomes measured precluded reliable comparison across studies to determine which models of care are most effective. However, among the 7 good-quality studies in which patient retention was more than 60% at 3 months, there was a pattern suggesting that successful interventions used coordinated, multidisciplinary models to support physicians in delivering medication. Thus, models that are closer to level 5 and 6 on the SAMHSA framework may be particularly effective.

The Substance Use, Motivation, Medication and Integrated Treatment (SUMMIT) randomized controlled trial sought to shed more light on the efficacy of these care coordination functions by comparing collaborative care for opioid and alcohol use disorder treatment in primary care with a standard care model, in which addiction services were colocated but not systematically integrated into the primary care practice.[76] SUMMIT enrolled patients who screened positive for alcohol and/or opioid use disorders at 2 federally qualified health centers. When patients arrived for primary care visits, medical assistants screened patients with the single-item drug and alcohol question followed by the ASSIST. Patients screening positive for alcohol or opioid use disorders were randomized to the intervention arm or usual care. In usual care, patients were told that the clinic provided addiction treatment and were given a number to call to schedule appointments for treatment as well as community referrals; they did not receive any care coordination. In the intervention arm, a care coordinator assessed substance use and arranged brief psychotherapy by clinic-based therapists and medications for SUD. The care coordinators (who had bachelor's degrees) monitored treatment progress and services received in a registry; alerts prompted care coordinators to communicate with patients after any missed appointments. Care coordinators and therapists met weekly as a team, led by a clinical psychologist, to discuss the progress of patients. More than half of patients enrolled had alcohol use disorders alone. At 6 months, intervention patients were more likely to report abstinence (33% vs 22%). Intervention patients were 3 times more likely than usual-care patients to have received brief psychotherapy (36% vs 11%). For unclear reasons, receipt of medication treatment was low in both groups, with only about 13% receiving this treatment in each study arm.

A 2014 Veterans Administration study also found a care management approach to be effective for alcohol use disorders, specifically. The study enrolled 126 veterans with alcohol use disorder who were referred by their PCPs. Patients were randomized to receive alcohol care management (ACM; including both counseling and naltrexone pharmacotherapy) from a behavioral health provider working within primary care, or to a control arm, which was a traditional outpatient substance use program. The behavioral health provider in ACM conducted regular assessments of alcohol use, and provided education, medication adherence support, and motivational interviewing, adapting the frequency of visits based on progress. ACM had a significantly higher proportion of participants engaged in treatment over the 26 weeks and a lower percentage of heavy drinking days, although overall self-reported abstinence did not differ between groups.[77] Notably, 66% of intervention patients received oral naltrexone, whereas only 12% of patients in the control arm received this medication.

However, a study examining a wider range of SUDs was negative. In the Alcohol Health Evaluation And Disease Management (AHEAD) study, Saitz and colleagues[56] recruited 563 people with alcohol or stimulant or opioid use disorders. Unlike the previous 2 studies, participants were recruited primarily from detoxification programs and asked to enroll at a new primary care setting. There, participants were randomly assigned to chronic care management or treatment as usual. The care management intervention was delivered by a team that included a social worker, nurse care manager, internist, and addiction psychiatrist. Components included an in-depth assessment, motivational enhancement therapy, relapse prevention counseling, a primary care appointment, referrals to specialty addiction treatment, medication for SUD, and active outreach by nurse care managers. Although patients in the intervention group were more likely to receive specialty addiction treatment and addiction medication, there were no differences between groups in the primary outcome of self-reported abstinence from stimulants, opioids, and heavy alcohol use.

In sum, primary care–based treatment of opioid use disorders can be highly effective, whereas primary care treatment of alcohol use disorders is at least modestly effective, and comparable with specialty-based care. There is particular promise for models that incorporate principles of collaborative care (eg, having care managers support physicians, and tracking patients' outcomes in a systematic way that allows care to be intensified as needed), although more data are needed to identify the highest-value parts of such models and allow the best use of resources. Patients already affiliated with the primary care clinic, and identified as having SUD in the primary care setting (rather than referred from an acute care setting, as in AHEAD) may be most likely to benefit. More data are needed regarding whether and how primary care settings can effectively manage nonopioid drug use disorders.

Implementation of Aspects of Collaborative Care for Substance Use Treatment

Many of the issues regarding implementation of SBIRT are relevant to the implementation of collaborative care models, or aspects thereof, for SUD treatment in primary care. In addition, depending on the breadth of services being considered, some of the most basic implementation considerations for collaborative care include:

- Buy-in from leadership and system reorganization. The practice must identify the high-level changes needed to lay the groundwork for the desired SUD treatment model. If possible, the practice may consider building on any existing model of collaborative care for depression or other behavioral health conditions. Financing considerations are pivotal in obtaining buy-in. In a fee-for-service model, leaders need to determine what services and activities are reimbursable, and which services are considered necessary even if not reimbursable (eg, team meetings). In accountable care organizations, estimating anticipated improvements in quality of care or reduced acute care use are vital; a successful business case will include a staffing model that is most likely to yield a return on investment. The SAMHSA Web site includes extensive relevant information.[78]
- Staffing and training. Who will be responsible for screening, care coordination, medication provision, and counseling? As noted earlier, existing

on-site behavioral health clinicians may be able to offer substance use counseling, but they may require additional training or supervision. If new staff need to be hired, leaders must determine the desired levels of licensure and available reimbursement options. A clinic may engage a consultant/specialist (such as a psychiatrist or addiction medicine specialist) to provide assistance with more difficult cases. Nurses, pharmacists, or other clinicians may serve as care managers and services may be reimbursable depending on the setting. Some practices are exploring the use of peer providers, also known as recovery coaches, to provide navigation and support behavior change.

- Care coordination. Registries can be a vital support in tracking patients who are identified with SUD and possibly risky substance use. Registries can allow staff to follow up with patients who do not engage with treatment and facilitate monitoring. However, the development of functional registries is not straightforward and may be resource intensive. Only in some cases can they be constructed from the EMR, and in other cases must be freestanding. Moreover, registries are only useful if there is adequate staffing for proactive use of the registry to guide outreach and care.
- Evidence-based guidelines. The practice should identify existing guidelines for the target problem and use these to determine workflows. Depending on the SUD being treated, these guidelines may include urine drug testing or checking state prescription monitoring programs. For all substances, guidelines are likely to include screening for mental health problems and particular related physical problems.
- Patient self-management. How will the team promote activated, involved patients? The practice may have education about self-management as a core function for the care manager. Practices should identify and provide preferred self-management tools to patients.
- Documentation requirements. A shared EMR facilitates shared care planning between all members of the primary care team. Clinic or hospital legal experts can help identify any confidentiality concerns and design a platform for communication that complies with federal regulations regarding protection of substance use treatment information.
- Decision support. Decision support tools in the EMR, such as best-practice alerts (BPAs), may enable evidence-based monitoring and treatment. For example, BPAs may prompt PCPs or staff that urine drug testing is due for a patient.
- Capacity to refer. As with SBIRT, collaborative care for SUD requires identification of and collaboration with local specialty addiction treatment sites to which patients can be referred if they need a different treatment setting, such as detoxification or methadone maintenance.
- Strategy for patients with co-occurring mental health disorder and SUD. All patients entering substance use treatment should be evaluated for co-occurring mental health conditions. In many cases, primary care physicians are able to prescribe psychiatric medications such as antidepressants. When available, on-site behavioral health clinicians may be able to do further assessment and therapy. A psychiatrist who is part of a collaborative care model can provide advice to primary care physicians and behavioral health clinicians and may be able to provide direct patient care to complex patients. If such a person is not available, it is important to identify psychiatrists to whom patients can be referred. A relationship with specialty psychiatry is important even if a psychiatrist is available on site, because some patients have more frequent mental health visits than a primary care–based team can provide.

- Performance management. As for SBIRT, the practice should identify intermediate and outcome metrics and a reporting mechanism that can drive quality improvement efforts.

For treatment models that include a focus on medication for opioid and/or alcohol use disorders, additional considerations include:

- Potential for the primary care site to participate in a larger regional medication treatment network that supports practices without prior expertise in treating patients, as has been modeled by the Massachusetts Model, the Vermont Hub-and-Spoke Model[79] or Project ECHO (Extension for Community Healthcare Outcomes).[80] Besides technical assistance and mentorship around clinical and operational challenges, these resources may help to build provider buy-in that medication treatment can and should be a PCP responsibility, and enhance PCP confidence.
- Staffing. Prescribers may either be the PCPs (physicians, nurse practitioners (NPs), or physician assistants [PAs]) themselves, or on-site addiction psychiatrists. PCPs may choose only to prescribe for their own primary care patients or may serve as consultants for their colleagues by prescribing for patients who are not in their own panel. Practices must also identify what level of support will be available to PCPs prescribing medication treatment. Collaborative care models typically have care managers (who may be nurses, pharmacists, or other clinicians) to track prescriptions, appointments, and monitoring results, and meet with patients for education and brief counseling.
- Medication and monitoring policies and workflows. The practice should develop standard policies regarding frequency of visits, urine drug testing, review of the state prescription drug monitoring program data, and response to inappropriate urine drug test results or other concerning behaviors.
- Counseling. The Drug Addiction Treatment Act of 2000 (DATA 2000), the law that allowed physicians to prescribe buprenorphine, requires that waivered providers have the capacity to refer patients for counseling.[81] For patients taking buprenorphine, it is unclear whether or for whom counseling provides additional benefit.[82] Therefore, sites need to determine their policies regarding the intensity and duration of counseling. Although on-site counseling is convenient for patients and consistent with a collaborative care model, it may be acceptable to refer patients elsewhere for counseling, particularly if the primary care site can develop a close relationship with off-site counselors. Psychotherapy and/or psychopharmacology treatment options are particularly important for people with co-occurring mental health conditions.
- Training. PCPs, NPs, and PAs require specific training to be waivered as buprenorphine providers, and providers may need training on medication for alcohol use disorders. For opioid use disorder treatment, the Providers' Clinical Support System for Medication-Assisted Treatment (PCSS-MAT, at pcssmat.org) provides training opportunities and online forums to discuss cases, and links new providers to clinical mentors. Care managers also require additional training in brief interventions and potentially use of a registry, depending on the model of care; they also need supervision about medication.

SUMMARY

SBIRT for unhealthy alcohol use and collaborative care models to manage SUD have promise as effective means for primary care to better identify and manage unhealthy substance use, although significant questions remain for future studies. Implementing these strategies requires planning, training, and a team approach. A cultural shift may also be needed, to encourage providers and staff to take on the diagnosis and management of conditions that are often stigmatized and/or seen as the responsibility of providers outside traditional medical settings. Despite these challenges, in our experience, primary care teams often find it deeply rewarding to engage with patients around unhealthy substance use, and to support patients in behavior change and recovery.

ACKNOWLEDGMENTS

The editors wish to thank Katherine Watkins, RAND Corporation, and Joji Suzuki, Brigham and Women's Hospital, Harvard Medical School, for providing a critical review of this article.

REFERENCES

1. Mokdad AH, Marks JS, Stroup DF, et al. Actual causes of death in the United States, 2000. JAMA 2004;291(10):1238–45.
2. Grant BF, Goldstein RB, Saha TD, et al. Epidemiology of DSM-5 alcohol use disorder: results from the national epidemiologic survey on alcohol and related conditions III. JAMA Psychiatry 2015;72(8):757–66.
3. Wu LT, McNeely J, Subramaniam GA, et al. DSM-5 substance use disorders among adult primary care patients: results from a multisite study. Drug Alcohol Depend 2017;179:42–6.
4. McLellan AT, Starrels JL, Tai B, et al. Can substance use disorders be managed using the chronic care model? Review and recommendations from a NIDA consensus group. Public Health Rev 2014;35(2).
5. Mauer BJ. Substance use disorders and the person-centered healthcare home. Washington, DC: National Council for Community Behavioral Healthcare; 2010.
6. Quinn AE, Rubinsky AD, Fernandez AC, et al. A research agenda to advance the coordination of care for general medical and substance use disorders. Psychiatr Serv 2017;68(4):400–4.
7. Manuel JK, Newville H, Larios SE, et al. Confidentiality protections versus collaborative care in the treatment of substance use disorders. Addict Sci Clin Pract 2013;8:13.
8. Ghitza UE, Tai B. Challenges and opportunities for integrating preventive substance-use-care services in primary care through the affordable care act. J Health Care Poor Underserved 2014;25(1 Suppl):36–45.
9. Walley AY, Alperen JK, Cheng DM, et al. Office-based management of opioid dependence with buprenorphine: clinical practices and barriers. J Gen Intern Med 2008;23(9):1393–8.
10. Urada D, Teruya C, Gelberg L, et al. Integration of substance use disorder services with primary care: health center surveys and qualitative interviews. Subst Abuse Treat Prev Policy 2014;9:15.
11. van Boekel LC, Brouwers EP, van Weeghel J, et al. Stigma among health professionals towards patients with substance use disorders and its consequences for healthcare delivery: systematic review. Drug Alcohol Depend 2013;131(1–2): 23–35.
12. Jones CM, Campopiano M, Baldwin G, et al. National and state treatment need and capacity for opioid agonist medication-assisted treatment. Am J Public Health 2015;105(8):e55–63.

13. Levey SM, Miller BF, Degruy FV 3rd. Behavioral health integration: an essential element of population-based healthcare redesign. Transl Behav Med 2012;2(3): 364–71.
14. National Institute on Alcohol Abuse and Alcoholism. Helping patients who drink too much: a clinician's guide. Bethesda (MD): National Institutes of Health; 2005. p. 1.
15. National Institute on Alcohol Abuse and Alcoholism. Alcohol facts and statistics. Overview of alcohol consumption 2017. Available at: https://www.niaaa.nih.gov/ alcohol-health/overview-alcohol-consumption/alcohol-facts-and-statistics. Accessed November 5, 2017.
16. Misuse of Prescription Drugs. National Institute on Drug Abuse Web site: NIDA; 2016.
17. McCabe SE, West BT, Jutkiewicz EM, et al. Multiple DSM-5 substance use disorders: a national study of US adults. Hum Psychopharmacol 2017;32(5). p.E2625.
18. Thakker KD. An overview of health risks and benefits of alcohol consumption. Alcohol Clin Exp Res 1998;22(7 Suppl):285S–98S.
19. Conroy DA, Arnett JT. Sleep and substance use disorders: an update. Curr Psychiatry Rep 2014;16(10):487.
20. Rosenblum A, Joseph H, Fong C, et al. Prevalence and characteristics of chronic pain among chemically dependent patients in methadone maintenance and residential treatment facilities. JAMA 2003;289(18):2370–8.
21. Zale EL, Maisto SA, Ditre JW. Interrelations between pain and alcohol: an integrative review. Clin Psychol Rev 2015;37:57–71.
22. Conway KP, Compton W, Stinson FS, et al. Lifetime comorbidity of DSM-IV mood and anxiety disorders and specific drug use disorders: results from the National Epidemiologic Survey on Alcohol and Related Conditions. J Clin Psychiatry 2006; 67(2):247–57.
23. McKnight-Eily LR, Liu Y, Brewer RD, et al. Vital signs: communication between health professionals and their patients about alcohol use–44 states and the District of Columbia, 2011. MMWR Morb Mortal Wkly Rep 2014;63(1):16–22.
24. SBIRT: screening, brief intervention, and referral to treatment. Available at: www. integration.samhsa.gov/clinical-practice/sbirt. Accessed October 24, 2017.
25. Jonas DE, Garbutt JC, Amick HR, et al. Behavioral counseling after screening for alcohol misuse in primary care: a systematic review and meta-analysis for the U.S. Preventive Services Task Force. Ann Intern Med 2012;157(9):645–54.
26. US Preventive Services Task Force. Final update summary: alcohol misuse: screening and behavioral counseling interventions in primary care. 2016. Available at: https:// www.uspreventiveservicestaskforce.org/Page/Document/UpdateSummaryFinal/ alcohol-misuse-screening-and-behavioral-counseling-interventions-in-primary-car.
27. Lanier D, Ko S. Screening in primary care settings for illicit drug use: assessment of screening instruments: a supplemental evidence update for the U.S. Preventive Services Task Force. U.S. Department of Health and Human Services. Rockville (MD): Agency for Healthcare Research and Quality; 2008.
28. Smith PC, Schmidt SM, Allensworth-Davies D, et al. Primary care validation of a single-question alcohol screening test. J Gen Intern Med 2009;24(7):783–8.
29. Frank D, DeBenedetti AF, Volk RJ, et al. Effectiveness of the AUDIT-C as a screening test for alcohol misuse in three race/ethnic groups. J Gen Intern Med 2008;23(6):781–7.
30. Johnson JA, Lee A, Vinson D, et al. Use of AUDIT-based measures to identify unhealthy alcohol use and alcohol dependence in primary care: a validation study. Alcohol Clin Exp Res 2013;37(Suppl 1):E253–9.

31. Smith PC, Schmidt SM, Allensworth-Davies D, et al. A single-question screening test for drug use in primary care. Arch Intern Med 2010;170(13):1155–60.

32. Resource guide: screening for drug use in general medical settings. 2012. Available at: https://www.drugabuse.gov/publications/resource-guide/preface. Accessed October 24, 2017.

33. National Institute on Drug Abuse. Resource guide: screening for drug use in general medical settings. National Institute on Drug Abuse Web site. Available at: http://www.drugabuse.gov/publications/resource-guide. Accessed September 5, 2017.

34. National Institute on Drug Abuse. NIDA-Quick Screen V1.0. National Institute on Drug Abuse Web site. Available at: http://www.drugabuse.gov/sites/default/files/pdf/nmassist.pdf. Accessed September 5, 2017.

35. Zgierska A, Amaza IP, Brown RL, et al. Unhealthy drug use: how to screen, when to intervene. J Fam Pract 2014;63(9):524–30.

36. Skinner HA. The drug abuse screening test. Addict Behav 1982;7:363–71.

37. WHO ASSIST Working Group. The alcohol, smoking and substance involvement screening test (ASSIST): development, reliability and feasibility. Addiction 2002; 97(9):1183–94.

38. McNeely J, Wu LT, Subramaniam G, et al. Performance of the Tobacco, Alcohol, Prescription Medication, and Other Substance Use (TAPS) tool for substance use screening in primary care patients. Ann Intern Med 2016;165(10):690–9.

39. Gryczynski J, McNeely J, Wu LT, et al. Validation of the TAPS-1: a four-item screening tool to identify unhealthy substance use in primary care. J Gen Intern Med 2017;32(9):990–6.

40. Fleming MF, Barry KL, Manwell LB, et al. Brief physician advice for problem alcohol drinkers. A randomized controlled trial in community-based primary care practices. JAMA 1997;277(13):1039–45.

41. Sullivan LE, Tetrault JM, Braithwaite RS, et al. A meta-analysis of the efficacy of nonphysician brief interventions for unhealthy alcohol use: implications for the patient-centered medical home. Am J Addict 2011;20(4):343–56.

42. Rooke S, Thorsteinsson E, Karpin A, et al. Computer-delivered interventions for alcohol and tobacco use: a meta-analysis. Addiction 2010;105(8):1381–90.

43. Glass JE, Andreasson S, Bradley KA, et al. Rethinking alcohol interventions in health care: a thematic meeting of the International Network on Brief Interventions for Alcohol & Other Drugs (INEBRIA). Addict Sci Clin Pract 2017;12(1):14.

44. Glass JE, Hamilton AM, Powell BJ, et al. Specialty substance use disorder services following brief alcohol intervention: a meta-analysis of randomized controlled trials. Addiction 2015;110(9):1404–15.

45. Roy-Byrne P, Bumgardner K, Krupski A, et al. Brief intervention for problem drug use in safety-net primary care settings: a randomized clinical trial. JAMA 2014; 312(5):492–501.

46. Saitz R, Palfai TP, Cheng DM, et al. Screening and brief intervention for drug use in primary care: the ASPIRE randomized clinical trial. JAMA 2014;312(5):502–13.

47. Kim TW, Bernstein J, Cheng DM, et al. Receipt of addiction treatment as a consequence of a brief intervention for drug use in primary care: a randomized trial. Addiction 2017;112(5):818–27.

48. Bernstein J, Bernstein E, Tassiopoulos K, et al. Brief motivational intervention at a clinic visit reduces cocaine and heroin use. Drug Alcohol Depend 2005;77(1):49–59.

49. Gelberg L, Andersen RM, Afifi AA, et al. Project QUIT (Quit Using Drugs Intervention Trial): a randomized controlled trial of a primary care-based multi-component brief intervention to reduce risky drug use. Addiction 2015;110(11):1777–90.

50. D'Onofrio G, Bernstein E, Rollnick S. Motivating patients for change: a brief strategy for negotiation. In: Bernstein E, Bernstein J, editors. Case studies in emergency medicine and the health of the public. Boston (MA): Jones and Bartlett; 1996.
51. Hendy J, Barlow J. The role of the organizational champion in achieving health system change. Soc Sci Med 2012;74(3):348–55.
52. Barbosa C, Cowell A, Bray J, et al. The cost-effectiveness of alcohol screening, brief intervention, and referral to treatment (SBIRT) in emergency and outpatient medical settings. J Subst Abuse Treat 2015;53:1–8.
53. Roussy V, Thomacos N, Rudd A, et al. Enhancing health-care workers' understanding and thinking about people living with co-occurring mental health and substance use issues through consumer-led training. Health Expect 2015; 18(5):1567–81.
54. Livingston JD, Milne T, Fang ML, et al. The effectiveness of interventions for reducing stigma related to substance use disorders: a systematic review. Addiction 2012;107(1):39–50.
55. Brener L, Cama E, Hull P, et al. Evaluation of an online injecting drug use stigma intervention targeted at health providers in New South Wales, Australia. Health Psychol Open 2017;4(1). 2055102917707180.
56. Saitz R, Cheng DM, Winter M, et al. Chronic care management for dependence on alcohol and other drugs: the AHEAD randomized trial. JAMA 2013;310(11): 1156–67.
57. Lipari RN, Park-Lee E, Van Horn S. America's need for and receipt of substance use treatment in 2015. Rockville (MD): Substance Use and Mental Health Services Administration; 2016.
58. Cicero TJ, Ellis MS, Surratt HL, et al. The changing face of heroin use in the United States: a retrospective analysis of the past 50 years. JAMA Psychiatry 2014;71(7):821–6.
59. Barry CL, Epstein AJ, Fiellin DA, et al. Estimating demand for primary care-based treatment for substance and alcohol use disorders. Addiction 2016;111(8):1376–84.
60. Martin GW, Rehm J. The effectiveness of psychosocial modalities in the treatment of alcohol problems in adults: a review of the evidence. Can J Psychiatry 2012; 57(6):350–8.
61. Lee NK, Rawson RA. A systematic review of cognitive and behavioural therapies for methamphetamine dependence. Drug Alcohol Rev 2008;27(3):309–17.
62. Rosner S, Hackl-Herrwerth A, Leucht S, et al. Opioid antagonists for alcohol dependence. Cochrane Database Syst Rev 2010;(12):CD001867.
63. Garbutt JC, Kranzler HR, O'Malley SS, et al. Efficacy and tolerability of long-acting injectable naltrexone for alcohol dependence: a randomized controlled trial. JAMA 2005;293(13):1617–25.
64. Anton RF, O'Malley SS, Ciraulo DA, et al. Combined pharmacotherapies and behavioral interventions for alcohol dependence: the COMBINE study: a randomized controlled trial. JAMA 2006;295(17):2003–17.
65. Laaksonen E, Koski-Jannes A, Salaspuro M, et al. A randomized, multicentre, open-label, comparative trial of disulfiram, naltrexone and acamprosate in the treatment of alcohol dependence. Alcohol Alcohol 2008;43(1):53–61.
66. Garbutt JC, West SL, Carey TS, et al. Pharmacological treatment of alcohol dependence: a review of the evidence. JAMA 1999;281(14):1318–25.
67. Mattick RP, Breen C, Kimber J, et al. Methadone maintenance therapy versus no opioid replacement therapy for opioid dependence. Cochrane Database Syst Rev 2009;(3):CD002209.

68. Mattick RP, Breen C, Kimber J, et al. Buprenorphine maintenance versus placebo or methadone maintenance for opioid dependence. Cochrane Database Syst Rev 2014;(2):CD002207.

69. Haddad MS, Zelenev A, Altice FL. Integrating buprenorphine maintenance therapy into federally qualified health centers: real-world substance abuse treatment outcomes. Drug Alcohol Depend 2013;131(1–2):127–35.

70. O'Connor PG, Oliveto AH, Shi JM, et al. A randomized trial of buprenorphine maintenance for heroin dependence in a primary care clinic for substance users versus a methadone clinic. Am J Med 1998;105(2):100–5.

71. Clinical guidelines for the use of buprenorphine in the treatment of opioid addiction. Treatment improvement protocol (TIP) series 40. Rockville (MD): Substance Abuse and Mental Health Services Administration; 2004 [DHHS Publication No. (SMA) 04–3939].

72. Krupitsky E, Nunes EV, Ling W, et al. Injectable extended-release naltrexone for opioid dependence: a double-blind, placebo-controlled, multicentre randomised trial. Lancet 2011;377(9776):1506–13.

73. Lagisetty P, Klasa K, Bush C, et al. Primary care models for treating opioid use disorders: what actually works? A systematic review. PLoS One 2017;12(10): e0186315.

74. Korthuis PT, McCarty D, Weimer M, et al. Primary care-based models for the treatment of opioid use disorder: a scoping review. Ann Intern Med 2017;166(4): 268–78.

75. Heath B, Wise Romero P, Reynolds KA. A review and proposed standard framework for levels of integrated healthcare. Washington, DC: SAMHSA-HRSA Center for Integrated Health Solutions; 2013.

76. Watkins KE, Ober AJ, Lamp K, et al. Collaborative care for opioid and alcohol use disorders in primary care: the SUMMIT randomized clinical trial. JAMA Intern Med 2017;177(10):1480–8.

77. Oslin DW, Lynch KG, Maisto SA, et al. A randomized clinical trial of alcohol care management delivered in Department of Veterans Affairs primary care clinics versus specialty addiction treatment. J Gen Intern Med 2014;29(1):162–8.

78. Integrating behavioral health into primary care. Available at: https://www.integration. samhsa.gov/integrated-care-models/behavioral-health-in-primary-care#business case. Accessed October 24, 2017.

79. Brooklyn JR, Sigmon SC. Vermont hub-and-spoke model of care for opioid use disorder: development, implementation, and impact. J Addict Med 2017;11(4): 286–92.

80. Komaromy M, Duhigg D, Metcalf A, et al. Project ECHO (extension for community healthcare outcomes): a new model for educating primary care providers about treatment of substance use disorders. Subst Abus 2016;37(1):20–4.

81. Substance Abuse and Mental Health Services Administration. Legislation, regulations, and guidelines. Programs & Campaigns. Available at: https://www. samhsa.gov/medication-assisted-treatment/legislation-regulations-guidelines. Accessed November 5, 2017.

82. Carroll KM, Weiss RD. The role of behavioral interventions in buprenorphine maintenance treatment: a review. Am J Psychiatry 2017;174(8):738–47.

Inpatient Addiction Consult Service

Expertise for Hospitalized Patients with Complex Addiction Problems

Zoe M. Weinstein, MD, MS[a],*, Sarah E. Wakeman, MD[b],
Seonaid Nolan, MD[c,d]

KEYWORDS

- Addiction • Inpatient management • Consult service • Withdrawal
- Hospitalized patient • Substance use disorder

KEY POINTS

- Hospitalized patients have a high prevalence of substance use; however, this problem often goes unaddressed.
- Inpatient addiction consult services are an important intervention to use the reachable moment of hospitalization to engage patients and initiate addiction treatment.
- Addiction consultation involves taking an addiction-specific history, motivational interviewing, withdrawal symptom management, and initiation of long-term pharmacotherapy.
- Addiction consult services have the potential to decrease readmissions and utilization costs for medical systems, improve substance use outcomes for patients, and increase provider knowledge.

INTRODUCTION: THE NEED FOR ADDICTION CONSULT SERVICES IN THE GENERAL HOSPITAL SETTING

Substance use disorders (SUDs) affect 40 million Americans and place an enormous burden on society, with a cost of $740 billion annually.[1,2] Hospitalization is an increasingly frequent and costly occurrence among individuals with an SUD, with almost

Disclosure Statement: The authors have nothing to disclose.
[a] Department of Medicine, Boston University School of Medicine, Boston Medical Center, 801 Massachusetts Avenue, Crosstown 2, Boston, MA 02118, USA; [b] Department of Medicine, Harvard Medical School, Massachusetts General Hospital, 50 Staniford Street, 9th Floor, Boston, MA 02114, USA; [c] British Columbia Centre on Substance Use, 608–1081 Burrard Street, Vancouver, BC V6Z 1Y6, Canada; [d] Department of Medicine, University of British Columbia, St. Paul's Hospital, 553B-1081 Burrard Street, Vancouver, British Columbia V6Z 1Y6, Canada
* Corresponding author.
E-mail address: zoe.weinstein@bmc.org

Med Clin N Am 102 (2018) 587–601
https://doi.org/10.1016/j.mcna.2018.03.001
0025-7125/18/© 2018 Elsevier Inc. All rights reserved.

one-quarter of hospitalized patients having an SUD, presenting a huge opportunity for intervention.[3,4] Despite this, only a minority of patients receive any treatment of SUDs in a hospital setting.[5]

Previous research has demonstrated not only the feasibility of providing addiction treatment to individuals in an acute care setting but also its efficacy. A recent meta-analysis demonstrated brief intervention for unhealthy alcohol use in the hospital as associated with a significant reduction in weekly alcohol consumption 6 months later.[6] Furthermore, hospitalized individuals with an alcohol use disorder have been shown more likely to participate in outpatient addiction treatment if they receive motivational interviewing and facilitated referral to treatment.[7] Similarly, pharmacotherapy initiation for alcohol, tobacco, or opioid use disorder in acute care settings has been associated with several positive outcomes, including a reduction in substance use, improvement in treatment retention, and a decrease in hospital readmission rates.[8–10] More specifically, 1 study of 302 individuals with an opioid use disorder initiated on methadone maintenance therapy in a hospital demonstrated an 82% follow-up rate to an outpatient methadone maintenance program.[11] Given the high prevalence of SUDs and recurring need to access medical care, hospitalization offers a critical opportunity for effective intervention and provision of evidence-based addiction treatment to dramatically reduce morbidity and mortality.

To date, an important barrier identified in the delivery of evidence-based addiction treatment pertains to many health care providers overall feeling ill equipped to accurately screen for, diagnose, or treat SUDs.[12,13] In an attempt to overcome this in hospital, 1 strategy has been the creation of an inpatient addiction consult service (ACS). Although varied in the nature and background of program clinical staff, patient recruitment strategies, and interventions offered, all ACSs share a common goal of reducing morbidity and mortality associated with SUDs by improving access to evidence-based addiction treatment while in a hospital and successfully transitioning individuals from acute to community settings. Hospital-based ACSs can further provide support, effective role modeling, and education about SUD interventions, which, in turn, may improve preparedness among health care providers in managing SUDs, reducing stigma associated with the condition, and ultimately improving clinical practice.[14]

CURRENT ADDICTION CONSULT SERVICE MODELS

To date, more than half a dozen hospital-based ACSs exist within North America. A range of model types, including different strategies of patient identification and team composition are described below.

Patient Identification

Although some hospitals use a universal screening approach for substance misuse or an SUD with validated tools, such as the Alcohol Use Disorders Identification Test, a majority of ACS referrals occur directly from the primary admitting medical or surgical team according to clinical judgment.

Team Composition

Although some pioneering consult services relied solely on a physician, current models often involve additional staffing, with compositions varying according to the needs and resources of each institution. A physician is essential to manage pharmacotherapy for withdrawal symptoms and long-term treatment. In addition, a nurse may assist with day-to-day clinical assessments and symptom management, whereas a social worker, nurse care manager, or resource specialist might assist with psychosocial interventions and community care transitions. A recovery coach or peer navigator may assist with motivational interviewing and patient navigation. Because many ACSs operate in an academic setting, often trainees are part of the team, including medical students, residents, and addiction fellows (medicine or psychiatry).

THE ADDICTION CONSULT

An individual who is referred for an addiction consult receives a comprehensive addiction history and physical examination (**Fig. 1**).

History

A complete addiction history is important for confirmation of a substance use disorder, to assess risk for withdrawal, and to evaluate an individual's readiness for addiction treatment. Patient medical comorbidities, number of active substance use disorders, and social circumstances have an impact on the ease and ability for providers to recommend and link patients to addiction treatment. An addiction history can be challenging to elicit, because it includes questions focused on stigmatized behaviors; accordingly, the establishment of a therapeutic relationship between patient and health care provider is of critical importance and can be aided by using nonjudgmental, stigma-free language.[15] In addition, much of this history may be obtained when a patient is actively in withdrawal and distress; thus, it is also essential to focus the consult on the components that most directly have an impact on treatment decision making (see **Table 1**).

Substance use disorder—diagnosis and severity

A positive screen for unhealthy substance use requires assessment for a SUD using the 11 criteria from the Diagnostic and Statistical Manual of Mental Disorders (DSM-5), including asking explicitly about cravings, tolerance, withdrawal, loss of control and consequences of use in the past 12 months.[16] Patients who meet 2-3 criteria have a mild use disorder, 4-5 a moderate use disorder and 6 or more a severe

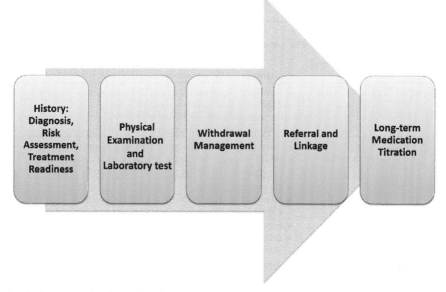

| History: Diagnosis, Risk Assessment, Treatment Readiness | Physical Examination and Laboratory test | Withdrawal Management | Referral and Linkage | Long-term Medication Titration |

Fig. 1. Components of an addiction consult.

Table 1
Questions to ask as part of the addiction consult history

- What age was your first use? How much and how frequently were you using? How did you use initially (e.g. inhalation, insufflation, oral, injection etc.)?
- How much are you using currently? How frequently and by what route?
- Are you requiring more of the substance (e.g. amount or frequency) to achieve the same effect compared to your time of first use?

- Do you currently have cravings to use?

- When you stop using, how do you feel?
- Do you spend a lot of your day using or recovering from its effects?

- Have you experienced any negative consequences from your use? This may include: inter-actions with law enforcement, development of a medical complication, deterioration of personal or professional relationships, loss of employment, cessation of hobbies or other activities previously important to you.
- Have you ever engaged in dangerous behavior while using? This may include: driving, operating heavy machinery etc.

- Have you ever previously tried to cut down or quit your use? Were you successful? If so, how did you achieve this and what was your longest period of abstinence? What caused you to relapse?

disorder.[16] Should an individual screen positive for more than one substance use disorder, the criteria should be assessed individually for each substance.

General risk assessment
A detailed assessment of associated risks should be undertaken as part of the addiction history. Specifically, patients should be asked about any previous or ongoing injection drug use, including inquiry about injection practices and risk for infectious diseases. Lastly, overdose risk and use of harm reduction services should be included (**Table 2**).

Readiness for addiction treatment Evaluating readiness for treatment is critical in developing an appropriate management plan. A good starting point is a patient's

Table 2
Risks associated with substance use and questions to ask as part of the addiction history

Substance Use—Associated Risks	Questions to Ask in the Addiction History
Injection drug use	• Have you ever injected drugs? If so, do you currently inject? Approximately how frequently? • Do you use clean injecting equipment? Have you ever pre-viously shared injecting equipment?
Infectious diseases (eg, HIV and hepatitis)	• Have you previously been tested for HIV or hepatitis? • When was your last test and what was the result? • Do you ever exchange sex for drugs or money?
Overdose risk	• Do you use alone? • Have you previously overdosed? If so, approximately how many times? When was your last overdose? • Have you ever witnessed anyone else overdose? • Do you have a naloxone kit? • Do you ever take a test dose before using to assess your drug's potency?
Harm reduction services	• Do you access needle exchange programs or supervised consumption sites?

previous treatment history, including treatment strategies (both pharmacologic and psychosocial) that were successful for a period of time and those that were unsuccessful, as an opportunity for discussion about a patient's current goals and treatment options. Furthermore, having a patient identify previous periods of abstinence or reduced substance use offers the health care provider the opportunity to enact motivational interviewing techniques to instill confidence in patients of their ability to achieve such an outcome again (**Table 3**).

Social history A detailed social history, specifically understanding if an individual is housed, on income assistance, and has a strong network of support (eg, friends and family), can provide helpful collateral when formulating a management plan.

Physical examination
All patients should be assessed for signs of withdrawal or intoxication as well as medical complications of use (**Table 4**).

Laboratory testing
Baseline laboratory assessment, including complete blood cell count, comprehensive metabolic panel, and coagulation studies, can help assess for safety of potential pharmacologic treatments (because some medications require dose adjustments or are contraindicated based on severity of liver or kidney disease) as well as sequelae of substance use.

Infectious disease testing, including HIV and hepatitis screening, should be offered.[17–19] Full sexually transmitted disease screening and HIV pre-exposure prophylaxis also may be offered.[20,21]

A comprehensive urine drug test, including synthetic and semisynthetic opioids (eg, buprenorphine and fentanyl), can assist in confirming recent substance use as well as reveal substances that a patient has not reported. Urine drug testing may be helpful in

---

Table 3
Readiness for addiction treatment and questions to ask in the addiction history

Readiness for Addiction Treatment	Questions to Ask in the Addiction History
Previous addiction treatment	• Have you previously received any addiction treatment? This may include detox, medications, support groups, or recovery homes. • If so, what types of treatment have you previously tried and approximately how many times? • How long ago was your last addiction treatment and what kind of treatment were you receiving?
Previous abstinence or reduced substance use	• Have you ever previously been able to cut down your substance use or stop all together? • If so, how many times? How did you achieve this and what was your longest period of abstinence or reduced substance use? • Was any or some of this time during a period of incarceration or other forced abstinence?
Relapse history	• If you have had periods of abstinence or reduced substance use previously, what caused you to relapse? Can you identify any potential triggers?
Current goals for treatment	• What are your current treatment goals (eg, total abstinence vs reduction in substance use vs harm reduction)?

Table 4
Addiction-focused physical examination

Vital signs	Pulse, blood pressure, respiratory rate, temperature, and oxygenation
Eye, ears, nose, and throat	Pupil size and scleral icterus
Cardiology	New or increased murmur
Pulmonary	Rales, wheeze, or decreased breath sounds
Abdominal	Hepatosplenomegaly, a nodular liver, and ascites
Genitourinary	Testicular size and gynecomastia
Lymph nodes	Lymphadenopathy
Skin	Diaphoresis, piloerection, abscesses, thrombophlebitis, Roth spots, Janeway lesions, jaundice, palmar erythema, and spider angioma
Neurologic/psychiatric	Mental status, delirium, hallucinations, restlessness, and anxiety

harm reduction counseling, if, for example, a patient was not aware of using heroin contaminated with fentanyl.

Withdrawal risk and management

Assessing a patient's risk for withdrawal and promptly treating the symptoms is a clinical priority. Suboptimal withdrawal symptom management has been shown a prominent reason for leaving a hospital against medical advice.[22] Conversely, appropriate withdrawal treatment and subsequent linkage to outpatient treatment are important strategies to help support patients to comply with their medical care.[23,24]

Nicotine withdrawal Nicotine cessation or a reduction in use may result in cravings and symptoms of the nicotine withdrawal syndrome (**Table 5**).[16] Nicotine dependence from cigarette smoking can be quantified using the Fagerstrom Test for Nicotine Dependence.[25] During hospitalization, a patient should be offered medications to treat nicotine withdrawal, including nicotine replacement therapy, with a starting dose chosen based on the Fagerstrom score and self-reported quantity of cigarettes used daily.

Alcohol withdrawal Alcohol cessation or a reduction in use may result in cravings and symptoms of the alcohol withdrawal syndrome (AWS). AWS ranges from minor withdrawal symptoms to seizures and delirium tremens. Minor withdrawal can begin within 6 hours of the last drink, and includes anxiety, headache diaphoresis nausea insomnia and tachycardia.[26,27] Severe AWS is associated with increased morbidity and mortality and may manifest as seizures, alcoholic hallucinosis and/or delirium tremens.

Table 5
Nicotine withdrawal syndrome—symptoms to ask about as part of the addiction history and predicted onset of symptoms following smoking cessation

Nicotine Withdrawal Syndrome Symptoms	Timing of Predicted Nicotine Withdrawal Syndrome
• Anxiety • Irritability • Restlessness • Increased appetite and weight gain • Changes in mood (dysphoria or depression) • Insomnia	After smoking cessation: • 72 h—peak • 3–4 wk—subside

Generalized tonic-clonic seizures can begin within 6 hours of the last drink. Alcohol hallucinosis presents after 12 hours from the last drink with visual, auditory and/or tactile hallucinations, but with intact orientation and normal vital signs.[26] Delirium tremens, including disorientation, confusion, hypertension fever and agitated can begin after 48 hours from the last drink.[26] Not all individuals with an alcohol use disorder experience severe symptoms of AWS. The Prediction of Alcohol Withdrawal Severity Scale is an instrument validated for use among hospitalized patients and may be used to assess the risk for developing severe, complicated withdrawal.[28]

The gold standard of treatment of individuals identified at high risk for severe, complicated alcohol withdrawal management is benzodiazepines to decrease the risk of delirium and seizures.[26,29,30] Benzodiazepines can be administered as a front-loading regimen, fixed-dose taper, or by symptom-triggered scale. Front-loading regimens include administering diazepam, 20 mg every 2 hours, until withdrawal symptoms have abated.[30] Fixed-dose tapers typically involve higher doses of benzodiazepines (eg, chlordiazepoxide, 100 mg, or diazepam, 20 mg) every 6 hours for at least 1 day, with scheduled decreasing doses over subsequent days and additional medication as needed. Symptom-triggered therapy can allow for shorter treatment duration and decreased amount of total medication required.[26] The revised Clinical Institute Withdrawal Assessment for Alcohol (CIWA-Ar) is the most commonly used scale to assess withdrawal symptoms, with medication administered as frequently as every hour when the CIWA-Ar score is greater than or equal to 8.[31] Not all patients, however, are medically appropriate for symptom-triggered monitoring. The evaluation of the CIWA-Ar scale does not include patients with a seizure history, thus these patients should receive at least 1 prophylactic benzodiazepine dose, even if asymptomatic.[32] Furthermore, patients who are unable to communicate easily with nursing staff (eg, non–English-speaking or dementia patients) may not be able to answer subjective questions reliably and thus may not be appropriate for CIWA-Ar. Phenobarbital may be used either in addition or instead of benzodiazepines, especially in the intensive care setting.[33,34]

Benzodiazepine withdrawal Benzodiazepine cessation after chronic use may cause a withdrawal syndrome with features similar to alcohol withdrawal.[35] Symptoms may be more severe when withdrawing from higher-dose or short-acting benzodiazepine formulations.[36] The window for benzodiazepine withdrawal can be highly variable, with onset occurring within 48 hours of discontinuing short-acting benzodiazepines and up to 10 days for long-acting benzodiazepines.[35] The primary treatment of benzodiazepine dependence and withdrawal is a slow taper of benzodiazepines.[35] Both fixed-dose and symptom triggered-tapering schedules are acceptable treatment modalities.[37] Additionally, a fixed-dose phenobarbital protocol can be used safely and effectively in the inpatient setting.[38]

Opioid withdrawal Opioid cessation, or a reduction in use, may result in cravings or symptoms of opioid withdrawal syndrome (OWS) (**Table 6**). The Clinical Opiate Withdrawal Scale (COWS) is a validated tool to assist with the diagnosis and severity of OWS.[39,40] During OWS treatment, the COWS helps guide therapy and monitor for symptom improvement. A detailed review of medications dispensed through an established prescription monitoring program can provide helpful collateral information about patterns of use and risk for overdose.

Opioid detoxification alone is associated with high relapse rates and increased HIV incidence[41] whereas maintenance opioid agonist therapy is associated with improved treatment retention, sustained abstinence, and a reduction in morbidity and

Table 6
Opioid withdrawal syndrome—symptoms to ask about as part of the addiction history and timing after opioid cessation

Addiction History—Opioid Withdrawal Syndrome Symptoms	Timing of Predicted Opioid Withdrawal Syndrome
• Nausea	Onset of symptoms
• Vomiting	• 6–12 h after last dose of short-acting opioid[a]
• Diarrhea	• 24–48 h after last dose of long-acting opioid[b]
• Sweating	Peak symptoms
• Irritability	• 24–48 h after onset
• Restlessness	Symptoms subside
• Tremor	• Days to weeks (short-acting vs long-acting,
• Yawning	respectively)

[a] Short-acting opioids: morphine, codeine, hydromorphone, oxycodone, hydrocodone, diacetylmorphine (heroin), meperidine, tramadol, and fentanyl.
[b] Long-acting opioid: methadone.

mortality.[42] Given this, maintenance opioid agonist treatment is recommended for the management of opioid withdrawal and the ACS should facilitate a seamless link to outpatient treatment programs posthospital discharge. The efficacy of methadone or buprenorphine is comparable with low rates of adverse effects.[43,44] An important consideration when prescribing buprenorphine is the potential for precipitated withdrawal, a syndrome of worsening withdrawal symptoms when buprenorphine, a partial opioid agonist with high affinity for the opioid receptor, is administered when a full opioid agonist is also systemically present. To avoid this, buprenorphine should not be administered until at least 12 hours after the last dose of a short-acting opioid and up to 48 hours after the last dose of a long-acting opioid.[42] A COWS score of 8 to 12, representing mild opioid withdrawal, should be obtained prior to starting buprenorphine if there are concerns regarding precipitated withdrawal (**Table 7**).

A common misconception in the United States is that hospitals or doctors need special licensing to provide methadone or buprenorphine in the inpatient setting; however, it is legal for both of these medications to be administered to manage withdrawal symptoms while patients complete their inpatient treatments.[45]

Adjuvant medications may be used for symptomatic management for patients who decline agonist treatment or while waiting to start buprenorphine. These medications may include α-agonists to treat anxiety or muscle spasms, antihistamines or benzodiazepines for anxiety, hypnotics for insomnia, anti-inflammatories for pain, and antidiarrheals or antispasmodics.

Table 7
Typical dosing schedule for methadone or buprenorphine for withdrawal

Medication	Initial Dose	Next Doses in First 24 h	Day 2
Methadone	20 mg oral	Reassess every 2–3 h, giving additional 10 mg until COWS <5 (40 mg maximum in 24 h)	Continue on total dose from first 24 h; can increase to 40 mg if not already reached
Buprenorphine	4 mg sublingual	Reassess every 2–3 h, giving additional 4 mg until COWS <5 (12 mg maximum in 24 h)	Continue on total dose from first 24 h; can increase up to 16 mg

Stimulant withdrawal Cocaine, methamphetamine, or other stimulant intoxication may present with hypertension, agitation, and anxiety, which should be managed symptomatically. Withdrawal from stimulants includes symptoms, such as depressed mood and somnolence, and does not routinely require medication management.[46]

Postwithdrawal management

After acute withdrawal has subsided, providers should engage patients in brief interventions and motivational interviewing to assess and enhance patients' readiness and motivation for long-term treatment of their SUDs.[6,7,47] All patients who are interested should receive a referral and connection to outpatient counseling as well as potentially residential treatment. Pharmacologic interventions should be offered as appropriate based on the substance use disorder.

Nicotine use disorder Despite approximately 70% of adult smokers in the United States expressing a desire to quit smoking,[48] only approximately half report being asked about their smoking by a health care provider in the previous 12 months.[49] Brief physician advice has been shown to have a significant effect on smoking cessation.[50] Medications can assist with quit rates 10-fold.[51] Drug therapies for nicotine use disorder include combination nicotine replacement therapy, varenicline, or bupropion. Behavioral interventions should be offered, because these provide significant benefit when combined with pharmacotherapy.[52,53]

Alcohol use disorder Among risky drinkers, brief intervention has proved effective in reducing alcohol consumption.[54,55] Patients should be offered pharmacologic treatment of alcohol use disorder with any of the 3 US Food and Drug Administration–approved medications: naltrexone, acamprosate, and disulfiram, based on a patient's medical characteristics and alcohol consumption goals.[56,57] Medications can be initiated in a hospital with patients and then linked to outpatient care.

Benzodiazepine use disorder The mainstay of treatment of benzodiazepine use disorder is a long-term taper over 1 month to 3 months.[35] In the inpatient setting, however, long-term taper is not always feasible. Inpatient teams should attempt to connect with an outpatient provider and assess the risks, benefits, and feasibility of continuing a taper beyond the inpatient period. If a taper must be completed while an inpatient, providers should complete the taper over the maximum number of days. There are no pharmacologic maintenance treatments of benzodiazepine use disorder. Counseling may provide additional benefit as well as treatment of underlying psychiatric disorders.[58]

Opioid use disorder Administration of opioids in-hospital and the timing of this influence a patient's management strategy (eg, choice of opioid agonist treatment and timing of induction with buprenorphine). Long-term opioid agonist treatment with either buprenorphine or methadone should be recommended (see **Table 7**). Furthermore, both medications should be titrated toward a therapeutic dose while a patient is in hospital. Buprenorphine can be increased by 2 mg to 4 mg daily until a patient achieves a therapeutic daily dose of approximately 16 mg. Methadone can be increased by 5 mg to 10 mg every 2 days to 3 days, with the goal of a dose that treats withdrawal symptoms, alleviates cravings, and minimizes or eliminates the euphoric effects of concurrent opioid use.[42] Before aggressive titration begins, efforts should be taken to ensure a patient has appropriate linkage to an outpatient buprenorphine or methadone provider who can continue treatment directly after hospital discharge.

If a patient presents who is not currently in withdrawal due to recent abstinence, but given concerns about relapse is otherwise motivated to be on pharmacologic treatment, this patient may be offered either naltrexone, which is an opioid antagonist, or opioid agonist therapy. If the patient elects agonist therapy, then buprenorphine or methadone can be slowly titrated.

If an outpatient prescriber cannot be located, the patient declines maintenance treatment, or maintenance is not possible (eg, incarceration), then the patient should be offered an opioid taper. Methadone may be tapered by 5 mg to 10 mg per day and buprenorphine tapered by 2 mg to 4 mg per day until discharge. Additionally, patients should be informed of the increased risk that exists for overdose in the setting of tapering and should be provided with overdose prevention education and naloxone at the time of discharge.

Stimulant use disorder There are no Food and Drug Administration–approved medications for stimulant use disorder because overall pharmacologic interventions have had mixed or negative results.[59–61] Counseling, especially contingency management, is the most evidence-based intervention.[62]

DEMONSTRATED BENEFITS OF ADDICTION CONSULT SERVICES: ONGOING RESEARCH AND EVALUATION

ACSs have been demonstrated as feasible across North America, are successful at engaging patients in care, provide evidence-based addiction treatment, and assist in transitioning patients from acute to community treatment settings.[63–68] Recipients of hospital-based ACSs have also been found to have higher rates of medical insurance coverage, increased engagement with primary care and HIV services, and decreased homelessness.[69] For example, at Johns Hopkins University, providers achieved a decrease in emergency department utilization and increase in ambulatory care visits for patients treated within an integrated addiction and medical treatment model in a day hospital setting.[70] In addition, inpatient addiction services can decrease addiction severity and increase self-reported abstinence rates at 30-days.[63]

Of importance, a challenge in the United States regarding the success of ACSs has been the restricted access of outpatient methadone or buprenorphine maintenance programs, limiting the ability to initiate long-term opioid agonist treatment in acute care settings.[69] In an attempt to overcome this, some ACSs have created a bridge clinic, where patients can obtain opioid agonist medications short-term while seeking a long-term placement. Inpatient addiction treatment with appropriate outpatient linkage has been shown beneficial to many health as well as care utilization outcomes. One study of an ACS, which offers linked services, demonstrated a self-reported reduction in substance-related hospitalizations and emergency room visits.[63] In both Vancouver, Canada, and Portland, Oregon, hospitalized patients with an SUD who require long-term antibiotics can choose to access a postdischarge residential care facility that includes harm reduction services in addition to maintenance addiction treatment.[64] Such a program can be cost-saving, allowing patients to leave the more expensive inpatient setting, while also facilitating completion of antibiotic therapy. An ACS model is estimated to yield significant savings, by reducing readmissions as well as length of stay, likely through linkage to appropriate outpatient services.[64]

In addition, an ACS can have an important educational role, increasing trainee knowledge of addiction medicine concepts[71] as well as creating a more patient-centered harm reduction culture within the hospital setting.

FUTURE CONSIDERATIONS

Although several positive outcomes have been reported with hospital-based ACSs, future research should focus on its impact on health outcomes, health care utilization, and health systems costs. Given the high prevalence of SUDs among hospitalized patients and their frequent need to access medical care on discharge, hospitalization offers a critical opportunity for effective intervention and evidence-based addiction treatment. Inpatient services alone are not sufficient, however, because having robust and available outpatient services for linkage seem critical to the successes of current consult service models. ACSs offer a feasible solution to address the intensive needs of patients with an SUD and consequently have immense potential to dramatically reduce the morbidity and mortality experienced by individuals with an SUD.

ACKNOWLEDGMENTS

The editors wish to thank Jan Gryczynski, Friends Research Institute, for providing a critical review of this article.

REFERENCES

1. National Institute on Drug Abuse. Trends & statistics. 2017. Available at: https://www.drugabuse.gov/related-topics/trends-statistics. Accessed July 10, 2017.
2. The National Center on Addiction and Substance Abuse. Addiction medicine: closing the gap between science and practice. 2012. Available at: https://www.centeronaddiction.org/addiction-research/reports/addiction-medicine-closing-gap-between-science-and-practice. Accessed July 10, 2017.
3. Brown RL, Leonard T, Saunders LA, et al. The prevalence and detection of substance use disorders among inpatients ages 18 to 49: an ppportunity for prevention. Prev Med 1998;27(1):101–10.
4. Weiss AJ, Elixhauser A, Barrett ML, et al. Opioid-related inpatient stays and emergency department visits by state, 2009–2014: statistical brief #219. In: healthcare Cost and Utilization Project (HCUP) Statistical Briefs. Rockville (MD): Agency for Healthcare Research and Quality (US); 2017. Available at: http://www.ncbi.nlm.nih.gov/books/NBK441648/. Accessed July 10, 2017.
5. Substance Abuse and Mental Health Services Administration. Reports and detailed tables from the 2015 National Survey on Drug Use and Health (NSDUH). Available at: https://www.samhsa.gov/samhsa-data-outcomes-quality/major-data-collections/reports-detailed-tables-2015-NSDUH. Accessed March 29, 2017.
6. McQueen J, Howe TE, Allan L, et al. Brief interventions for heavy alcohol users admitted to general hospital wards. Cochrane Database Syst Rev 2011;(8):CD005191.
7. Pecoraro A, Horton T, Ewen E, et al. Early data from project engage: a program to identify and transition medically hospitalized patients into addictions treatment. Addict Sci Clin Pract 2012;7:20.
8. Liebschutz JM, Crooks D, Herman D, et al. Buprenorphine treatment for hospitalized, opioid-dependent patients: a randomized clinical trial. JAMA Intern Med 2014;174(8):1369–76.
9. Rigotti NA, Regan S, Levy DE, et al. Sustained care intervention and postdischarge smoking cessation among hospitalized adults: a randomized clinical trial. JAMA 2014;312(7):719–28.
10. Wei J, Defries T, Lozada M, et al. An inpatient treatment and discharge planning protocol for alcohol dependence: efficacy in reducing 30-Day readmissions and emergency department visits. J Gen Intern Med 2015;30(3):365–70.
11. Shanahan CW, Beers D, Alford DP, et al. A transitional opioid program to engage hospitalized drug users. J Gen Intern Med 2010;25(8):803–8.

12. Wakeman SE, Pham-Kanter G, Donelan K. Attitudes, practices, and preparedness to care for patients with substance use disorder: Results from a survey of general internists. Subst Abus 2016;37(4):635–41.

13. Wakeman SE, Baggett MV, Pham-Kanter G, et al. Internal medicine residents' training in substance use disorders: a survey of the quality of instruction and residents' self-perceived preparedness to diagnose and treat addiction. Subst Abus 2013;34(4):363–70.

14. Wakeman SE, Kanter GP, Donelan K. Institutional substance use disorder intervention improves general internist preparedness, attitudes, and clinical practice. J Addict Med 2017;11(4):308–14.

15. Kelly JF, Wakeman SE, Saitz R. Stop talking 'dirty': clinicians, language, and quality of care for the leading cause of preventable death in the United States. Am J Med 2015;128(1):8–9.

16. American Psychiatric Association. Diagnostic and statistical manual of mental disorders. 5th edition. Washington (DC): American Psychiatric Association Publishing Co; 2013.

17. Hutchinson AB, Farnham PG, Sansom SL, et al. Cost-effectiveness of frequent HIV testing of high-risk populations in the United States. J Acquir Immune Defic Syndr 1999 2016;71(3):323–30.

18. Thakarar K, Weinstein ZM, Walley AY. Optimising health and safety of people who inject drugs during transition from acute to outpatient care: narrative review with clinical checklist. Postgrad Med J 2016;92(1088):356–63.

19. Walsh N, Verster A, Rodolph M, et al. WHO guidance on the prevention of viral hepatitis B and C among people who inject drugs. Int J Drug Policy 2014; 25(3):363–71.

20. Centers for Disease Control and Prevention (CDC). Update to interim guidance for Preexposure Prophylaxis (PrEP) for the prevention of HIV infection: PrEP for injecting drug users. MMWR Morb Mortal Wkly Rep 2013;62(23):463–5.

21. Günthard HF, Saag MS, Benson CA, et al. Antiretroviral drugs for treatment and prevention of HIV infection in adults: 2016 recommendations of the International Antiviral Society–USA panel. JAMA 2016;316(2):191–210.

22. McNeil R, Small W, Wood E, et al. Hospitals as a 'risk environment': An ethno-epidemiological study of voluntary and involuntary discharge from hospital against medical advice among people who inject drugs. Soc Sci Med 2014; 105:59–66.

23. Fanucchi L, Lofwall MR. Putting parity into practice — integrating opioid-use disorder treatment into the hospital setting. N Engl J Med 2016;375(9):811–3.

24. Wakeman SE, Ghoshhajra BB, Dudzinski DM, et al. Case records of the Massachusetts General Hospital. Case 35-2014: a 31-year-old woman with fevers, chest pain, and a history of HCV infection and substance-use disorder. N Engl J Med 2014;371(20):1918–26.

25. Heatherton TF, Kozlowski LT, Frecker RC, et al. The fagerström test for nicotine dependence: a revision of the fagerström tolerance questionnaire. Br J Addict 1991;86(9):1119–27.

26. Bayard M, McIntyre J, Hill K, et al. Alcohol withdrawal syndrome. Am Fam Physician 2004;69(6):1443–50.

27. Gortney JS, Raub JN, Patel P, et al. Alcohol withdrawal syndrome in medical patients. Cleve Clin J Med 2016;83(1):67–79.

28. Maldonado JR, Sher Y, Ashouri JF, et al. The "Prediction of Alcohol Withdrawal Severity Scale" (PAWSS): systematic literature review and pilot study of a new

scale for the prediction of complicated alcohol withdrawal syndrome. Alcohol 2014;48(4):375–90.

29. Mayo-Smith MF. Pharmacological management of alcohol withdrawal: a meta-analysis and evidence-based practice guideline. JAMA 1997;278(2):144–51.

30. Saitz R, O'Malley SS. Pharmacotherapies for alcohol abuse: withdrawal and treatment. Med Clin North Am 1997;81(4):881–907.

31. Sullivan JT, Sykora K, Schneiderman J, et al. Assessment of alcohol withdrawal: the revised clinical institute withdrawal assessment for alcohol scale (CIWA-Ar). Br J Addict 1989;84(11):1353–7.

32. Saitz R, Mayo-Smith MF, Roberts MS, et al. Individualized treatment for alcohol withdrawal: a randomized double-blind controlled trial. JAMA 1994;272(7): 519–23.

33. Askgaard G, Hallas J, Fink-Jensen A, et al. Phenobarbital compared to benzodiazepines in alcohol withdrawal treatment: a register-based cohort study of subsequent benzodiazepine use, alcohol recidivism and mortality. Drug Alcohol Depend 2016;161:258–64.

34. Mo Y, Thomas MC, Karras GE Jr. Barbiturates for the treatment of alcohol withdrawal syndrome: a systematic review of clinical trials. J Crit Care 2016;32:101–7.

35. Soyka M. Treatment of benzodiazepine dependence. N Engl J Med 2017; 376(24):2399–400.

36. Pétursson H. The benzodiazepine withdrawal syndrome. Addiction 1994;89(11): 1455–9.

37. Mcgregor C, Machin A, White JM. In-patient benzodiazepine withdrawal: comparison of fixed and symptom-triggered taper methods. Drug Alcohol Rev 2003;22(2):175–80.

38. Kawasaki SS, Jacapraro JS, Rastegar DA. Safety and effectiveness of a fixed-dose phenobarbital protocol for inpatient benzodiazepine detoxification. J Subst Abuse Treat 2012;43(3):331–4.

39. Tompkins DA, Bigelow GE, Harrison JA, et al. Concurrent validation of the Clinical Opiate Withdrawal Scale (COWS) and single-item indices against the Clinical Institute Narcotic Assessment (CINA) opioid withdrawal instrument. Drug Alcohol Depend 2009;105(1):154–9.

40. Wesson DR, Ling W. The clinical opiate withdrawal scale (COWS). J Psychoactive Drugs 2003;35(2):253–9.

41. MacArthur GJ, Minozzi S, Martin N, et al. Opiate substitution treatment and HIV transmission in people who inject drugs: systematic review and meta-analysis. BMJ 2012;345:e5945.

42. Schuckit MA. Treatment of opioid-use disorders. N Engl J Med 2016;375(4): 357–68.

43. Amato L, Davoli M, Minozzi S, et al. Methadone at tapered doses for the management of opioid withdrawal. Cochrane Database Syst Rev 2013;(2):CD003409.

44. Gowing L, Ali R, White JM, et al. Buprenorphine for managing opioid withdrawal. Cochrane Database Syst Rev 2017;(5):CD002021.

45. Noska A, Mohan A, Wakeman S, et al. Managing opioid use disorder during and after acute hospitalization: a case-based review clarifying methadone regulation for acute care settings. J Addict Behav Ther Rehabil 2015;4(2) [pii:1000138].

46. Donroe JH, Tetrault JM. Substance use, intoxication, and withdrawal in the critical care setting. Crit Care Clin 2017;33(3):543–58.

47. Velez CM, Nicolaidis C, Korthuis PT, et al. "It's been an experience, a life learning experience": a qualitative study of hospitalized patients with substance use disorders. J Gen Intern Med 2017;32(3):296–303.

48. Babb S, Malarcher A, Schauer G, et al. Quitting smoking among adults — United States, 2000–2015. MMWR Morb Mortal Wkly Rep 2017;65(52):1457–64.

49. Nugent CN, Schoenborn CA, Vahratian A. Discussions between health care providers and their patients who smoke cigarettes: NCHS Data Brief No. 174. 2014. Available at: https://www.cdc.gov/nchs/data/databriefs/db174.pdf. Accessed July 10, 2017.

50. Stead LF, Buitrago D, Preciado N, et al. Physician advice for smoking cessation. Cochrane Database Syst Rev 2013. https://doi.org/10.1002/14651858.CD000165.pub4. Accessed July 10, 2017.

51. Cahill K, Stevens S, Perera R, et al. Pharmacological interventions for smoking cessation: an overview and network meta-analysis. Cochrane Database Syst Rev 2013;(5):CD009329.

52. Stead LF, Koilpillai P, Fanshawe TR, et al. Combined pharmacotherapy and behavioural interventions for smoking cessation. Cochrane Database Syst Rev 2016;(3):CD008286.

53. Stead LF, Koilpillai P, Lancaster T. Additional behavioural support as an adjunct to pharmacotherapy for smoking cessation. Cochrane Database Syst Rev 2015;(10):CD009670.

54. Kaner EFS, Beyer F, Dickinson HO, et al. Effectiveness of brief alcohol interventions in primary care populations. Cochrane Database Syst Rev 2007;(2):CD004148.

55. Makdissi R, Stewart SH. Care for hospitalized patients with unhealthy alcohol use: a narrative review. Addict Sci Clin Pract 2013;8(1):11.

56. Addolorato G, Mirijello A, Leggio L, et al. Management of alcohol dependence in patients with liver disease. CNS Drugs 2013;27(4):287–99.

57. Friedmann PD. Alcohol use in adults. N Engl J Med 2013;368(4):365–73.

58. Darker CD, Sweeney BP, Barry JM, et al. Psychosocial interventions for benzodiazepine harmful use, abuse or dependence. Cochrane Database Syst Rev 2015;(5):CD009652.

59. Castells X, Cunill R, Pérez-Mañá C, et al. Psychostimulant drugs for cocaine dependence. Cochrane Database Syst Rev 2016;(9):CD007380.

60. Pettinati HM, Kampman KM, Lynch KG, et al. A pilot trial of injectable, extended-release naltrexone for the treatment of co-occurring cocaine and alcohol dependence. Am J Addict 2014;23(6):591–7.

61. Singh M, Keer D, Klimas J, et al. Topiramate for cocaine dependence: a systematic review and meta-analysis of randomized controlled trials. Addiction 2016;111(8):1337–46.

62. Minozzi S, Saulle R, De Crescenzo F, et al. Psychosocial interventions for psychostimulant misuse. Cochrane Database Syst Rev 2016;(9):CD011866.

63. Wakeman SE, Metlay JP, Chang Y, et al. Inpatient addiction consultation for hospitalized patients increases post-discharge abstinence and reduces addiction severity. J Gen Intern Med 2017;32(8):909–16.

64. Englander H, Weimer M, Solotaroff R, et al. Planning and designing the Improving Addiction Care Team (IMPACT) for hospitalized adults with substance use disorder. J Hosp Med 2017;12(5):339–42.

65. O'Toole DTP, Conde-Martel A, Young JH, et al. Managing acutely ill substance-abusing patients in an integrated day hospital outpatient program. J Gen Intern Med 2006;21(6):570–6.

66. Murphy MK, Chabon B, Delgado A, et al. Development of a substance abuse consultation and referral service in an academic medical center: challenges, achievements and dissemination. J Clin Psychol Med Settings 2009;16(1):77–86.

67. McDuff DR, Solounias BL, Beuger M, et al. A substance abuse consultation service. Am J Addict 1997;6(3):256–65.
68. Trowbridge P, Weinstein ZM, Kerensky T, et al. Addiction consultation services – Linking hospitalized patients to outpatient addiction treatment. J Subst Abuse Treat 2017;79:1–5.
69. Aszalos R, McDuff DR, Weintraub E, et al. Engaging hospitalized heroin-dependent patients into substance abuse treatment. J Subst Abuse Treat 1999;17(1–2):149–58.
70. O'Toole TP, Pollini RA, Ford DE, et al. The effect of integrated medical-substance abuse treatment during an acute illness on subsequent health services utilization. Med Care 2007;45(11):1110–5.
71. Klimas J, Ahamad K, Fairgrieve C, et al. Impact of a brief addiction medicine training experience on knowledge self-assessment among medical learners. Subst Abuse 2017;38(2):141–4.

Addressing Adolescents' and Young Adults' Substance Use Disorders

Nicholas Chadi, MD[a],*, Sarah M. Bagley, MD, MSc[b,c,d,e],
Scott E. Hadland, MD, MPH, MS[b,c]

KEYWORDS

- Adolescents • Young adults • Substance use disorders • Prevention • Intervention

KEY POINTS

- Adolescents and young adults (AYAs) have unique needs and important biopsychosocial differences when compared with older adults who use substances.
- As their brains continue to develop, youth are especially susceptible to the reinforcing effects of substances in the context of a still-developing capacity for executive control and decision making.
- In this article, the authors highlight key differences in the neurobiologic, epidemiologic, and relational aspects of substance use found in AYA.
- The authors also discuss how best to engage with youth who use substances and how prevention and intervention can be adapted for optimal effectiveness for this distinct and high-risk population.

INTRODUCTION

Most people who use substances start using in their teen and young adult years,[1] and a common misconception is that most do not experience the consequences of substance use until later in adulthood. Although this is true for some people, adolescents and young adults (AYAs) are disproportionately represented in substance-related hospital admissions and are at high risk for injury and acute health problems related to substance use.[2,3] There has also been an increasing awareness of

[a] Adolescent Substance Use and Addiction Program, Division of Developmental Medicine, Department of Pediatrics, Boston Children's Hospital, Harvard Medical School, 300 Longwood Avenue, Boston, MA 02115, USA; [b] Division of General Pediatrics, Department of Pediatrics, Boston University School of Medicine, 88 East Newton Street, Vose Hall Room 322, Boston, MA 02118, USA; [c] Section of General Internal Medicine, Department of Medicine, Boston University School of Medicine, 801 Massachusetts Avenue, 2nd Floor, Boston, MA 02118, USA; [d] Department of Pediatrics, Boston Medical Center, Grayken Center for Addiction, 850 Harrison Avenue, Boston, MA 02118, USA; [e] Department of Medicine, Boston Medical Center, Grayken Center for Addiction, 850 Harrison Avenue, Boston, MA 02118, USA
* Corresponding author.
E-mail address: nicholas.chadi@childrens.harvard.edu

Med Clin N Am 102 (2018) 603–620
https://doi.org/10.1016/j.mcna.2018.02.015
0025-7125/18/© 2018 Elsevier Inc. All rights reserved.
medical.theclinics.com

medical complications among AYAs who inject drugs.[4] Addressing substance use among youth provides both a challenge and an opportunity for health care providers.

AYAs have unique needs and important biopsychosocial differences compared with older adults who use substances.[5,6] Understanding these differences is essential to tailoring strategies to address substance use disorders and associated harms. Care should be developmentally appropriate and youth-focused and should not only aim to address the substance use itself but also provide an overarching understanding of the biopsychosocial context in which it occurs.[7] Historically, treatments for substance use disorders have often been punitive in nature; these "traditional" approaches may result in poor treatment engagement and retention in care and represent a lost opportunity to address substance use problems at an earlier stage.[8] A developmentally appropriate approach that incorporates parents, other caregivers, school support, and for adolescents less than the age of 18, state agencies responsible for child protection when appropriate, requires careful coordination and providers who are aware of the issues specific to this age group.

After describing key differences in the neurobiologic and psychosocial aspects and patterns of substance use among AYAs when compared with older adults, the authors discuss how prevention and intervention can be adapted for optimal effectiveness for AYAs.

UNIQUE CONSIDERATIONS FOR ADOLESCENTS AND YOUNG ADULTS
Neurobiologic and Neuropsychiatric Considerations

Functional neuroimaging provides robust evidence that the adolescent brain continues to develop late into the third decade of life.[9] In AYAs, the developmental process of synaptic pruning and myelination (responsible for strengthening and improving the efficiency of existing neuronal pathways) is particularly active in the prefrontal cortex, an area of the brain central to decision making and impulse control. The relative immaturity of this executive functioning center contrasts with an already developed dopaminergic system (the "reward pathway," involving the nucleus accumbens, ventral tegmental area, and other structures), which stems from more primitive areas of the brain. In AYAs, this results in a vulnerability to the reinforcing pleasurable effects of psychoactive substances, combined with potentially limited insight into the harmful consequences of substance use.[10] A well-established body of literature shows that substances like nicotine, alcohol, marijuana, and illicit drugs have long-lasting effects on brain function, suggesting that there is no safe level of substance use during the neural development of adolescence and young adulthood.[11]

Not only are AYAs more vulnerable to the immediate rewarding effects of drugs and alcohol, but substance use during adolescence can also increase susceptibility to addiction later in life.[12] For instance, youth who start drinking alcohol before age 15 are 6 times more likely to develop an alcohol use disorder in their adult years than youth who start drinking at age 21.[13] Substance use during critical periods of adolescent brain development may underlie this long-term risk for addiction.[14] There are still many unanswered questions concerning the interplay between inherited and acquired factors and how they can impact a young person's brain's response to substances.[15] Nevertheless, AYAs with a family history of substance use disorder should be aware that their vulnerability to addiction may be higher than that of their peers, and that earlier onset of substance use may further amplify this risk.[12]

Puberty and Developmental Considerations

Adolescence, and especially puberty, is a period of rapid physical growth and development. During this period, the body is rapidly changing, and as youth develop decision-making and reasoning capacities, they also further refine interpersonal and coping skills.[16] Adolescence and early adulthood is also an important period for acquiring independence from parents through prosocial and positive risk activities. Substance use poses a challenge because it can be perceived by youth as a positive opportunity to seek further independence from the family unit, and in many settings, substance use among young people is normalized. Although the exploration of risk-seeking behaviors is a normal part of adolescence, the use of substances during critical windows of development can easily interrupt or delay the attainment of key developmental milestones.[17] For instance, youth who use substances heavily may delay completing school, obtaining a first job, or forming healthy relationships, all of which may make meeting later developmental milestones more challenging. AYAs are thus placed in a challenging position whereby substance use can act as a response to biological and developmental impulses while at the same time posing a risk of delaying healthy transition into adulthood.[18]

Risk Factors for Substance Use

As with older adults, AYAs have individual risk and predisposing factors that impact their vulnerability to substance use disorders.[12] It can be helpful to categorize these factors in 3 categories: developmental (as described above), genetic, and environmental. A thorough review of genetic risk factors for substance use in adolescents is beyond the scope of this article, but it should be noted that genes have been found to explain more than half of the total variance between individuals with and without substance use disorders.[19] Several candidate genes have also been identified as either increasing risk of misusing substances or of developing adverse health effects related to their use.[20]

AYAs are faced with unique psychosocial issues that can have a strong influence on their perception and attitudes related to substances. Three important risk factors for adolescent substance use are family history of substance use (to which genetics is also a contributor); family perceptions and opinions about substance use; and history of childhood maltreatment, unhealthy use, and neglect.[21] In the context of rapidly evolving policies on marijuana, tobacco, and e-cigarettes in North America, parents and health care providers are faced with new challenges in choosing how to discuss and set rules around licit and illicit substances with youth.[22] Recent research suggests that parenting styles have an impact on rates of substance use in youth. In general, parenting styles that are more authoritative, where parents set high expectations, establish clear rules, and provide support to achieve goals, are protective, and adolescents of parents who are less involved are more likely to use substances.[23] In addition, a dose-response association has been shown between the number of adverse childhood experiences and rates of alcohol, tobacco, and illicit drug use and subsequent risk of developing a substance use disorder in AYAs. This association suggests that historical and contextual elements, such as trauma, economic disadvantage, and early exposure to substance use in the family or environment, should always be considered in prevention and treatment strategies involving young people and that childhood adversity has long-term consequences on the risk of developing a substance use disorder.[24,25]

Although adolescents are in the process of forming their own identity and confirming their own personal values, the influence of peers and family members plays an important role in shaping what is considered normative, healthy, and acceptable.[26] It is important to understand that friendships and friends' behaviors both online and offline have a direct impact on adolescent risk behaviors and substance use and across studies are a consistent predictor of substance use among AYAs.[27,28] In addition, certain sociodemographic subgroups of youth exhibit higher rates of substance use and medical and mental health complications related to tobacco, drug, and alcohol use.[29] Although belonging to certain racial or ethnic groups may be protective (eg, Asian American youth typically have lower rates of substance use), other characteristics (ie, mental illness, unstable housing, foster care, and identifying as lesbian, gay, bisexual, transgender, or queer/questioning) have historically had higher rates of substance use disorders and complications related to their drug use, in part owing to stigma and its contributions to adverse health outcomes.[30,31]

PATTERNS OF SUBSTANCE USE
Use Versus Addiction

Adolescence is often a period of experimentation. A central limitation of many national surveys seeking to measure the prevalence of substance use among AYAs is that they focus on frequency of use rather than on problems resulting from the use of substances. For instance, most large national surveys compiling data on substances use the concept of lifetime, past-year, or past-month use but do not further inquire about consequences related to substance use.[13,29] As a result, national data tend to center on measuring experimentation and use rather than on describing the true burden of "addiction." The distinctions between use and addiction, that is, a clinically significant substance use disorder, are important. Substance use disorder, as defined by the *Diagnostic and Statistical Manual* (Fifth Edition), encompasses not only use of a substance but also interpersonal, social, or professional problems; use despite ongoing psychological or physical harm; and/or cravings, tolerance, or withdrawal.[32] As such, national screening and survey studies reporting prevalence rates of substance use should be taken for what they are: an indication of national trends warranting further discussion and investigation. Another important limitation of large national youth surveys is that they are often school or household based and thus do not capture youth who are absent from school or homeless and likely represent a high-risk group for substance use.

Epidemiologic Trends

According to recent data from *Monitoring the Future*, a representative epidemiologic survey collecting data annually on behaviors and attitudes from approximately 50,000 American students in the 8th, 10th, and 12th grades, use of nearly all substances by adolescents has trended downwards since the late 1990s.[29] This trend is also shown by the *National Survey on Drug Use and Health*, an annual survey that provides national data on the rates of tobacco, alcohol, and illicit drugs use in individuals 12 years and older in the United States.[13] Two exceptions are the prevalence of marijuana use, which has remained relatively stable among youth, and the misuse of prescription opioids, which peaked in the early 2000s, but has been trending downwards, particularly during the mid-2010s.[33] Some experts think that decreasing perceptions of risk of use are contributing to continued increases in the prevalence of daily marijuana use, which has increased from 2% to 6% in grade 12 students between 1991 and 2016.[29,34]

In 2016, approximately half of all high school seniors had ever used an illegal drug (including marijuana), and this percentage decreases to 20% when marijuana is excluded.[29] Data from Canadian surveys show similar rates of drug use as in the

United States,[35] but important differences exist as compared with European countries.[36] For instance, the incidence of alcohol use in the past 30 days (22% vs 48%) and daily cigarette use (3% vs 12%) is much higher in Europe, whereas rates of marijuana, cocaine, opioids, and stimulants are much lower in Europe (approximately half compared with North American rates) except for a few countries (eg, France and Czech Republic) that have similar rates of marijuana use and illicit drug use to the United States.[36]

It is also important to note that data from national surveys do not reliably capture the increasing incidence of person who injects drugs and overdose-related medical complications and deaths among AYAs, which have received much attention in recent years.[37,38] Indeed, overdose deaths and hospitalizations (most related to opioids, including heroin and prescription pills) have continued to climb despite declining self-reported use in *Monitoring the Future*.[39] Nevertheless, the *National Survey on Drug Use and Health* shows that young adults aged 18 to 25 are disproportionately affected by heroin and prescription opioid use disorders with rates that are almost twice as high as in older adults with marked increase in rates since the beginning of the current decade.[40]

Most Commonly Used Substances by Age Group

Multiple factors influence which substances young people decide to use at different times in their adolescent and young adult years. Access is an important factor, which might explain why young children of age 12 and younger are overly represented in the prevalence of inhalant and domestic product use (including, for example, nitrous oxide, amyl nitrite, gasoline, bath salts, cough syrup, cleaning fluids, spray paint, computer keyboard cleaner, felt-tip pens, and glue).[29] Although use of alcohol, tobacco, marijuana, and stimulants increases throughout adolescence, alcohol is by far the most commonly used substance among adolescents, followed by marijuana[13]; a marked increase in the incidence of binge drinking and tobacco use is observed epidemiologically among youth when they reach 13 to 14 years of age. It is notable that the pattern of intermittent heavy use common among adolescents differs quite significantly from use among adults, for whom regular daily use is much more common than for AYAs.[13] Although infrequent, the use of Ecstasy and injectable drugs is much more predominant among older adolescents than young adolescents.[29]

In response to an increase in misuse by AYAs of prescription medications (now second only to cannabis as the most common illicit drug use issue in the United States), the *National Survey on Drug Use and Mental Health* started tracking detailed data on the use and misuse of 4 categories of medications in 2015 (pain relievers, tranquilizers, stimulants, and sedatives).[13] The survey revealed that 15.3% of 18 to 25 year olds, 7.2% of 12 to 17 year olds, and 5.8% of adults 26 or older misused at least one of these 4 categories of medications in the last year, thus demonstrating a particular burden among young adults.[41] It is worth noting that the average age of onset of prescription drug misuse was 26 years for pain relievers and tranquilizers and 22 years for stimulants.[29]

Legal access to substances and recent changes in legislation around tobacco and marijuana are important factors influencing risk perception, and ultimately, use of these substances. In the past decade, since the first American states have legalized recreational marijuana, there has been a steady decrease in risk perception associated with its use.[29] For tobacco, more stringent policies are emerging, with several jurisdictions considering raising the legal age of cigarette sales to 21. Overall, the effects of legislative changes on marijuana and tobacco availability along with changes in risk perception on substance use in AYAs remain a controversial topic requiring caution and further investigation.[42]

Adverse Effects Linked to Substance Use

Substance use among AYAs is associated with multiple negative health consequences. In addition, important gender differences exist between male and female AYAs, with girls who use substances tending to have more associated internalizing and traumatic stress disorders and with boys who use substances tending to have more associated juvenile justice problems and externalizing disorders.[43] Despite relatively successful public health education campaigns on youth alcohol use over the past 3 decades, rates of alcohol-related motor vehicle crash fatalities remain highest among young people.[2] Recent research has shown that more restrictive policies can be effective in reducing the burden of deaths related to this issue.[44] Driving while under the influence of marijuana has also been shown to contribute to the burden of motor vehicle crashes.[45] Because of the immaturity of the prefrontal cortex, youth are disproportionately vulnerable to the disinhibition effect of substances, especially in sexuality and relationships. Rates of unprotected sex, sexually transmitted infections, and relationship violence are relatively high among AYAs, but are even higher among youth who use alcohol, marijuana, or illicit substances compared with AYAs who do not.[46,47] In addition, research has suggested that AYAs may experience less severe withdrawal symptoms than older adults and as a result may experience less of a deterring effect from substance use.[48–50] These factors are important elements to consider in planning comprehensive prevention and intervention strategies with youth.

SCREENING AND PREVENTION
Taking a Substance Use History

Approaching the topic of substance use with AYAs in a youth-friendly way is a skill that requires practice. Leaders in adolescent medicine have developed a structured approach to facilitate the formation of a therapeutic alliance with adolescents with the rationale that AYAs will share much more accurate information with providers they can trust, especially when it comes to sensitive topics such as substance use.[7] Providers caring for adolescents need to have an open-minded and nonjudgmental attitude with their patients and show that they are genuinely interested in them. In a safe and supportive setting, most AYAs will willingly share the details of their substance use.

The HEADSS mnemonic (H for home, E for education/work, A for activities, D for drug/ substance use, S for sexuality, and S for suicidality/mood) is a clinical tool that allows clinicians to explore topics that might be more challenging to discuss (ie, drug/substance use, sexuality, and suicidality) after reviewing more casual conversation topics (ie, home, education, and activities).[51] Clinicians should ask several open-ended questions related to each of the different domains outlined in the HEADSS mnemonic while also remaining attentive to verbal and nonverbal language cues that might reveal the adolescent's willingness to share more sensitive information. The HEADSS approach has also been adapted into a strength-based model, with the acronym SHADESS where the first "S" encourages the clinician to inquire about patient strengths in a way that is conducive to the development of a therapeutic alliance between patient and provider.[52] The HEADSS/SHADESS mnemonic has also been modified to tailor to the needs of specific populations, such as youth with chronic illness, who are at particular risk of experiencing negative health consequences related to substance use.[53,54]

Addressing Substance Use in General Medical Care

Longitudinal follow-up in the context of primary care often offers an optimal setting for discussions about substance use. Signs and symptoms of substance use can be subtle and difficult to detect in adolescents, especially in youth who use only intermittently or in small amounts. Most of the time, there are no physical symptoms, but clinicians and parents should keep a high level of suspicion for youth reporting behavioral changes, mood changes, changes in appetite, sleep, or level of alertness, new difficulties at school, or loss of interest in hobbies and activities.[16] In addition, some of these signs may indicate other mental health conditions, such as depression or even bullying at school.[55] In heavier or more experienced users, providers need to be ready to inquire about how youth access or pay for their substances. In patients who are less than 18 years old, this may uncover high-risk sexual or criminal activity or situations where unhealthy use or trafficking is present, which may need to be reported to child protective services. In addition, helping AYAs reflect upon how much money they are spending on substances can be a motivating factor for them to reduce their use.

There are several barriers that can come in the way of addressing substance use disorders in primary care. These barriers include perceived lack of time, alignment with other priorities, physician discomfort, need for confidentiality and removing parents from room, and issues related to reimbursement.[56,57] However, several facilitators also exist, such as computer, tablet, or mobile-based screening methods,[58] integration of screening questions in electronic medical records, and new models for integrated behavioral health, which can reduce the burden on providers when patients have positive screens.[59]

Screening, Brief Intervention, and Referral to Treatment

Whereas the US Preventive Services Task Force does not currently recommend the regular use of Screening, Brief Intervention, and Referral to Treatment (SBIRT) for adolescents younger than the age of 18 (grade I) due to insufficient evidence, both the American Academy of Pediatrics and the Substance Abuse and Mental Health Services Administration recommend that all AYAs receive SBIRT as part of routine health care.[7] Considering that adolescents have the highest level of risk of experiencing adverse consequences related to substance use, they may be the most likely to benefit from SBIRT.[7] Some experts recommend that health providers provide SBIRT at every health maintenance visit or at an acute visit if a routine health visit has been missed, as well as when youth present with behavioral or mental health symptoms.[60]

Developmentally appropriate screening for substance use is important for all adolescents and will help guide the delivery of effective behavioral intervention according to the youth's past experiences and situation on the continuum of substance use. Several brief screening and assessment tools taking no longer than a few minutes to complete have been developed and validated for adolescents. The S2BI (Screening to Brief Intervention) model (**Table 1**) allows clinicians to screen for tobacco, alcohol, marijuana, and other illicit drugs and is endorsed by the American Academy of Pediatrics.[7] Other screening tools, such as the CRAFFT (Car, Relax, Alone, Forget, Friends, Trouble),[61] BSTAD (Brief Screener for Tobacco, Alcohol, and Other Drugs),[62] and the NIAAA Youth Alcohol Screen,[63] have also been shown effective for AYAs. Research comparing screening and assessment responses between emerging and older adults has shown significant differences in the sensitivity and specificity of validated screening when used in these 2 groups, providing further evidence for the need to tailor SBIRT not only for adolescents but also for young adults.[62,64,65]

Brief intervention with youth should be tailored to the frequency of use, the type of substances used, and associated risky behaviors. As a primary focus, brief intervention should aim to reinforce healthy choices with the aim of preventing, reducing, or stopping risky behaviors related to substances. For youth who are abstinent, this

Table 1
Adolescent screen and assessment tool questions (Screening to Brief Intervention)

Screening Questions (Asked of All Participants)	Response Items
In the past year, how many times have you used [X]?	Never
Tobacco products	Once or twice
Alcohol	Monthly
Marijuana	Weekly
Illegal drugs (such as cocaine or Ecstasy)	Daily
Prescription drugs that were not prescribed for you (such as pain medication or Adderall)	Almost daily
Over-the-counter medications (such as cough medicine) for nonmedical reasons	
Inhalants (such as nitrous oxide)	
Herbs or synthetic drugs (such as salvia, K2, or bath salts)	
Brief assessment questions (asked of participants who answered "yes" to screening questions, contingent on frequency):	Yes/No
RAFFT (for any past-year alcohol, marijuana, or other drug use)	
Do you ever use alcohol or drugs to relax, feel better about yourself, or fit in?	
Do you ever use alcohol or drugs while you are by yourself, alone?	
Do you ever forget things you did while using alcohol or drugs?	
Do your family or friends ever tell you that you should cut down on your drinking or drug use?	
Have you ever gotten into trouble while you were using alcohol or drugs?	
Alcohol (if once or more):	
Have you had [X] or more drinks on one occasion on 3 or more days?	
Had an alcoholic "blackout" (periods that you could not remember due to drinking), "passed out," or had an emergency department visit due to substance use?	
Had 10 or more drinks on one occasion?	
Combined any of the following: alcohol, sedatives such as barbiturates (such as phenobarbital or pentobarbital), benzodiazepines (such as Klonopin, Ativan, or Xanax), opiates, or a prescription pain medication?	
If weekly or monthly:	
Have you used alcohol 5 or more days per week for 2 or more weeks?	
Marijuana (if weekly or monthly):	
Have you used marijuana one or more times per day for 2 or more weeks?	
Tobacco products (if weekly or monthly):	
Have you used tobacco one or more times per day for 2 or more weeks?	
Other substances (if once or more):	
Have you used [X] in the past 30 d?	
Prescription medications (not prescribed for you)	
Over-the-counter medications (not for medical purposes)	
Inhalants	
Herbal supplements	
Synthetic drugs	

could include positive reinforcement, some education about the effects of drugs and alcohol on the adolescent brain, and discussion of risks associated with substance use; for youth with infrequent use, a short motivational interviewing session promoting patient strengths and providing information about the medical harms of substance use; and for youth with frequent use and/or a substance use disorder, a discussion centered around harm reduction and referral to treatment. Here, the authors use the term "harm reduction" to refer to an approach that supports reductions in use falling short of full abstinence and that can be associated with a partial decrease in impairment and increases in psychosocial function. This approach serves as an initial interim goal that is part of a broader motivational enhancement strategy seeking patient engagement and with the eventual goal of encouraging abstinence from all substances. The 2016 US Surgeon General's report emphasizes the importance of early intervention for adolescents aged 12 to 17 years who binge drink due to their elevated risk for future substance use disorders owing to their young age.[66] Many researchers have also looked at the effectiveness of brief interventions provided in the school setting. Although several studies have shown a reduction in alcohol and marijuana use with brief school-based interventions, evidence for long-term effects remains limited.[67]

Referral to treatment is a critical yet challenging step in SBIRT as a result of relatively poorer availability of adolescent-friendly services. According to the 2016 *National Survey on Drug Use and Health*, only 6.3% of adolescents and 7.7% of young adults with severe substance use disorders receive the treatment they need compared with 12.3% of adults over 25 years of age.[68] To maximize chances of success, clinicians should emphasize to AYAs and their families the importance of substance use treatment for the health and well-being of the young person. The clinician should also provide guidance and support with the referral process and ensure that the family has access to the right contact and follow-up information while continuing to see the young person throughout treatment to promote retention in care and support recovery.[7] Finally, given the limited number and availability of evidence-based treatment options for youth, communication with specialty providers and expectation of reciprocal communication back from those providers to whom referrals are made should be encouraged.

EFFECTIVE INTERVENTION
Differences in Treatment Approaches

AYAs offer unique challenges when it comes to substance use treatment. Of these, issues surrounding consent, capacity, and decision making are perhaps the most important and complex.[69] In the United States, adolescents younger than the age of 18 generally must rely on their parents to consent to medical care, unless they are found to be mature or emancipated minors, or in the case of an emergency situation.[70] However, in many states, a minor younger than the age of 18 can consent for his or her own substance use treatment; providers should be aware of the policies in the state in which they practice. Even for minors whose parents consent for treatment, providers should also seek assent from the young person whenever possible, given the voluntary nature of many outpatient substance use treatment programs and in order to promote a strong patient-clinician relationship.[8] Nonetheless, nearly half of all adolescent admissions to substance use disorder treatment services are mandated by the criminal justice system.[1] Regardless of the referral source and motivations that bring youth to seek treatment, every encounter with an adolescent should begin with a discussion of the limits of confidentiality. Although any sensitive information not directly pertaining to an adolescent's safety should not be disclosed to parents (for instance, parents need not be told all the details of a young person's substance use), treatment-related decisions most commonly benefit from parental involvement and information sharing.

It is particularly important to have a good understanding of a young person's psychosocial history and support network before considering different treatment settings and modalities. Treatments requiring frequent medical appointments or administration of medication under direct supervision may require additional planning for youth with unstable housing or lack of support from parents and family; nevertheless, frequent clinical follow-up may promote recovery. For AYAs who are in a precontemplative state regarding treatment of their substance use, harm reduction strategies are critical.[66] In cases where youth are not willing to commit to completely abstaining from substance use, reduction in amount or frequency of use may be a central goal.

It is also important to address medical and mental health comorbidities, such as mood and anxiety disorders, attention deficit/hyperactivity disorder (ADHD), and chronic pain, which may place AYAs at risk of developing or further increasing their substance use. When untreated, these comorbid conditions can significantly interfere with abstinence or harm reduction goals.[71] For example, it has been shown that youth with ADHD whose symptoms are treated with psychostimulants have significantly lower risks of developing a substance use disorder and that the younger the initiation of medication treatment, the higher the protective effect.[72,73] All AYAs with substance use problems should also be tested for sexually transmitted infections, including human immunodeficiency virus and hepatitis B and C because of the high prevalence of high-risk sexual behaviors in the AYA population and possibility of person who injects drugs, which may result in acquisition of blood-borne infection.[43] Vaccination for hepatitis A and B should also be ensured.

Treatment

As with older adults, treatment of substance use disorders falls on a spectrum of intensity ranging from outpatient and community-based treatment to intensive outpatient, partial hospitalization programs, and residential programs. Regardless of the intensity of treatment, a combination of behavioral and pharmacologic treatments should be considered for AYAs with substance use disorders. Treatments need to address the unique needs of this population and should be determined by the types of substances used and the young person's developmental stage.[43]

Behavioral Approaches

Behavioral approaches represent a cornerstone of substance use disorder treatment in youth, and compared with other age groups, have the strongest evidence base in this population.[43,48] Cognitive-behavioral therapy (CBT) has been shown to be effective for the reduction of tobacco, alcohol, and marijuana use in adolescents, with improved efficacy when combined with other approaches, such as medication or technology-driven interventions.[74] Typically, a course of CBT for youth will include at least 6 to 8 sessions and contain concrete and actionable content delivered in a youth-friendly and developmentally adapted fashion. Motivational enhancement therapy, an approach that encourages individuals to resolve their ambivalence about engaging in treatment by evoking rapid and internally motivated changes, is also efficacious for youth and can be combined with CBT.[71] Sessions can be short, problem focused, and goal directed, an approach that has proven useful in AYAs, including those with limited attention capacity. The Adolescent Community Reinforcement Approach (A-CRA), which uses cognitive and behavioral techniques to replace environmental cues supporting substance use with prosocial activities promoting recovery, is another modality that is increasingly used and has shown promise in adolescents, particularly for youth with externalizing and internalizing emotional problems.[75,76] Finally, contingency management, an approach based on the creation of incentives and rewards to encourage patients to adopt healthy behaviors, has shown promise in youth, especially in youth with cannabis use disorders,[77–79] and can be combined with other behavioral treatments.

Treatment engagement is a key element of substance use disorder therapy for youth and requires the combination of multiple elements to maximize outcomes. Dunne and colleagues[80] have grouped critical elements into 6 categories: youth participation in treatment program development, relationship with parents, use of technology, health visits, school support, and social marketing. For instance, it has been shown that individual behavioral strategies work best for youth when combined with family and community-based interventions, because they can better address the complex needs of young people.[71] Family-based therapy and A-CRA with or without family training are particularly useful.[81,82] Although youth participation in 12-step programs (such as *Alcoholics Anonymous* or *Narcotics Anonymous*) has been traditionally limited, some youth may find participation a helpful adjunct to the clinically based substance use care they receive.[83] Youth-friendly community groups offering opportunities for socialization and identity formation are especially helpful for AYAs who are seeking independence from their families transitioning into adulthood.[84] Finally, several private residential programs, such as wilderness programs, offer opportunities for alternative treatment environments for AYAs, often away from usual clinical sites. Clinicians should exercise caution in recommending these programs because they can be very costly, are generally not covered by insurance, lack evidence of outcomes, and may be harmful in some cases.[85]

Medication

Medication should be considered in the treatment of AYAs with moderate to severe tobacco, opioid, marijuana, and alcohol use disorders. Although there are still few US Food and Drug Administration–approved pharmacologic treatments for adolescents younger than the age of 18, there is an increasing body of literature showing that medications used in older adults are safe and effective in young people and can be an important component of substance use disorder management.[86]

Tobacco
Over-the-counter nicotine replacement products (gums, lozenges, and patches) are currently the only pharmaceutical treatment approved for nicotine use disorder for adolescents younger than the age of 18. These products have been shown to be most effective in youth who smoke daily and more heavily.[87] In addition, medications approved for adults (bupropion and varenicline) that have been used off-label among adolescents have shown some effectiveness and received the support of pediatric societies in Canada and the United States.[88,89]

Opioids
Only 1 in 4 AYAs with opioid use disorder receives medication treatment, and the proportion is even lower among adolescents younger than the age of 18, even though offering medication is clearly encouraged by the American Academy of Pediatrics and the US Substance Abuse and Mental Health Services Administration.[90,91] For opioid use disorder, the American Academy of Pediatrics supports the use of methadone or buprenorphine (opioid agonists) as well as naltrexone (an opioid antagonist) to support and maintain recovery.[92] AYAs and their families should also be offered overdose education and naloxone. Recent research has shown high uptake of naloxone among family members of individuals at high risk of opioid overdose.[93]

Marijuana
Although research is limited, the use of *N*-acetylcysteine (NAC) for the treatment of moderate to severe cannabis use disorders has shown some promising results in a

study of AYAs aged 15 to 21[94] and could be considered a helpful adjunct to behavioral interventions.[86] Also, a large multicenter trial of NAC, including young adults, is currently underway.[95] At this time, however, evidence is lacking, and NAC is not yet recommended for routine use for adolescents or adults. In addition, in a small pilot study, gabapentin has been found to reduce cannabis use in adults ages ≥18 years, but there is currently no evidence for adolescents younger than the age of 18.[96]

Alcohol

Medication treatment of alcohol use disorders in adolescents less than 18 years of age remains poorly studied, but there have been some accounts of successful use of disulfiram and naltrexone in this population.[97,98] Medication should be routinely offered to young adults ≥18 years of age.

Recovery Support Services

Although less well studied, in the United States, an important network of mutual help groups, peer recovery services, and recovery high schools and collegiate programs provides opportunities for youth to find constructive opportunities to increase their level of function and participation in education and employment. Recent studies have shown that peer-delivered recovery services are not only effective, but highly appreciated by youth.[99] Several medium to large cities in the United States offer adapted programs for youth who are recovering from substance use disorders. These programs may include sober living environments and easy access to community groups.[100] Although recovery schools show high success and graduation rates, there are still too few of them to address the needs of the American population, and many of them have limited funding, posing an important threat to their long-term sustainability.[101]

SUMMARY

In conclusion, AYAs represent a distinct population at high risk for substance use disorders. During periods of rapid brain development, youth are especially susceptible to the reinforcing effects of substances amid a still-developing capacity for executive control and decision making. AYAs have different substance use patterns from older adults and place a high level of importance on experimentation and social inclusiveness, which increases their vulnerability to peer pressure and high-risk behaviors. Busy clinicians should integrate SBIRT into their routine practice to help with early recognition and effective mobilization of youth and their families. Although there are still important gaps in the youth substance use literature, several behavioral-, family-, and community-based interventions as well as medications and recovery support treatments provide evidence-based options for AYAs with substance use disorders. The importance of supporting preventive efforts, research, and intervention in young people cannot be overstated. Substance use causes important losses of time and productivity in young people, resulting in serious societal repercussions. The healthy future of North Americans is directly related to upstream interventions that can address substance use issues before they become enrooted and are more difficult to treat later in life.

ACKNOWLEDGMENTS

The editors wish to thank Marc Fishman, Maryland Treatment Centers, for providing a critical review of this article.

REFERENCES

1. Substance Abuse and Mental Health Services Administration. Treatment episode data set (TEDS): 2002-2012. Rockville (MD): National Admissions to Substance Abuse Treatment Services; 2015.
2. National Center for Statistics and Analysis. Alcohol-impaired driving: 2015 data. Washington, DC: National Highway Traffic Safety Administration; 2016.
3. Gaither JR, Leventhal JM, Ryan SA, et al. National trends in hospitalizations for opioid poisonings among children and adolescents, 1997 to 2012. JAMA Pediatr 2016;170(12):1195-201.
4. Chatterjee S, Tempalski B, Pouget ER, et al. Changes in the prevalence of injection drug use among adolescents and young adults in large U.S. metropolitan areas. AIDS Behav 2011;15(7):1570-8.
5. Arnett JJ. The developmental context of substance use in emerging adulthood. J Drug Issues 2005;35(2):235-54.
6. Sussman S, Skara S, Ames SL. Substance abuse among adolescents. Subst Use Misuse 2008;43(12-13):1802-28.
7. Levy SJ, Williams JF. Substance use screening, brief intervention, and referral to treatment. Pediatrics 2016;138(1) [pii:e20161211].
8. McWhirter PT. Enhancing adolescent substance abuse treatment engagement. J Psychoactive Drugs 2008;40(2):173-82.
9. Winters KC, Arria A. Adolescent brain development and drugs. Prev Res 2011; 18(2):21-4. Available at: https://www.ncbi.nlm.nih.gov/pubmed/22822298.
10. Casey BJ, Jones RM, Hare TA. The adolescent brain. Ann N Y Acad Sci 2008; 1124(1):111-26.
11. Volkow ND, Swanson JM, Evins AE, et al. Effects of cannabis use on human behavior, including cognition, motivation, and psychosis: a review. JAMA Psychiatry 2016;73(3):292-7.
12. Leyton M, Stewart S. Substance abuse in Canada: childhood and adolescent pathways to substance use disorders. Ottawa (ON): Canadian Centre on Substance Abuse; 2014.
13. Center for Behavioral Health Statistics and Quality (CBHSQ). 2015 national survey on drug use and health: detailed tables. Rockville (MD): Substance Abuse and Mental Health Services Administration; 2016.
14. Hanson KL, Medina KL, Padula CB, et al. Impact of adolescent alcohol and drug use on neuropsychological functioning in young adulthood: 10-year outcomes. J Child Adolesc Subst Abuse 2011;20(2):135-54.
15. Jacobus J, Tapert SF. Effects of cannabis on the adolescent brain. Curr Pharm Des 2014;20(13):2186-93.
16. Sherer S, Radzik M. Psychosocial Development in Normal Adolescents and Young Adults, Neinstein's adolescent and young adult health care: a practical guide, 6th edition, chapter 3. Philadelphia: Wolters Kluwer; 2016.
17. Brown SA, McGue M, Maggs J, et al. A developmental perspective on alcohol and youths 16 to 20 years of age. Pediatrics 2008;121(Suppl 4):S290-310.
18. Casey BJ, Jones RM. Neurobiology of the adolescent brain and behavior: implications for substance use disorders. J Am Acad Child Adolesc Psychiatry 2010; 49(12):1189-201.
19. Verweij KJH, Zietsch BP, Lynskey MT, et al. Genetic and environmental influences on cannabis use initiation and problematic use: a meta-analysis of twin studies. Addiction 2010;105(3):417-30.

20. Pelayo-Terán JM, Suárez-Pinilla P, Chadi N, et al. Gene-environment interactions underlying the effect of cannabis in first episode psychosis. Curr Pharm Des 2012;18(32):5024–35.

21. Whitesell M, Bachand A, Peel J, et al. Familial, social, and individual factors contributing to risk for adolescent substance use. J Addict 2013;2013:9.

22. Hsiao RC-J, Walker LR. Understanding adolescent substance use disorders in the era of marijuana legalization, opioid epidemic, and social media. Child Adolesc Psychiatr Clin N Am 2016;25(3):xiii–xiv.

23. Calafat A, Garcia F, Juan M, et al. Which parenting style is more protective against adolescent substance use? Evidence within the European context. Drug Alcohol Depend 2014;138:185–92.

24. Goncalves H, Soares AL, Santos AP, et al. Adverse childhood experiences and consumption of alcohol, tobacco and illicit drugs among adolescents of a Brazilian birth cohort. Cad Saude Publica 2016;32(10):e00085815.

25. LeTendre ML, Reed MB. The effect of adverse childhood experience on clinical diagnosis of a substance use disorder: results of a nationally representative study. Subst Use Misuse 2017;52(6):689–97.

26. Hemovich V, Lac A, Crano WD. Understanding early-onset drug and alcohol outcomes among youth: the role of family structure, social factors, and interpersonal perceptions of use. Psychol Health Med 2011;16(3):249–67.

27. Huang GC, Unger JB, Soto D, et al. Peer influences: the impact of online and offline friendship networks on adolescent smoking and alcohol use. J Adolesc Health 2014;54(5):508–14.

28. Leung RK, Toumbourou JW, Hemphill SA. The effect of peer influence and selection processes on adolescent alcohol use: a systematic review of longitudinal studies. Health Psychol Rev 2014;8(4):426–57.

29. Johnston LD, Miech RA, Bachman JG, et al. Monitoring the future national survey results on drug use, 1975-2016: overview, key findings on adolescent drug use. Ann Arbor (MI): University of Michigan Institute for Social Research; 2017.

30. Goldbach JT, Tanner-Smith EE, Bagwell M, et al. Minority stress and substance use in sexual minority adolescents: a meta-analysis. Prev Sci 2014;15(3): 350–63.

31. Patrick ME, Schulenberg JE. Prevalence and predictors of adolescent alcohol use and binge drinking in the United States. Alcohol Res 2014;35(2):193–200. Available at: http://www.ncbi.nlm.nih.gov/pmc/articles/PMC3908711/.

32. American Psychiatry Association. Substance-related and addictive disorders. Diagnostic and statistical manual of mental disorders, 5th edition. Washington, DC: American Psychiatric Association; 2013.

33. McCabe SE, West BT, Veliz P, et al. Trends in medical and nonmedical use of prescription opioids among US adolescents: 1976-2015. Pediatrics 2017; 139(4):e20162387.

34. Yeomans-Maldonado G, Patrick ME. The effect of perceived risk on the combined used of alcohol and marijuana: results from daily surveys. Addict Behav Rep 2015;2:33–6.

35. Boak A, Hamilton HA, Adlaf EM, et al. Drug use among Ontario students 1977–2015. Detailed findings form the Ontario Student Drug Use and Health Survey. Toronto (ON): Centre for Addiction and Mental Health; 2015.

36. Kraus L, Guttormsson U, Leifman H, et al. ESPAD report 2015-results from the European School Survey Project on Alcohol and other drugs. Luxembourg: 2016.

37. Wurcel AG, Anderson JE, Chui KKH, et al. Increasing infectious endocarditis admissions among young people who inject drugs. Open Forum Infect Dis 2016; 3(3):ofw157.
38. Rudd RA, Seth P, David F, et al. Increases in Drug and Opioid-Involved Overdose Deaths — United States, 2010–2015. Morb Mortal Wkly Rep 2016;65: 1445–52.
39. Curtin SC, Tejada-Vera B, Warner M. Drug overdose deaths among adolescents aged 15–19 in the United States: 1999–2015. NCHS Data Brief No. 282. 2017. Available at: https://www.cdc.gov/nchs/products/databriefs/db282.htm. Accessed October 17, 2017.
40. Key substance use and mental health indicators in the United States: results from the 2016 national survey on drug use and health (HHS Publication No. SMA 17-5044 NSH-52), ed.. Rockville (MD): Center for Behavioral Health Statistics and Quality, Substance Abuse and Mental Health Services Administration; 2017
41. Hughes A, Lipari RN, Bose J, et al. Prescription drug use and misuse in the United States: results from the 2015 national survey on drug use and health. Rockville (MD): Substance Abuse and Mental Health Services Administration; 2016.
42. Keyes KM, Wall M, Cerdá M, et al. How does state marijuana policy affect US youth? Medical marijuana laws, marijuana use and perceived harmfulness: 1991–2014. Addiction 2016;111(12):2187–95.
43. National Institute on Drug Abuse. Principles of adolescent use disorder treatment: a research-based guide, 3rd edition. Rockville (MD): National Institute on Drug Abuse; 2018.
44. Hadland SE, Xuan Z, Sarda V, et al. Alcohol policies and alcohol-related motor vehicle crash fatalities among young people in the US. Pediatrics 2017;139(3) [pii:e20163037].
45. Asbridge M, Hayden JA, Cartwright JL. Acute cannabis consumption and motor vehicle collision risk: systematic review of observational studies and meta-analysis. BMJ 2012;344:e536. Available at: https://www.ncbi.nlm.nih.gov/pubmed/22323502.
46. Decker MR, Miller E, McCauley HL, et al. Recent partner violence and sexual and drug-related STI/HIV risk among adolescent and young adult women attending family planning clinics. Sex Transm Infect 2014;90(2):145–9.
47. Senn TE, Carey MP, Vanable PA. The intersection of violence, substance use, depression, and STDs: testing of a syndemic pattern among patients attending an Urban STD Clinic. J Natl Med Assoc 2010;102(7):614–20.
48. Simpson AK, Magid V. Cannabis use disorder in adolescence. Child Adolesc Psychiatr Clin N Am 2016;25(3):431–43.
49. O'Dell LE. A psychobiological framework of the substrates that mediate nicotine use during adolescence. Neuropharmacology 2009;56(Suppl 1):263–78.
50. DiFranza JR, Savageau JA, Fletcher K, et al. Symptoms of tobacco dependence after brief intermittent use: the development and assessment of nicotine dependence in youth-2 study. Arch Pediatr Adolesc Med 2007;161(7):704–10.
51. Cohen E, Mackenzie RG, Yates GL. HEADSS, a psychosocial risk assessment instrument: implications for designing effective intervention programs for runaway youth. J Adolesc Health 1991;12(7):539–44.
52. Ginsburg KR. Viewing our adolescent patients through a positive lens. Contemp Pediatr 2007;24(11):65–76.

53. Chadi N, Amaria K, Kaufman M. Expand your HEADS, follow the THRxEADS! Paediatr Child Health 2017;22(1):23–5.

54. Goldenring JM, Rosen DS. Getting into adolescent heads: an essential update. Contemp Pediatr 2004;21(1):64–90.

55. Bradshaw CP, Waasdorp TE, Goldweber A, et al. Bullies, gangs, drugs, and school: understanding the overlap and the role of ethnicity and urbanicity. J Youth Adolesc 2013;42(2):220–34.

56. Levy S, Ziemnik RE, Harris SK, et al. Screening adolescents for alcohol use. J Addict Med 2017;1. https://doi.org/10.1097/ADM.0000000000000340.

57. Rahm AK, Boggs JM, Martin C, et al. Facilitators and barriers to implementing screening, brief intervention, and referral to treatment (SBIRT) in primary care in integrated health care settings. Subst Abuse 2015;36(3):281–8.

58. Harris SK, Csémy L, Sherritt L, et al. Computer-facilitated substance use screening and brief advice for teens in primary care: an international trial. Pediatrics 2012;129(6):1072–82.

59. Sterling S, Valkanoff T, Hinman A, et al. Integrating substance use treatment into adolescent health care. Curr Psychiatry Rep 2012;14(5):453–61.

60. Levy S, Shrier L. Adolescent screening, brief intervention, and referral for treatment for alcohol and other drug use - Toolkit for providers. Boston (MA): 2015. Available at: https://www.mcpap.com/pdf/S2BI Toolkit.pdf. Accessed October 9, 2017.

61. Knight JR, Sherritt L, Harris SK, et al. Validity of brief alcohol screening tests among adolescents: a comparison of the AUDIT, POSIT, CAGE, and CRAFFT. Alcohol Clin Exp Res 2003;27(1):67–73.

62. Kelly SM, Gryczynski J, Mitchell SG, et al. Validity of brief screening instrument for adolescent tobacco, alcohol, and drug use. Pediatrics 2014;133(5):819–26.

63. National Institute on Alcohol Abuse and Alcoholism. Alcohol screening and brief intervention for youth: a practical guide. Bethesda (MD): National Institutes of Health; 2011.

64. Bagley SM, Anderson BJ, Stein MD. Usefulness of the CRAFFT to diagnose alcohol or cannabis use disorders in a sample of emerging adults with past-month alcohol or cannabis use. J Child Adolesc Subst Abuse 2017;26(1):18–23.

65. Kelly TM, Donovan JE, Chung T, et al. Brief screens for detecting alcohol use disorder among 18-20 year old young adults in emergency departments: comparing AUDIT-C, CRAFFT, RAPS4-QF, FAST, RUFT-Cut, and DSM-IV 2-Item Scale. Addict Behav 2009;34(8):668–74.

66. Office of the Surgeon General (US). Facing addiction in America: the surgeon general's report on alcohol, drugs, and health. [Chapter 4, ed]. Washington, DC: Substance Abuse and Mental Health Services Administration (US); 2016.

67. Carney T, Myers BJ, Louw J, et al. Brief school-based interventions and behavioural outcomes for substance-using adolescents. Cochrane Database Syst Rev 2016;(1):CD008969.

68. Lipari RN, Park-Lee W, Van Horn S. America's need for and receipt of substance use treatment in 2015. Substance Abuse and Mental Health Services Administration; 2016.

69. Harrison C. Treatment decisions regarding infants, children and adolescents. Pediatr Child Health 2004;9(2):99–103.

70. National District Attorneys Association. Minor Consent to Medical Treatment Laws. 2013. Available at: http://www.ndaa.org/pdf/Minor Consent to Medical Treatment (2).pdf. Accessed March 27, 2018.

71. Brewer S, Godley MD, Hulvershorn LA. Treating mental health and substance use disorders in adolescents: what is on the menu? Curr Psychiatry Rep 2017;19(1):5.

72. Schoenfelder EN, Faraone SV, Kollins SH. Stimulant treatment of ADHD and cigarette smoking: a meta-analysis. Pediatrics 2014;133(6):1070–80.

73. Dalsgaard S, Mortensen PB, Frydenberg M, et al. ADHD, stimulant treatment in childhood and subsequent substance abuse in adulthood — a naturalistic long-term follow-up study. Addict Behav 2014;39(1):325–8.

74. Wu SS, Schoenfelder E, Hsiao RC. Cognitive behavioral therapy and motivational enhancement therapy. Child Adolesc Psychiatr Clin N Am 2016;25(4): 629–43.

75. Godley SH, Hunter BD, Fernández-Artamendi S, et al. A comparison of treatment outcomes for adolescent community reinforcement approach participants with and without co-occurring problems. J Subst Abuse Treat 2014;46(4): 463–71.

76. Dennis M, Godley SH, Diamond G, et al. The Cannabis Youth Treatment (CYT) Study: main findings from two randomized trials. J Subst Abuse Treat 2004; 27(3):197–213.

77. Stanger C, Budney AJ, Kamon JL, et al. A randomized trial of contingency management for adolescent marijuana abuse and dependence. Drug Alcohol Depend 2009;105(3):240–7.

78. Stanger C, Budney AJ. Contingency management approaches for adolescent substance use disorders. Child Adolesc Psychiatr Clin N Am 2010;19(3): 547–62.

79. Stanger C, Lansing AH, Budney AJ. Advances in research on contingency management for adolescent substance use. Child Adolesc Psychiatr Clin N Am 2016;25(4):645–59.

80. Dunne T, Bishop L, Avery S, et al. A review of effective youth engagement strategies for mental health and substance use interventions. J Adolesc Health 2017;60(5):487–512.

81. Das JK, Salam RA, Arshad A, et al. Interventions for adolescent substance abuse: an overview of systematic reviews. J Adolesc Health 2016;59(4S): S61–75.

82. Godley SH, Smith JE, Karvinen T, et al. The adolescent community reinforcement approach for adolescent cannabis users. Silver Spring (MD): Substance Abuse and Mental Health Services Administration; 2001.

83. Sussman S. A review of alcoholics anonymous/narcotics anonymous programs for teens. Eval Health Prof 2010;33(1):26–55.

84. Staff J, Schulenberg JE, Maslowsky J, et al. Substance use changes and social role transitions: proximal developmental effects on ongoing trajectories from late adolescence through early adulthood. Dev Psychopathol 2010;22(4):917–32.

85. Bettmann JE, Gillis HL, Speelman EA, et al. A meta-analysis of wilderness therapy outcomes for private pay clients. J Child Fam Stud 2016;25(9):2659–73.

86. Hammond CJ. The role of pharmacotherapy in the treatment of adolescent substance use disorders. Child Adolesc Psychiatr Clin N Am 2016;25(4):685–711.

87. King JL, Pomeranz JL, Merten JW. A systematic review and meta-evaluation of adolescent smoking cessation interventions that utilized nicotine replacement therapy. Addict Behav 2016;52:39–45.

88. Harvey J, Chadi N, Di Meglio G, et al. Strategies to promote smoking cessation among adolescents. Paediatr Child Health 2016;21(4):201–8.

89. Farber HJ, Groner J, Walley S, et al. Protecting children from tobacco, nicotine, and tobacco smoke. Pediatrics 2015. https://doi.org/10.1542/peds.2015-3110.

90. Hadland SE, Wharam J, Schuster MA, et al. Trends in receipt of buprenorphine and naltrexone for opioid use disorder among adolescents and young adults, 2001-2014. JAMA Pediatr 2017. https://doi.org/10.1001/jamapediatrics.2017.0745.

91. Liebling EJ, Yedinak JL, Green TC, et al. Access to substance use treatment among young adults who use prescription opioids non-medically. Subst Abuse Treat Prev Policy 2016;11(1):38.

92. Committee on Substance Use and Prevention. Medication-assisted treatment of adolescents with opioid use disorders. Pediatrics 2016;138(3). https://doi.org/10.1542/peds.2016-1893.

93. Bagley SM, Forman LS, Ruiz S, et al. Expanding access to naloxone for family members: the Massachusetts experience. Drug Alcohol Rev 2017. https://doi.org/10.1111/dar.12551.

94. Gray KM, Carpenter MJ, Baker NL, et al. A double-blind randomized controlled trial of N-acetylcysteine in cannabis-dependent adolescents. Am J Psychiatry 2012;169(8):805–12.

95. McClure EA, Sonne SC, Winhusen T, et al. Achieving cannabis cessation – evaluating N-acetylcysteine treatment (ACCENT): design and implementation of a multi-site, randomized controlled study in the National Institute on Drug Abuse Clinical Trials Network. Contemp Clin Trials 2014;39(2):211–23.

96. Mason BJ, Crean R, Goodell V, et al. A proof-of-concept randomized controlled study of gabapentin: effects on cannabis use, withdrawal and executive function deficits in cannabis-dependent adults. Neuropsychopharmacology 2012;37(7):1689–98.

97. De Sousa A, De Sousa A. An open randomized trial comparing disulfiram and naltrexone in adolescents with alcohol dependence. J Subst Use 2008;13(6):382–8.

98. Niederhofer H, Staffen W. Comparison of disulfiram and placebo in treatment of alcohol dependence of adolescents. Drug Alcohol Rev 2003;22(3):295–7.

99. Bassuk EL, Hanson J, Greene RN, et al. Peer-delivered recovery support services for addictions in the United States: a systematic review. J Subst Abuse Treat 2016;63:1–9.

100. Laudet A, Harris K, Kimball T, et al. Collegiate recovery communities programs: what do we know and what do we need to know? J Soc Work Pract Addict 2014;14(1):84–100.

101. Finch AJ, Moberg DP, Krupp AL. Continuing care in high schools: a descriptive study of recovery high school programs. J Child Adolesc Subst Abuse 2014;23(2):116–29.

Preventing Opioid Overdose in the Clinic and Hospital
Analgesia and Opioid Antagonists

Stephanie Lee Peglow, DO, MPH[a],*,
Ingrid A. Binswanger, MD, MPH, MS[b,c]

KEYWORDS

- Opioid overdose • Naloxone • Overdose education • Harm reduction
- Opioid prescribing • Prevention of overdose

KEY POINTS

- Tailor opioid overdose preventive efforts to patients' individual stage of opioid therapy or involvement; not all interventions are universally appropriate.
- Consider risk stratification when treating pain with opioids.
- Apply appropriate harm-reduction strategies, such as prescribing naloxone, to patients as risk for overdose.
- Consider treatment of opioid use disorders with pharmacotherapy in your own practice.

INTRODUCTION

North America has experienced an overdose epidemic linked across countries related to increased opioid pharmaceutical marketing, opioid prescribing, prescribed and illicit opioid use, and opioid trafficking.[1] As a result, greater than 2 million United States inhabitants met criteria for opioid use disorder (OUD) and nearly 5% of US adults reported nonmedical use of opioids in 2013.[2] US opioid advertising campaigns and prescribing patterns have spread to Canada.[3] In 2012 it was estimated 75,000 to 125,000

Disclosure Statement: Dr S.L. Peglow was supported by the Veterans Administration Mental Illness, Research, Education and Clinical Center and by Research in Addiction Medicine Scholars Program-R25DA033211. Dr I.A. Binswanger is supported by the National Institute On Drug Abuse of the National Institutes of Health under Award Number R01DA042059. The content is solely the responsibilities of the authors and does not necessarily represent the official views of the National Institutes of Health. Dr I.A. Binswanger is currently employed by the Colorado Permanente Medical Group.

[a] Department of Psychiatry and Behavioral Sciences, Eastern Virginia Medical School, 825 Fairfax Avenue Suite 710, Norfolk, VA 23507, USA; [b] Institute for Health Research, Kaiser Permanente Colorado, 2550 South Parker Road, Suite 200, Aurora, CO 80014, USA; [c] Division of General Internal Medicine, Department of Medicine, University of Colorado, 12631 East 17th Avenue, Academic Office One, Campus Box B180, Aurora, CO 80045, USA
* Corresponding author.
E-mail address: Peglowsl@evms.edu

Canadians injected drugs, and another 200,000 had OUDs because of pharmaceutical opioids.[4] In Mexico, estimates suggest that 100,000 people use illicit opioids and an increasing number of those use heroin.[1]

In the United States, a large proportion of individuals who use illicit pharmaceutical opioids (68%) report they received the prescription drug from a friend or family member who was prescribed it by their doctor.[5] Those that reported heavy, nonmedical opioid use reported that their primary source was direct physician prescribing.[6] Thus, physicians have the responsibility to prevent the potential harms of opioids by using sound preventive strategies.

This article describes opioid overdose preventive strategies for medical providers (**Fig. 1**), with a particular focus on special populations, such as youth and pregnant women. Opioid overdose can occur in any point along the continuum of use, from opioid naivety to long-term opioid use for pain to OUD (**Box 1**). Furthermore, overdose is caused by a range of factors, including drug interactions, use via injection route, and intentional overdose. We summarize current preventive strategies medical providers in primary care may use to reduce risk throughout the continuum of opioid use and across a range of contributing factors.

We highlight opioid prescribing guidelines from the Veterans Affairs/Department of Defense, Centers for Disease Control and Prevention (CDC), and Canadian Guidelines, last updated February 2017, March 2016, and 2017, respectively.[7–9] The recommendations within these guidelines are largely based on observational data; hence the quality of the evidence supporting many recommendations is still moderately weak.[10] In addition, overdose prevention research is evolving and recommendations may change based on results from ongoing and new studies. Importantly, existing guidelines focus heavily on limiting prescribing, but a one-size-fits-all approach may not be appropriate or feasible, nor address other facets of the opioid epidemic, such as increasing heroin and nonprescribed fentanyl use. Furthermore, we acknowledge that counseling patients about overdose risk and meeting all opioid prescribing guidelines may be difficult in busy primary care practices, particularly in the face of other competing demands.[11]

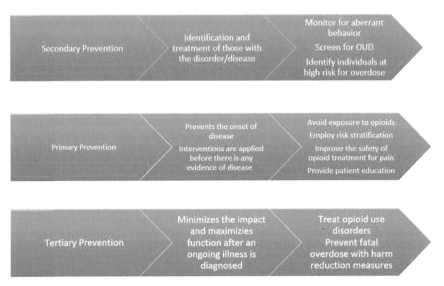

Fig. 1. Levels of overdose prevention.

Box 1
Definitions

Chronic opioid use: "Daily or near-daily use of opioids for at least 90 days, often indefinitely."[12] Chronic opioid use should be distinguished from an OUD; although it may be associated with tolerance and/or physiologic withdrawal, it does not necessarily involve the other social, behavioral, and compulsive characteristics of an OUD.

Nonmedical use of opioids (or misuse): "Use of a medication (for a medical purpose) other than as directed or as indicated, whether willful or unintentional, and whether harm results or not."[12] Nonmedical use may occur in individuals with or without an OUD.

Aberrant use: "A behavior outside the boundaries of the agreed on treatment plan which is established as early as possible in the doctor-patient relationship."[12] Aberrant use by someone prescribed opioids does not necessarily define an OUD but may raise a provider's concerns that that individual is developing an OUD.

Diversion: "The intentional transfer of a controlled substance from legitimate distribution and dispensing channels."[12] Individuals with and without OUDs may engage in diversion.

PRIMARY PREVENTION MEASURES
Minimizing Exposure to Opioids Among People Who Are Opioid Naive or Do Not Have an Opioid Use Disorder

Prescribed opioids are associated with an overall 5.5% risk of addiction[8] and a 0.2% risk of fatal overdose at a mean of 2.6 years after initial opioid prescription.[13] Even opioids prescribed at hospital discharge are associated with an increased risk of chronic opioid use 1 year later.[14] Avoiding exposure to opioids may reduce incidence of addiction and death from overdose, hence the first strong recommendation in all three guidelines is nonpharmacologic therapy for pain, such as physical therapy, and, when medications are needed, nonopioid pharmacotherapy, such as acetaminophen or nonsteroidal anti-inflammatory drugs.[7–9,15]

History Taking and Risk Evaluation and Mitigation

If opioids are needed for pain, then providers should conduct a thorough history and evaluate the risk of aberrant behavior and overdose (**Box 2**). The Substance Abuse

---

Box 2
Risk groups for overdose

- Chronic medical illness (pulmonary, renal, or hepatic)[18]
- History of substance use disorder[19]
- History of psychiatric disorder[20]
- Controlled substance prescriptions from multiple providers[21]
- Prescribed a combination of opioids and benzodiazepines[21]
- High daily dosages of opioids[21]
- Long-acting and extended-released opioid formulations[22]
- Illicit drug use[23]
- Recent history of incarceration[24]
- History of prior overdose[23]

and Mental Health Services Administration[5] toolkit for providers suggests including specific questions about alcohol and over-the-counter medications.[5] To help evaluate the risk of aberrant behavior, commonly used tools are the Screener and Opioid Assessment for Patients with Pain[16] and the Opioid Risk Tool.[9] Prescription opioids taken in combination with benzodiazepines were found in 30% of opioid overdoses,[6] and coprescribing increases the risk of fatal and nonfatal overdose.[17] Thus, to mitigate risk, providers should consider alternatives to either benzodiazepines or opioids when coprescribing both medications.[8,15]

Patient Education and Informed Consent

If opioids are used, it is helpful to establish treatment goals, discuss risks and realistic benefits, and consider how opioids will be discontinued if benefits do not outweigh risks.[8,9] This discussion should include the responsibilities of the patient and the doctor; potential side effects including sedation, addiction, motor vehicle accidents, and death; limited evidence showing long-term benefits for chronic pain; and the risk of respiratory depression when combined with sedatives.[8,9]

Considerations on Prescribing Practices to Reduce Overdose Risk

Both dose and duration have a dose-dependent effect on development of overdose, but duration seems to be a stronger predictor of OUD.[8,25] Partially because of this, Canadian, Veterans Affairs/Department of Defense, and CDC recommend an upper limit to opioid prescribing (90-mg morphine equivalent dosing). Although research consensus is lacking, there is some evidence that extended-release or long-acting formulations may increase risk of unintentional overdose[22]; thus the Veterans Affairs and CDC guidelines advise against using longer acting formulations.[9] A recent intervention that combined nursing care management, an electronic registry, academic detailing, and electronic decision support tools demonstrated increased adherence to opioid guidelines compared with the group receiving electronic decision support only.[26]

Safe Storage Practices and Reducing Household Exposure

Parents are an important source of pharmaceutical opioids to children. Exposure may occur through two routes: intentional sharing of opioids for a treatment of a child's minor aches and pains, or by diversion of pills by an adolescent from their parent's prescription.[27] Counseling on safe storage and disposal practices when providing opioids to an adult with children in the home is also important to protect household members from risky, inadvertent, or recreational exposure.[27]

Educational Strategies to Prevent Risky Use in Adolescents

Brief universal preventive interventions administered during middle school have been shown to reduce prescription drug misuse among adolescents and young adults.[28] The American Academy of Pediatrics suggests providers echo these clear and consistent nonuse messages and provide Screening, Brief Intervention, and Referral to Treatment to their adolescent patients.[29] CRAFFT, an age-appropriate Screening, Brief Intervention, and Referral to Treatment intervention, can be used as a screener.[30] In those found to be of low risk, brief negotiated interviews may be helpful to reduce risky use of opioids; those of higher risk should be referred to treatment.[29]

SECONDARY PREVENTION MEASURES
Urine Drug Test

Substance misuse has been shown to be 30% or greater in patients prescribed long-term opiates.[31] Although urine drug testing has not been robustly shown to reduce opioid misuse as a stand-alone intervention,[31] urine toxicology at initiation of opioids and periodically throughout treatment with appropriate confirmatory testing can help identify patients who warrant further education about opioid safety, evaluation for a substance use disorder (SUD), and referral for treatment.[32] Barriers to use of urine toxicology include provider discomfort discussing results, lack of access to testing, inadequate knowledge on how to interpret results, and belief that one's patients are not at risk of misuse or illicit use.[31] In addition, misinterpretation of results or lack of confirmatory testing may lead to falsely accusing patients of diversion or illicit use, hence restricting care to patients and breaking down the therapeutic alliance.[31]

Prescription Monitoring Programs

Evidence on state-wide prescription monitoring programs (PMP) suggests that they have potential to change prescribing behaviors and identify patients at risk for overdose.[15] Although it is still not known if implementation or use decreases overdose deaths, research has suggested some positive effects in isolated states.[33–35] Thus, the CDC guidelines suggest checking PMP at the initiation of opioid therapy and at intervals of no greater than 3 months while on treatment.[9] The utility of PMPs can be limited. Providers may be unaware of their existence and have difficulty accessing data from other states. In addition, reporting to these systems can be limited.[36] These systems also have the potential to lead to inadequate pain care. For example, providers may inappropriately label patients as "doctor shoppers" or become uncomfortable prescribing opioids because they are required to access the system and face risks of criminal sanctions for overprescribing.[36]

Identifying Nonmedical Opioid Use and Opioid Use Disorders

Aberrant behavior has an estimated prevalence of 11.5% among patients prescribed chronic opioid therapy,[37] but patients on chronic opioid therapy may be reluctant to disclose risk behavior to their prescribing providers.[38] Integrating loved ones into follow-up can bring the provider's attention to worrisome behaviors and medication use practices. Two screeners have been shown to help identify potential nonmedical use, the Pain Assessment and Documentation Tool and the Current Opioid Misuse Measure.[39,40] Providers should evaluate those patients identified with nonmedical or aberrant use for OUD and refer those with OUD to treatment, or initiate OUD treatment in their practices.

Continued Evaluation of Opioid Risk/Benefit Profile and Considering Tapering

The CDC suggests that the marker of clinical improvement is a 30% improvement in *both* pain and function.[9] If these milestones are not achieved with opioid treatment optimization, the physician may consider opioid discontinuation.[9] These functional outcomes can be measured with the Pain Average, Interference with Enjoyment of Life[41] and Interference with General Activity Assessment Scale.[42]

When the risks of long-term opioid therapy outweigh benefits, opioid tapering may be considered. Although there are concerns about patients transitioning to heroin after being discontinued or rapidly tapered from opioids,[43] several strategies are successful in tapering opioids, such as weekly dose reductions of 10% to 50% of total daily dose.[9] To address patients' concerns of increased pain and withdrawal, support from a trusted health care provider and social support can facilitate a successful opioid taper.[44] One review suggested improvement in pain severity, function, and quality of life after dose tapering.[45]

TERTIARY PREVENTION
Naloxone

Naloxone is an effective, short-acting opioid antagonist that is used for overdose reversal. Based on the successful experience of community-based overdose education and naloxone distribution programs,[18,46] which have traditionally targeted people using heroin and other illicit opioids, naloxone is increasingly being prescribed to patients at risk in medical settings. There is evidence to support community-based overdose education and naloxone distribution programs.[18] For example, in Massachusetts, communities with high concentrations of naloxone distribution to lay bystanders seemed to have reduced overdose rates.[47] Studies have shown that educating lay bystanders about naloxone increases knowledge about how to identify and treat an opioid overdose, with scores that were similar to those of medical experts.[48,49] Trained individuals have been able to successfully diffuse this information within their communities.[50] Outside of community settings, naloxone has been feasibly implemented in community emergency department settings[51] and primary care.[41,52]

Although the optimal patient groups for naloxone prescription have not yet been determined, naloxone may be considered for patients started on chronic opioid therapy and those who are in the process of tapering or have recently discontinued opioid therapy. Providers may opt to prescribe naloxone to individuals with risk factors for opioid overdose (see **Box 2**). **Table 1** shows groups suggested for naloxone by recent guidelines. In US states where laws allow for it, physicians may prescribe naloxone to family members and lay persons (**Fig. 2**). For medical providers, the liability risks of prescribing naloxone seem limited.[53] Furthermore, some states have implemented standing orders, under which individuals can obtain naloxone from a pharmacy without getting an individual prescription from their provider.

Providers may be concerned about increasing risk behavior as a result of naloxone prescribing,[11] whereas patients may be concerned about the stigma associated with receiving naloxone.[38] In one study, coprescribing naloxone with chronic opioid therapy for noncancer pain was associated with reduced opioid-related emergency department visits.[52] Although the reasons for this reduction are unknown, it may be partially caused by the education provided with naloxone, because overdose education combined with motivational interviewing has been shown to reduce self-reported opioid overdose risk behaviors and nonmedical use of prescription opioids.[54]

Table 1
Patient groups to consider for naloxone prescribing, by guidelines

CDC[9]	Veterans Affairs/ Department of Defense[7]	Canadian[8]
• Prescribed doses of greater or equal to 50-mg morphine equivalents • Personal history of previous overdose • History of substance use disorder or concurrent use of benzodiazepines • Relatives of family members with OUD in states where third party prescribing is allowed	• Starting chronic opioid therapy • Tapering or have recently discontinued opioid therapy	• High-dose opioid therapy • Comorbidities • During opioid rotation • OUD • Recreational opioid use • Intravenous drug use

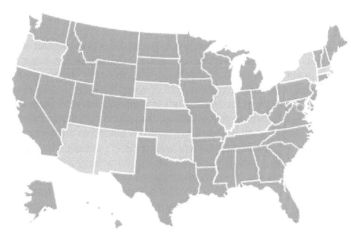

Fig. 2. States that give immunity to prescribers for prescribing naloxone to lay persons (in *green*) as of July 1, 2017. This figure was created under a Creative Commons Attribution-4.0 International License. (*Adapted from* Prescription drug abuse policy system (PDAPS). Legal Science, LLC. Naloxone overdose prevention laws. Available at: http://j.mp/2hDyf2N. Accessed September 30, 2017; with permission.)

Naloxone is available in different formulations. Although the auto-injector and nasal spray are easy to use and avoid the risk of needle stick injuries, the auto-injector is costly and both have variable insurance coverage.[55] Substance Abuse and Mental Health Services Administration has issued an Opioid Overdose Prevention Toolkit[56] and Prescribe to Prevent (prescribetoprevent.org) provides Continuing Medical Education for medical providers.

Treatment of Opioid Use Disorders

Opioid agonist treatment (including methadone and buprenorphine) effectively decreases opioid use and reduces the risk of overdose and death in those with OUDs.[57] However, these modalities are vastly underused.[58] For buprenorphine, management may occur in primary care settings. In the United States, a buprenorphine Drug Enforcement Administration[28] waiver is required for health care practitioners. In Canada, specialized training is suggested but not required.[59] Buprenorphine provided in primary care has been shown to be safe and effective.[60] In the United States, providers have to refer to specialized methadone treatment centers for their patients to access methadone for addiction.[61] Primary care providers can prescribe the opioid antagonist naltrexone in daily oral or monthly injectable form without special licenses, although evidence for reduced overdose rates with naltrexone is currently lacking.

Reducing Risk After Nonfatal Overdose

Those with a previous overdose are commonly considered a high-risk group for repeat overdose; of those prescribed opioids, most continue to be prescribed opioids after overdose.[62] The CDC recommends clinicians work with these patients to reduce opioid dosage and prescribe naloxone.[9] If opioids are continued, providers should consider incorporating risk mitigation strategies and carefully considering the risks versus benefits of ongoing opioid therapy.[9]

SPECIAL POPULATIONS
Patients with Psychiatric Disorders

Patients with comorbid psychiatric disorders are more likely to receive an opioid for pain than those without mental health diagnoses,[63] and are more likely to receive higher dose opioids, multiple opioids, and benzodiazepines with opioids.[64,65] Patients with psychiatric disorders are also less likely to benefit from opioids,[66] are more likely to misuse opioids and develop an OUD,[67] and are more likely to attempt suicide.[68] Guidelines suggest caution in prescribing opioids to those with active, uncontrolled psychiatric illness.[7–9] Alternative therapies are preferred, such as tricyclic or serotonin and norepinephrine reuptake inhibitor antidepressants for patient with chronic pain and depression/anxiety. Opioid therapy in this population necessitates more frequent follow-up, monitoring, and observation.[8,9] When available, consider referring patients with psychiatric conditions to addiction medicine/psychiatry or other behavioral health specialists.[7] Complimentary treatment of chronic pain with movement, exercise, and cognitive-behavioral therapy for pain may help pain and mood outcomes and reduce suicide risk.[69]

Adolescents and Young Adults

Opioid use is common among adolescents.[61,70] Adolescents prescribed opioids had a 33% increase in misuse of opiates after high school[71]; the earlier the exposure to opioids the higher the risk of developing misuse and dependence.[7,25,72] All guidelines suggest avoiding opioids in adolescents when possible, and when it is not possible, frequent monitoring and dispensing, close monitoring for aberrancies, and tapering as early as clinically appropriate.[7–9]

Elderly Patients

Pain management is difficult in the elderly because of increased risks of opioid and nonopioid therapies.[73] Because of physiologic changes, opioids may accumulate and increase risk of respiratory depression and overdose.[74] Polypharmacy may increase risk of medication interactions and cognitive errors may lead to medication dosages beyond what is prescribed.[9,59,75] In patients greater than 65 years of age, additional caution and increased monitoring is suggested when prescribing opioids.[9] Prescribers might consider exercise or bowel regimes to prevent constipation, assessing for risk of falls, and monitoring for cognitive impairment.[9] Suggestions to improve safety among the elderly include starting at half the starting dose of younger populations, and considering codeine or tramadol first.[7,8]

Women of Reproductive Age and Pregnant Women

Opioids used in pregnancy are associated with low birth weight, stillbirth, poor fetal growth, preterm delivery, birth defects, cardiac abnormalities, and neonatal abstinence syndrome.[76] Severe withdrawal from opioids has been associated with premature labor and spontaneous abortion.[8] If a woman is planning to become pregnant, providers may consider opioid tapering and discontinuation before pregnancy.[8] For women already taking opioids and pregnant, providers may consider referral or specialized consultation before considering tapering/discontinuing opioids because of potential fetal risks. If a pregnant woman is determined to have an OUD, urgent referral to buprenorphine or methadone management is especially important because these therapies have been associated with improved outcomes.[77] However, naltrexone is not recommended.[9,78] Codeine is be avoided in breastfeeding mothers, because of possibility of neonatal toxicity and death,[8] but breastfeeding is encouraged in mothers prescribed buprenorphine or methadone.[79]

Patients with Active Substance Use Disorders

Patients with untreated SUDs have significant risk of developing an OUD or experiencing and overdose, suicide, and other cause of mortality.[8,19,63,80] Patients with past SUD history, especially if recent, prolonged, or severe, also have elevated risk.[8,80,81] Screening for recent SUDs is as simple as a single question "How many times in the past year have you used an illegal drug or used a prescription medication for nonmedical reasons?"[82] Other options for screening include the Drug Abuse Screening Test or the Alcohol Use Disorders Identification Test.[9,59,83,84] Guidelines strongly suggest against opioids for chronic noncancer pain in people with an active SUD[7,8] because of the risk of addiction to opioids. After nonpharmacologic or nonopioid options, codeine and tramadol are first line for patients with SUD. If higher potency is required, morphine is preferred to oxycodone or hydromorphone.[8,59] Referrals are encouraged for patients with continued pain despite buprenorphine and minimal counseling in the primary care setting and for those with comorbid active SUDs when available.[7] Unfortunately, successful referral is difficult in clinical practice because access to these services is limited.[85]

SUMMARY

Prescribers have an important role in prevention of OUDs and opioid overdose. These strategies include minimizing opioid exposure for opioid-naive patients, using risk-mitigation and harm-reduction strategies, and treating OUD. Given that not all interventions are universally appropriate, it is important to consider tailoring preventive efforts to match the individual's stage of opioid involvement.

ACKNOWLEDGMENT

The editors thank Antonio Quidgley-Nevares, Eastern Virginia Medical School, for providing a critical review of this article.

REFERENCES

1. Vashishtha D, Mittal ML, Werb D. The North American opioid epidemic: current challenges and a call for treatment as prevention. Harm Reduct J 2017;14(1):7.
2. Han B, Compton WM, Jones CM, et al. Nonmedical prescription opioid use and use disorders among adults aged 18 through 64 years in the United States, 2003-2013. JAMA 2015;314(14):1468–78.
3. Van Zee A. The promotion and marketing of oxycontin: commercial triumph, public health tragedy. Am J Public Health 2009;99(2):221–7.
4. Nosyk B, Anglin MD, Brissette S, et al. A call for evidence-based medical treatment of opioid dependence in the United States and Canada. Health Aff (Millwood) 2013;32(8):1462–9.
5. Administration SAaMHS. SAMSHA opioid overdose prevention toolkit: opioid overdose prevention TOOLKIT: information for prescribers. 2013. Available at: https://store.samhsa.gov/product/SAMHSA-Opioid-Overdose-Prevention-Toolkit/SMA16-4742. Accessed August 1, 2017.
6. Jones CM, Mack KA, Paulozzi LJ. Pharmaceutical overdose deaths, United States, 2010. JAMA 2013;309(7):657–9.
7. The Opioid Therapy for Chronic Pain Work Group. VA/DoD Clinical Practice Guidelines for Opioid Therapy for Chronic Pain. Version 3.0- February 2017. Available at: https://www.healthquality.va.gov/guidelines/Pain/cot/VADoDOTCPG022717.pdf. Accessed August 1, 2017.

8. Busse JW, Craigie S, Juurlink DN, et al. Guideline for opioid therapy and chronic noncancer pain. CMAJ 2017;189(18):E659–66.

9. Dowell D, Haegerich TM, Chou R. CDC guideline for prescribing opioids for chronic pain: United States, 2016. JAMA 2016;315(15):1624–45.

10. Chou R, Turner JA, Devine EB, et al. The effectiveness and risks of long-term opioid therapy for chronic pain: a systematic review for a National Institutes of Health Pathways to Prevention Workshop. Ann Intern Med 2015;162(4):276–86.

11. Binswanger IA, Koester S, Mueller SR, et al. Overdose education and naloxone for patients prescribed opioids in primary care: a qualitative study of primary care staff. J Gen Intern Med 2015;30(12):1837–44.

12. Chou R, Fanciullo GJ, Fine PG, et al. Clinical guidelines for the use of chronic opioid therapy in chronic noncancer pain. J Pain 2009;10(2):113–30.

13. Kaplovitch E, Gomes T, Camacho X, et al. Sex differences in dose escalation and overdose death during chronic opioid therapy: a population-based cohort study. PLoS One 2015;10(8):e0134550.

14. Calcaterra SL, Yamashita TE, Min SJ, et al. Opioid prescribing at hospital discharge contributes to chronic opioid use. J Gen Intern Med 2016;31(5):478–85.

15. Office of he Assistant Secretary for Planning and Evaluation; US Department of Health & Human Services. Opioid abuse in the US and HHS actions to address opioid-drug related overdoses and death 2015. Available at: https://aspe.hhs.gov/basic-report/opioid-abuse-us-and-hhs-actions-address-opioid-drug-related-overdoses-and-deaths. Accessed August 1, 2017.

16. Butler SF, Budman SH, Fernandez K, et al. Validation of a screener and opioid assessment measure for patients with chronic pain. Pain 2004;112(1–2):65–75.

17. Turner BJ, Liang Y. Drug overdose in a retrospective cohort with non-cancer pain treated with opioids, antidepressants, and/or sedative-hypnotics: interactions with mental health disorders. J Gen Intern Med 2015;30(8):1081–96.

18. Mueller SR, Walley AY, Calcaterra SL, et al. A review of opioid overdose prevention and naloxone prescribing: implications for translating community programming into clinical practice. Subst Abus 2015;36(2):240–53.

19. Bohnert AS, Valenstein M, Bair MJ, et al. Association between opioid prescribing patterns and opioid overdose-related deaths. JAMA 2011;305(13):1315–21.

20. Toblin RL, Paulozzi LJ, Logan JE, et al. Mental illness and psychotropic drug use among prescription drug overdose deaths: a medical examiner chart review. J Clin Psychiatry 2010;71(4):491–6.

21. U S Department of Health And Human Services. Opioid abuse in the United States and Department of Health and Human Services actions to address opioid-drug-related overdoses and deaths. J Pain Palliat Care Pharmacother 2015;29(2):133–9.

22. Miller M, Barber CW, Leatherman S, et al. Prescription opioid duration of action and the risk of unintentional overdose among patients receiving opioid therapy. JAMA Intern Med 2015;175(4):608–15.

23. Coffin PO, Tracy M, Bucciarelli A, et al. Identifying injection drug users at risk of nonfatal overdose. Acad Emerg Med 2007;14(7):616–23.

24. Binswanger IA, Stern MF, Deyo RA, et al. Release from prison: a high risk of death for former inmates. N Engl J Med 2007;356(2):157–65.

25. Edlund MJ, Martin BC, Russo JE, et al. The role of opioid prescription in incident opioid abuse and dependence among individuals with chronic noncancer pain: the role of opioid prescription. Clin J Pain 2014;30(7):557–64.

26. Liebschutz JM, Xuan Z, Shanahan CW, et al. Improving adherence to long-term opioid therapy guidelines to reduce opioid misuse in primary care: a cluster-randomized clinical trial. JAMA Intern Med 2017;177(9):1265–72.
27. Binswanger IA, Glanz JM. Pharmaceutical opioids in the home and youth: implications for adult medical practice. Subst Abus 2015;36(2):141–3.
28. Spoth R, Trudeau L, Shin C, et al. Longitudinal effects of universal preventive intervention on prescription drug misuse: three randomized controlled trials with late adolescents and young adults. Am J Public Health 2013;103(4):665–72.
29. Levy SJ, Kokotailo PK. Substance use screening, brief intervention, and referral to treatment for pediatricians. Pediatrics 2011;128(5):e1330–40.
30. Knight JR, Sherritt L, Shrier LA, et al. Validity of the CRAFFT substance abuse screening test among adolescent clinic patients. Arch Pediatr Adolesc Med 2002;156(6):607–14.
31. Starrels JL, Becker WC, Alford DP, et al. Systematic review: treatment agreements and urine drug testing to reduce opioid misuse in patients with chronic pain. Ann Intern Med 2010;152(11):712–20.
32. Jarvis M, Williams J, Hurford M, Lindsay D, Lincoln P, Giles L, Luongo P, Safarian T. Appropriate use of drug testing in clinical addiction medicine. J addict med. 2017;11(3):163–73.
33. Brown R, Riley MR, Ulrich L, et al. Impact of New York prescription drug monitoring program, I-STOP, on statewide overdose morbidity. Drug Alcohol Depend 2017;178:348–54.
34. Haegerich TM, Paulozzi LJ, Manns BJ, et al. What we know, and don't know, about the impact of state policy and systems-level interventions on prescription drug overdose. Drug Alcohol Depend 2014;145:34–47.
35. Paulozzi LJ, Kilbourne EM, Desai HA. Prescription drug monitoring programs and death rates from drug overdose. Pain Med 2011;12(5):747–54.
36. Deyo RA, Irvine JM, Millet LM, et al. Measures such as interstate cooperation would improve the efficacy of programs to track controlled drug prescriptions. Health Aff (Millwood) 2013;32(3):603–13.
37. Fishbain DA, Cole B, Lewis J, et al. What percentage of chronic nonmalignant pain patients exposed to chronic opioid analgesic therapy develop abuse/addiction and/or aberrant drug-related behaviors? A structured evidence-based review. Pain Med 2008;9(4):444–59.
38. Mueller SR, Koester S, Glanz JM, et al. Attitudes toward naloxone prescribing in clinical settings: a qualitative study of patients prescribed high dose opioids for chronic non-cancer pain. J Gen Intern Med 2017;32(3):277–83.
39. Meltzer EC, Rybin D, Saitz R, et al. Identifying prescription opioid use disorder in primary care: diagnostic characteristics of the current opioid misuse measure (COMM). Pain 2011;152(2):397–402.
40. Passik SD, Kirsh KL, Whitcomb L, et al. Monitoring outcomes during long-term opioid therapy for noncancer pain: results with the pain assessment and documentation tool. J Opioid Manag 2005;1(5):257–66.
41. Spelman JF, Peglow S, Schwartz AR, et al. Group visits for overdose education and naloxone distribution in primary care: a pilot quality improvement initiative. Pain Med 2017;18(12):2325–30.
42. Krebs EE, Lorenz KA, Bair MJ, et al. Development and initial validation of the PEG, a three-item scale assessing pain intensity and interference. J Gen Intern Med 2009;24(6):733–8.
43. Compton WM, Jones CM, Baldwin GT. Relationship between nonmedical prescription-opioid use and heroin use. N Engl J Med 2016;374(2):154–63.

44. Frank JW, Levy C, Matlock DD, et al. Patients' perspectives on tapering of chronic opioid therapy: a qualitative study. Pain Med 2016;17(10):1838–47.

45. Frank JW, Lovejoy TI, Becker WC, et al. Patient outcomes in dose reduction or discontinuation of long-term opioid therapy: a systematic review. Ann Intern Med 2017;167(3):181–91.

46. Wheeler E, Jones TS, Gilbert MK, et al. Opioid overdose prevention programs providing naloxone to laypersons—United States, 2014. MMWR Morb Mortal Wkly Rep 2015;64(23):631–5.

47. Walley AY, Xuan Z, Hackman HH, et al. Opioid overdose rates and implementation of overdose education and nasal naloxone distribution in Massachusetts: interrupted time series analysis. BMJ 2013;346:f174.

48. Strang J, Manning V, Mayet S, et al. Overdose training and take-home naloxone for opiate users: prospective cohort study of impact on knowledge and attitudes and subsequent management of overdoses. Addiction 2008;103(10):1648–57.

49. Green TC, Heimer R, Grau LE. Distinguishing signs of opioid overdose and indication for naloxone: an evaluation of six overdose training and naloxone distribution programs in the United States. Addiction 2008;103(6):979–89.

50. Sherman SG, Gann DS, Tobin KE, et al. "The life they save may be mine": diffusion of overdose prevention information from a city sponsored programme. Int J Drug Policy 2009;20(2):137–42.

51. Dwyer K, Walley AY, Langlois BK, et al. Opioid education and nasal naloxone rescue kits in the emergency department. West J Emerg Med 2015;16(3):381–4.

52. Coffin PO, Behar E, Rowe C, et al. Nonrandomized intervention study of naloxone coprescription for primary care patients receiving long-term opioid therapy for pain. Ann Intern Med 2016;165(4):245–52.

53. Davis CS, Burris S, Beletsky L, et al. Co-prescribing naloxone does not increase liability risk. Subst Abus 2016;37(4):498–500.

54. Bohnert AS, Bonar EE, Cunningham R, et al. A pilot randomized clinical trial of an intervention to reduce overdose risk behaviors among emergency department patients at risk for prescription opioid overdose. Drug Alcohol Depend 2016; 163:40–7.

55. Kerensky T, Walley AY. Opioid overdose prevention and naloxone rescue kits: what we know and what we don't know. Addict Sci Clin Pract 2017;12(4):1–7.

56. Substance Abuse and Mental Health Services Administration. SAMHSA opioid overdose prevention toolkit. Rockville (MD): US Department of Health and Human Services; 2013. HHS Publication No. (SMA) 13-4742.

57. Potter JS, Marino EN, Hillhouse MP, et al. Buprenorphine/naloxone and methadone maintenance treatment outcomes for opioid analgesic, heroin, and combined users: findings from Starting Treatment With Agonist Replacement Therapies (START). J Stud Alcohol Drugs 2013;74(4):605–13.

58. Volkow ND, Frieden TR, Hyde PS, et al. Medication-assisted therapies: tackling the opioid-overdose epidemic. N Engl J Med 2014;370(22):2063–6.

59. Kahan M, Wilson L, Mailis-Gagnon A, et al, National Opioid Use Guideline Group. Canadian guideline for safe and effective use of opioids for chronic noncancer pain: clinical summary for family physicians. Part 2: special populations. Can Fam Physician 2011;57(11):1269–76, e1419–28.

60. Fiellin DA, Pantalon MV, Pakes JP, et al. Treatment of heroin dependence with buprenorphine in primary care. Am J Drug Alcohol Abuse 2002;28(2):231–41.

61. McCabe SE, West BT, Boyd CJ. Leftover prescription opioids and nonmedical use among high school seniors: a multi-cohort national study. J Adolesc Health 2013;52(4):480–5.

62. Larochelle MR, Liebschutz JM, Zhang F, et al. Opioid prescribing after nonfatal overdose and association with repeated overdose. Ann Intern Med 2016; 165(5):376–7.
63. Edlund MJ, Martin BC, Devries A, et al. Trends in use of opioids for chronic non-cancer pain among individuals with mental health and substance use disorders: the TROUP study. Clin J Pain 2010;26(1):1–8.
64. Nielsen S, Lintzeris N, Bruno R, et al. Benzodiazepine use among chronic pain patients prescribed opioids: associations with pain, physical and mental health, and health service utilization. Pain Med 2015;16(2):356–66.
65. Seal KH, Shi Y, Cohen G, et al. Association of mental health disorders with pre-scription opioids and high-risk opioid use in US veterans of Iraq and Afghanistan. JAMA 2012;307(9):940–7.
66. Wasan AD, Davar G, Jamison R. The association between negative affect and opioid analgesia in patients with discogenic low back pain. Pain 2005;117(3): 450–61.
67. Edlund MJ, Steffick D, Hudson T, et al. Risk factors for clinically recognized opioid abuse and dependence among veterans using opioids for chronic non-cancer pain. Pain 2007;129(3):355–62.
68. Im JJ, Shachter RD, Oliva EM, et al. Association of care practices with suicide attempts in US veterans prescribed opioid medications for chronic pain management. J Gen Intern Med 2015;30(7):979–91.
69. Davidson CL, Babson KA, Bonn-Miller MO, et al. The impact of exercise on sui-cide risk: examining pathways through depression, PTSD, and sleep in an inpa-tient sample of veterans. Suicide Life Threat Behav 2013;43(3):279–89.
70. Mazer-Amirshahi M, Mullins PM, Rasooly IR, et al. Trends in prescription opioid use in pediatric emergency department patients. Pediatr Emerg Care 2014; 30(4):230–5.
71. Miech R, Johnston L, O'Malley PM, et al. Prescription opioids in adolescence and future opioid misuse. Pediatrics 2015;136(5):e1169–77.
72. McCabe SE, West BT, Morales M, et al. Does early onset of non-medical use of prescription drugs predict subsequent prescription drug abuse and depen-dence? Results from a national study. Addiction 2007;102(12):1920–30.
73. Bernabei R, Gambassi G, Lapane K, et al. Management of pain in elderly patients with cancer. SAGE Study Group. Systematic Assessment of Geriatric Drug Use via Epidemiology. JAMA 1998;279(23):1877–82.
74. Wilder-Smith OH. Opioid use in the elderly. Eur J Pain 2005;9(2):137–40.
75. Le Roux C, Tang Y, Drexler K. Alcohol and opioid use disorder in older adults: ne-glected and treatable illnesses. Curr Psychiatry Rep 2016;18(9):87.
76. Broussard CS, Rasmussen SA, Reefhuis J, et al. Maternal treatment with opioid analgesics and risk for birth defects. Am J Obstet Gynecol 2011;204(4): 314.e1-11.
77. ACOG Committee on Health Care for Underserved Women, American Society of Addiction Medicine. ACOG committee opinion no. 524: opioid abuse, depen-dence, and addiction in pregnancy. Obstet Gynecol 2012;119(5):1070–6.
78. Administration SAaMHS. Clinical use of extended-release injectable naltrexone in the treatment of opioid use disorder: a brief guide. Rockville (MD): US Department of Health and Human Services; 2015. HHS Publication No. (SMA) 14-4892R.
79. American College of Obstetricians and Gynecologists. Patient education Fact Sheet: Important information about opioid use disorder and pregnancy 2016. Available at: https://www.acog.org/Patients/FAQs/Important-Information-About-Opioid-Use-Disorder-and-Pregnancy. Accessed August 4, 2017.

80. Huffman KL, Shella ER, Sweis G, et al. Nonopioid substance use disorders and opioid dose predict therapeutic opioid addiction. J Pain 2015;16(2):126–34.
81. Hser YI, Evans E, Grella C, et al. Long-term course of opioid addiction. Harv Rev Psychiatry 2015;23(2):76–89.
82. Smith PC, Schmidt SM, Allensworth-Davies D, et al. A single-question screening test for drug use in primary care. Arch Intern Med 2010;170(13):1155–60.
83. Yudko E, Lozhkina O, Fouts A. A comprehensive review of the psychometric properties of the drug abuse screening test. J Subst Abuse Treat 2007;32(2):189–98.
84. Reinert DF, Allen JP. The alcohol use disorders identification test: an update of research findings. Alcohol Clin Exp Res 2007;31(2):185–99.
85. Jones CM, Campopiano M, Baldwin G, et al. National and state treatment need and capacity for opioid agonist medication-assisted treatment. Am J Public Health 2015;105(8):e55–63.

Office-Based Addiction Treatment in Primary Care
Approaches That Work

E. Jennifer Edelman, MD, MHS[a],*, Benjamin J. Oldfield, MD[b],
Jeanette M. Tetrault, MD[c]

KEYWORDS

- Primary health care • Opioid use disorder • Alcohol use disorder • Buprenorphine
- Naltrexone

KEY POINTS

- Primary care practices are well-suited for implementing evidence-based treatments to address alcohol and other substance use disorders.
- Effective approaches to treatment largely focus on provision of pharmacotherapy (eg, buprenorphine, naltrexone) in conjunction with counseling-based treatments.
- Studies to identify effective approaches for treating vulnerable populations are needed.

INTRODUCTION

Of the roughly 22 million individuals in the United States suffering from addiction, only 11% receive specialty care.[1] Reasons cited for the treatment gap include lack of provider education with regard to substance use and substance use disorders, perceived lack of need for treatment on the part of the patient, and lack of access to evidence-based treatment.[1,2] Integrating addiction treatment into office-based primary care is an important approach to improving access to care.[3] Primary care settings, including those providing primary care to special populations, offer several advantages to treatment of substance use disorder over specialty settings. These advantages include

Disclosure Statement: The authors have no conflicts of interest. Dr B.J. Oldfield was supported as a Yale National Clinician Scholar with additional support from the Veterans Health Administration during the conduct of this work. Dr J.M. Tetrault was supported as a Macy Foundation Faculty Scholar during the conduct of this work.

[a] Department of Medicine, Yale University School of Medicine and Public Health, 367 Cedar Street, E.S. Harkness Memorial Hall, Building A, Suite 401, New Haven, CT 06510, USA; [b] National Clinician Scholars Program, Yale University School of Medicine, PO Box 208088, New Haven, CT 06520, USA; [c] Department of Internal Medicine, Yale University School of Medicine, 367 Cedar Street, Suite 305, New Haven, CT 06510, USA
* Corresponding author.
E-mail address: ejennifer.edelman@yale.edu

https://doi.org/10.1016/j.mcna.2018.02.007
medical.theclinics.com

accessibility to patients, ability to tailor services to patient need, reduction of stigma associated with accessing treatment, and the ability to provide many services in one location. Additionally, clinical preventive services are an integral part of primary care medicine, with screening and provision of brief counseling for alcohol use and treatment of tobacco use among the top priorities for the provision of high-quality care.[4]

Through primary care settings, patients may receive a range of evidence-based addiction treatment services, in addition to treatment for tobacco use. These services include US Food and Drug Administration (FDA)-approved medications for alcohol (ie, disulfiram, acamprosate and oral and extended-release [XR] naltrexone) and opioid use disorder (ie, buprenorphine alone or coformulated with naloxone by a certified provider; and oral and XR naltrexone; **Table 1**). Additionally, primary care settings may lend themselves well to the implementation of counseling-based strategies. Specifically, brief counseling may be provided and the Affordable Care Act has supported the integration of additional behavioral health services into primary care. Efforts at treatment expansion have resulted in several proposed approaches for office-based addiction treatment in primary care.

Based on a PubMed and Ovid MEDLINE search designed to identify articles published since 2007 that reported on behavioral and/or medical treatments used in outpatient settings to address alcohol, opioid, and/or stimulant (cocaine, amphetamine) use, we identified office-based approaches to addiction treatment. Herein, we highlight office-based treatment approaches within primary care and a specialty treatment setting (**Box 1**) to address alcohol, opioid, and other substance use.

PRIMARY CARE-BASED APPROACHES
Alcohol

The prevalence of alcohol use disorder in the US population is increasing and has been termed a public health crisis. Certain groups, such as women, older adults, racial/ethnic minorities, and the socioeconomically disadvantaged, are particularly affected.[5] For decades, primary care settings have been considered important sites for the delivery of care to people with alcohol use and related disorders.[6] However,

Table 1	
Pharmacotherapy options for alcohol use disorder and opioid use disorder	
Generic Name	**Usual Daily Dose**
FDA approved for alcohol use disorder	
Acamprosate	666 mg orally 3 times daily
Disulfiram	250–500 mg orally daily
Naltrexone	50 mg orally daily
Extended-release Naltrexone	380 mg intramuscularly every 4 wk
Not FDA approved for alcohol use disorder	
Gabapentin	300–600 mg orally 3 times daily
Topiramate	100 mg orally twice daily
FDA approved for opioid use disorder	
Buprenorphine (with and without naloxone)	2–24 mg sublingually daily
Methadone	60–80 mg orally daily
Naltrexone	50 mg orally daily
Extended-release Naltrexone	380 mg intramuscularly every 4 wk

Abbreviation: FDA, US Food and Drug Administration.

Box 1
Approaches to care for addiction treatment

Primary care settings

- Alcohol
  - Brief intervention
  - Clinic-based counseling
  - Pharmacotherapy
  - Technological interventions
- Opioids
  - Pharmacotherapy with variable levels of counseling
  - Primary care based treatment
  - FQHC based treatment
  - Midlevel practitioner models
  - Hub and spoke models
  - Shared medical appointments
  - Improved provider education through Internet-based audiovisual networks to improve care access
- Stimulants
  - Contingency management
  - Cognitive–behavioral therapy with harm reduction framework

Specialty settings

- HIV clinics
  - Alcohol
    - Pharmacotherapy
    - Stepped care
  - Opioids
    - Pharmacotherapy
    - Rapid treatment access programs
  - Stimulants
- Transitions clinics
  - Alcohol
    - Pharmacotherapy
  - Opioids
    - Pharmacotherapy

Abbreviations: FQHC, federally qualified health center; HIV, human immunodeficiency virus.

---

uptake of these treatments remains low: overall only 7.8% of US adults with alcohol use disorder received treatment in 2013.[7] A menu of evidence-based treatments are available in the office setting, including brief interventions by primary providers and other clinicians, clinic-based counseling, pharmacotherapy, referral for specialized treatment, or combinations thereof.

Screening and brief intervention (SBI) is widely recommended for prevention and early intervention of unhealthy alcohol use[8] in primary care settings based on high-quality evidence.[9] SBI, designed to suit the time constraints of primary care, consists of alcohol screening with a validated instrument[10,11] followed by a brief intervention[12] for those who exceed recommended drinking limits. For those who drink alcohol, the National Institute on Alcohol Abuse and Alcoholism recommends screening for unhealthy alcohol use with a single question: "How many times in the past year have you had five or more drinks in a day (for men) or four or more drinks in a day (for women)?"[13] Weekly average (in drinks per week) alcohol intake should be calculated and documented in the medical record. Those who screen positive for at-risk drinking but do not meet criteria for an alcohol use disorder should undergo a brief intervention (**Table 2**). The sequence of Screening, Brief Intervention, and Referral to Treatment (SBIRT) is associated with improvements in alcohol use severity, clinical efficiency, cost, and also is associated with a reduction of disparities in treatment of alcohol use disorder.[14] These interventions can be performed effectively by nurses[15] and other nonphysician clinicians in primary care settings.[16]

Table 2	
How to conduct a brief intervention for unhealthy alcohol use	
1. Raise subject	• Hello, I am _____. Would you mind taking a few minutes to talk with me about your alcohol/drug use? <<**PAUSE**>>
2. Provide feedback	
Review screen	• From what I understand you are drinking/using [insert screening data]... We know that drinking above certain levels or using... can cause problems, such as [insert facts]... I am concerned about your drinking/drug use.
Make connection	• What connection, if any, do you see between your drinking/drug use and this medical visit or other medical issue? **If patient sees connection**: reflect/reiterate what patient has said. **If patient does not see connection**: make one using facts.
Show NIAAA guidelines	• These are what we consider the upper limits of low risk drinking for your age and sex. You would be less likely to experience illness or injury if you stayed within these guidelines.
3. Enhance motivation	
Readiness to change	• **[Show readiness ruler]** On a scale from 1 to 10, how ready are you to change any aspect of your drinking or drug use... Or seek treatment?
Develop discrepancy	• **If patient says**: ≥2 **ask**: Why did you choose that number and not a lower one? ≤1 **or unwilling ask**: What would it take for you to become a "2"? What would make this a problem for you? How important would it be for you to prevent that from happening? Have you ever done anything you wish you hadn't while drinking?
Reflective listening	• Reflect/reiterate patients reasons for making a change
4. Negotiate and advise	
Negotiate goal	• What's the next step? *(If a positive next step, reflect it; if not, suggest one.)*
Give advice	• If you can stay within these limits...or reduce or abstain from your drug use... you will be less likely to experience illness/injury related to your use of...
Summarize	• Overall, this is what I've heard you say... *(reflect on reasons for change)*... You have agreed to... *(state actual amounts of reduction of drinking/drug use or to seek treatment.)* I have included this in your discharge instructions that you are signing. This is an agreement between you and yourself.
Suggest follow-up with primary care	• **Suggest follow-up to discuss drinking/drug use.**
Thank patient	• **Thank patient for their time.**

Abbreviation: NIAAA, National Institute on Alcohol Abuse and Alcoholism.
Adapted from D'Onofrio G, Pantalon MV, Degutis LC, et al. Development and implementation of an emergency practitioner-performed brief intervention for hazardous and harmful drinkers in the emergency department. Acad Emerg Med 2005;12(3):252; with permission.

The Substance Abuse and Mental Health Services Administration (SAMHSA) allocated significant resources into expanding the continuum of care for unhealthy alcohol and other substance use through demonstration projects and cooperative agreements. Over 5 years, these SAMHSA–funded projects screened more than 1 million patients. Although decreases in substance use were observed, this effort also raised questions about the optimal ways to proceed with SBIRT as a public health intervention. Assessment of another SBIRT implementation project within 5 Veterans Administration Hospital Primary Care clinics found that key informants and stakeholders thought that further training or academic detailing of providers may address SBIRT implementation barriers.[17] Additional data further questions the usefulness of widespread SBIRT implementation for substances other than unhealthy alcohol use, including data suggesting that SBIRT did not improve engagement in specialty treatment.[18,19] Which elements of the counseling provided may be efficacious remains unknown, however,[20,21] and recent evidence suggests SBIRT may not be effective in certain populations (such as people living with human immunodeficiency virus [HIV, PLWH]), or delivered in certain settings.[22] Repeated brief counseling by a registered nurse has been shown to engage patients in alcohol-related care (including the use of pharmacotherapy for alcohol use disorder), but not to improve drinking outcomes at 12 months.[23]

Pharmacotherapy for alcohol use disorder does not require specialized training to prescribe, is efficacious, and is grossly underused,[24–28] and can be prescribed as part of a standard medical management approach (**Table 3**).[29] Naltrexone (in oral and XR forms), acamprosate, and disulfiram are FDA approved for the treatment of alcohol use disorder,[25] and topiramate[24,30,31] and gabapentin[32] have shown efficacy in randomized clinical trials (see **Table 1**). Pharmacotherapy need not be combined with intensive behavioral interventions to be efficacious.[29,33] In medical management, a patient attends office visits with a licensed health professional (physician, nurse, physician assistant, or clinical pharmacist) weekly at first, then spacing to monthly visits. These sessions include a review of drinking, overall level of functioning, medication adherence, and adverse effects. External supports, such as group treatment, can be offered within this approach.[29] The clinician should be prepared to make appropriate counseling referrals if the patient requires a greater intensity of services. With alcohol pharmacotherapy grossly underprescribed, especially by primary care providers, expanding access to these medications will add to the nationwide efforts to address a critical unmet need with an evidence-based approach and further decrease stigma related to treatment.

Technology-delivered interventions can also be incorporated into outpatient practices and have demonstrated feasibility for those with unhealthy alcohol use. Emerging digital technologies (eg, treatment-based digital kiosk) show promise for helping to both hone therapies to patients' individual needs and to support them in settings beyond the clinic, but how to integrate them successfully into outpatient treatment settings remains unknown.[34]

Opioids

The cornerstone of treatment for opioid use disorder is pharmacotherapy[35,36] and models for integrating pharmacotherapy into office-based settings vary in structure.[37] FDA-approved medications include a full opioid agonist (methadone), which can be only delivered in specialty treatment settings for treatment of opioid use disorder; partial opioid agonists (buprenorphine sublingual, buprenorphine-naloxone sublingual or buccal, and implantable buprenorphine); and opioid antagonists (oral and XR naltrexone).[37] Naltrexone may be an attractive option for patients with mild opioid

Table 3
Counseling and adjunctive considerations in the provision of pharmacotherapy for AUD and OUD in office-based settings

Pharmacotherapy for AUD	Office-Based Pharmacotherapy for OUD
Counseling	
Medical management	Addiction counseling
• Weekly to monthly 20-min visits with licensed health care professional (physician, nurse, physician assistant, clinical pharmacist)	• Weekly 15- to 30-min visits with licensed health care professional or behavioral health specialist with periodic, longer counseling sessions (30–60 min)
• Review drinking, overall functioning, medication adherence, and adverse effects	• Individual or group therapies that may include elements of cognitive, behavioral, insight-oriented, and/or supportive psychotherapies
• Encourage attendance at support groups and other community resources	Cognitive–behavioral therapy
Combined behavioral intervention	• Weekly to biweekly 50-min visits with licensed behavioral health specialist
• Weekly to biweekly 50-min visits with licensed behavioral health specialist	
• Integrates aspects of cognitive behavioral therapy, 12-step facilitation, motivational interviewing, and support system involvement	
Patient education	
Medication interactions	Medication interactions
• Naltrexone should not be used concurrently with opioids	• Concurrent use of alcohol, benzodiazepines, or gabapentin with buprenorphine may increase risk of sedation, respiratory depression, and death
	• Naltrexone should not be used concurrently with opioids
	Pain syndromes
	• Strategies should be offered regarding how to manage pain syndromes without misusing opioids or other drugs
Laboratory testing	
Hepatic aminotransferases	Urine toxicology
• For patients receiving naltrexone, aspartate aminotransferase and alanine aminotransferase should be checked before initiation and periodically; elevations >3–5 times the upper limit of normal should prompt discontinuation or transition to another option	• Periodic urine drug testing to assess risk of medication interaction (eg, risk of overdose with buprenorphine and concurrent benzodiazepine use)
	Hepatic aminotransferases
	• For patients receiving naltrexone, aspartate aminotransferase and alanine aminotransferase should be checked before initiation and periodically; elevations >3–5 times the upper limit of normal should prompt discontinuation or transition to another option

Abbreviations: AUD, alcohol use disorder; OUD, opioid use disorder.

use disorder, those in situations where medication administration can be supervised, and those with occupations that do not permit opioid agonist treatment. However, data to compare the efficacy of opioid agonists versus naltrexone are just beginning to emerge.[38,39] These pharmacotherapies more effectively reduce opioid use than behavioral treatment alone, translating into improved health outcomes and survival, and the Office of National Drug Control Policy and the US Department of Health and Human Services have recently prioritized increasing access to pharmacotherapy for opioid use disorder, with a focus on primary care providers.[40] With the goal of initiating treatment for opioid use disorder as soon as possible, patients are increasingly initiated on pharmacotherapy in emergency department and inpatient settings.[41–44] Additionally, new treatment options now include XR buprenorphine.

The advent of buprenorphine and the passage of the Drug Addiction Treatment Act in 2000 transformed the opioid use disorder delivery system by granting physicians the ability to administer office-based opioid agonist treatment.[45] Although fixed-dose buprenorphine, in most studies, is considered noninferior to moderate doses of methadone in terms of retention in treatment and illicit opioid use,[36] buprenorphine is generally considered a safer alternative to methadone.[46] In primary care settings, ongoing maintenance treatment in patients with prescription opioid use disorder who receive buprenorphine is more efficacious than tapering.[47] Concurrent counseling along with buprenorphine pharmacotherapy need not be extensive: brief, once-weekly counseling with once-weekly medication dispensing is no less efficacious than extended weekly counseling and more frequent dispensing.[48] Primary care-based options are available for counseling provided concurrently with buprenorphine (see **Table 3**). Patients who also take benzodiazepines, have severe alcohol use disorder, or have severe respiratory diseases are at risk of respiratory depression with buprenorphine[49] and, therefore, may benefit from specialist referral for a higher level of monitoring.

Given that a great deal of additional resources are not needed to provide buprenorphine in primary care, Federally Qualified Health Centers are an ideal clinical setting to offer office-based addiction treatment.[50] Buprenorphine may be successfully initiated by primary providers, but approaches in which a specialist performs initial psychological evaluation and initiates buprenorphine, then transitions patients once stabilized to community health centers, also show efficacy.[51] Collaborative care consisting of generalist clinicians working alongside nurse care managers, who perform patient education, obtain informed consent, develop treatment plans, oversee medication management, refer to specialty care, and monitor adherence, provides successful treatment to most patients with opioid and/or alcohol use disorder and makes effective use of time for physicians who prescribe buprenorphine.[52–54] The recent passage of legislation allowing advance practice nurse practitioners and physician assistants the ability to provide buprenorphine after 24 hours of training will open the door for the development of new and innovative models of care delivery. On a health systems level, hub-and-spoke models allow for centralized intake at a "hub," and then patients are connected to "spokes" in primary care settings for ongoing management.[55,56]

Group visit models (ie, shared medical appointments) can be important and efficient sites of primary care for patients with opioid use disorder, including pharmacotherapy with buprenorphine. Group visit models allow providers to see many patients at once, decrease relapse rates and craving, and increase treatment retention rates.[57,58] They may also foster group-specific communication behaviors that uniquely support patients through treatment.[59] Groups, described and offered to patients during individual visits, are typically hour-long sessions that occur weekly with rolling enrollment, and thus continually welcome new patients in varying stages of treatment. Urine drug testing samples are taken weekly, and the previous week's results may be posted for the group to see if all consent. Patients check in about their week and engage in psychoeducation related to addiction self-management skills.[59] Internet-based, audiovisual networks for provider education can increase access to buprenorphine in rural areas, and can emphasize and empower the physician assistants and nurse practitioners in the primary care of those with opioid use disorder. In the Project Extension for Community Healthcare Outcomes model (ECHO), an MD/DO primary care provider, nurse practitioner, or physician assistant performs an initial evaluation and screening and then refers to a collaborating physician for mentored buprenorphine prescribing.[60] Telemedicine models, in which a patient presents at a secure videoconferencing site under the supervision of a nurse and videoconferences with a buprenorphine provider, have successfully increased access to buprenorphine in Canada.[61] Text message interventions can foster patients' self-efficacy and facilitate unobserved, home initiation of buprenorphine.[62]

XR naltrexone can be successfully integrated into some of the models of care described herein, including the collaborative care between generalists and nurse care managers.[52,53] One-stop shop models, or integrated centers in mental health clinics that provide psychosocial services, primary care, care for comorbid conditions such as HIV and hepatitis C virus, and harm reduction services such as syringe exchange, are well-suited to offer naltrexone and other pharmacotherapies as treatment options.[63]

As with treatment of alcohol use disorder, approaches focusing on the movement of the treatment of opioid use disorder out of specialty settings and into office-based care, with delivery of a medical model by an interdisciplinary team, offers the greatest potential for patient success. Additionally, this approach increases treatment access and decreases treatment-related stigma. Based on resources, alternative models such as those that rely on a hub-and-spoke model or telemedicine may also be appropriate.

Other Drugs

There is limited evidence for effective treatment of cocaine and other stimulants, as well as other drug use disorders in office-based settings. Current data do not support the use of anticonvulsants,[64] dopamine agonists,[65] antipsychotics,[66] or antidepressants[67] in the management of cocaine use disorder. Some evidence supports the effectiveness of disulfiram for cocaine use disorder, but large-scale, randomized trials are lacking.[68] Contingency management (CM), a psychosocial treatment that offers rewards and incentives for demonstration of reduced use or abstinence, show positive but short-lived efficacy and likely represents the best currently available treatment option (**Table 4**).[69,70]

Methamphetamine use disorder presents a similar conundrum to office-based providers. No pharmacotherapies are currently FDA approved for methamphetamine use disorder.[71–73] CM again may be an efficacious option.[73–76] In addition, community-based cognitive–behavioral therapy that uses a harm reduction framework has been effective in the treatment of methamphetamine use disorder in men who have sex with men, but large or randomized studies of these interventions are lacking.[77,78]

Given the limited evidence for managing these disorders in primary care settings, patients with these disorders, particularly those with complex withdrawal, psychiatric comorbidity, or medical comorbidity, should be considered for referral to higher levels of care.

SPECIALTY SETTINGS AND POPULATIONS
Human Immunodeficiency Virus Clinics

Among PLWH, alcohol and other substance use adversely impacts care along the HIV care continuum, resulting in uncontrolled HIV with negative consequences for the individual and public health. To address this problem, the integration of addiction

Table 4
Prize-based contingency management: Rewarded behaviors

Behavior	Comments/Examples
Health-related activities	• Scheduling a medical or nutritionist appointment • Obtaining medications • Recording medication or food consumption daily • Exercising.
General goal-related activities	Activities that focused on • Abstinence • Recreation • Transportation • Housing • Legal • Education or employment • Psychiatric or personal improvement
Submission of a test to assess for abstinence	• Submission of urine and breath samples to assess for drug and alcohol use, respectively
Evidence of abstinence	• Negative urine and breath samples, with potential for increased earnings if abstinence from both drugs and alcohol demonstrated and over time

Data from Petry NM, Weinstock J, Alessi SM, et al. Group-based randomized trial of contingencies for health and abstinence in HIV patients. J Consult Clin Psychol 2010;78(1):89–97.

treatment and HIV care is recommended by national and international organizations.[79,80] Several approaches have been developed and evaluated to promote addiction treatment in HIV clinics, and others are actively being investigated.

Alcohol

XR naltrexone decreases heavy drinking days among those with alcohol use disorder[33] and is safe for use in PLWH, including those on antiretroviral therapy.[81,82] The availability of an injectable formulation with monthly administration avoids adding to pill burden, an important consideration for this population. A recent study demonstrated the feasibility and acceptability of XR naltrexone for alcohol use disorder in combination with medical management when delivered in HIV clinics.[83] These findings were supported by a separate randomized clinical trial that evaluated the impact of XR naltrexone versus placebo on HIV-related and drinking outcomes among PLWH with heavy alcohol use and suboptimal antiretroviral therapy adherence.[84] In this study, participants in both treatment groups also received counseling, which incorporated medical management and medication coaching.[29,85] By combining these 2 efficacious behavioral treatments, participants received counseling and advice to decrease alcohol use by health care practitioners with referral to mutual help groups (eg, Alcoholics Anonymous) and education regarding the importance of and strategies to promote antiretroviral medication adherence. Compared with the placebo group, those randomized to XR naltrexone demonstrated a decrease in heavy alcohol use; this result, however, did not translate into improved antiretroviral therapy adherence or other HIV-related outcomes (ie, HIV viral load, CD4 cell count, and VACS Index score [a validated measure of morbidity and mortality based on routinely collected laboratory data]).[84]

In the STEP Trials (*S*tarting *T*reatment for *E*thanol in *P*rimary Care), the effectiveness of integrated stepped care to address unhealthy alcohol use among PLWH when delivered in HIV clinics is being evaluated.[86] In this approach to care and consistent with approaches used for the treatment of medical conditions routinely treated in office-based settings (eg, depression, diabetes mellitus, and hypertension), individuals receive an increasing intensity of services depending on their treatment response and level of alcohol use, including a social worker-delivered brief negotiation interview with a follow-up telephone booster at 2 weeks, 4 sessions of psychologist-delivered motivational enhancement therapy, addiction physician management with consideration of alcohol pharmacotherapy, and/or referral to a higher level of care (eg, detoxification, intensive outpatient program). This approach holds promise for addressing unhealthy alcohol use among patients with moderate alcohol and liver disease[87]; however, the impact of this approach on addressing at-risk drinking and alcohol use disorder is actively being studied.

Findings that PLWH are 14% less likely than uninfected patients to receive evidence-based alcohol-related care after a positive screen for unhealthy alcohol use[88] underscore the need for ongoing research and implementation efforts. Given the lack of training and comfort with delivering alcohol-related care among HIV providers,[89] approaches that include multidisciplinary care as applied in the STEP Trials or include targeted training, are likely to be most effective in specialty settings.

Opioids

The BHIVES Collaborative (Buprenorphine HIV Evaluation and Support), a 10-site demonstration project, led to the implementation and evaluation of integration HIV care and buprenorphine/naloxone for opioid use disorder. Before patient enrollment, physicians and clinical staff participated in an 8-hour training on buprenorphine, which was followed by the opportunity for sites to participate in monthly 1-hour-long technical assistance conference calls to discuss issues related to clinical management and access to a restricted access listserv to allow for discussion of clinical issues via email and dissemination of appropriate clinical support material. In addition, technical assistance was provided as needed during annual meetings, site visits, and individually via phone and email.[90] This demonstration project revealed the importance of multidisciplinary teams for implementing buprenorphine/naloxone in HIV clinics. Specifically, these programs had multiple prescribers (ie, 2–5 depending on patient census) to ensure sufficient coverage coupled with a nonphysician "buprenorphine/naloxone coordinator." This coordinator, who had varying credentials across sites (ie, licensed practice nurse, registered nurse, nurse practitioner, certified substance use counselor, health educator, or pharmacist) was essential and offered counseling and case management services, and served as a link between the patients and providers; in some clinics, this individual also performed outreach services.[91] This approach to care is associated with improvements in HIV and substance use-related outcomes, as well as other important outcomes.[90,92–96]

In the FAST PATH program (Facilitated Access to Substance abuse Treatment with Prevention And Treatment for HIV), which has been implemented in both HIV and general medical clinics, a physician, nurse care manager, and licensed addiction counselor together deliver care to address addiction treatment needs to people living with and at increased risk for HIV. Physicians provided addiction care along with primary care (if primary care was not already provided by another provider). FAST PATH included the following services: an initial multidisciplinary team visit including the physician, nurse, and addiction counselor, addiction pharmacotherapy with medication monitoring with treatment agreements, urine drug testing and pill counts, weekly individual and group addiction counseling with the addiction counselor, HIV risk reduction and overdose prevention counseling, case management and facilitated referral for higher level of services as needed, and ongoing coordination with the primary care team. On-site face-to-face buprenorphine inductions were conducted by the nurse.

Counseling provided by addiction counselors included cognitive behavioral therapy, with the addition of motivational interviewing–based therapy for those with ongoing substance use, plus encouragement of engagement in 12-step programs. In this approach to care, buprenorphine receipt was associated with improved treatment engagement and qualitative data revealed patient endorsement of this approach.[97,98]

In addition to the provision of buprenorphine, XR naltrexone may offer a future potential treatment option to address opioid use disorder in isolation or in combination with comorbid alcohol use disorder. However, larger studies are first needed to evaluate its efficacy and effectiveness in HIV treatment settings.[83]

In specialty HIV settings, on-site addiction treatment provided by a multidisciplinary team and linkage to enhanced clinical services offers the best approach for patient success. Other public health benefits of this approach include improvement in access to care and destigmatization of opioid use disorder and its treatment.

Other substances

Similar to primary care settings, few treatment approaches have shown efficacy for the treatment of other substance use disorders in specialty treatment settings. CM is an effective intervention to address stimulant use with similar benefits in individuals with and without HIV.[99] Offered through a HIV drop-in center and involving a sample of PLWH in which the majority had cocaine dependence, prize-based CM increased the number of consecutive drug-free urine specimens, and decreased HIV viral load and HIV risk behaviors during the treatment period when compared with a 12-step treatment approach.[100] In this study, specific behaviors were reinforced (see **Table 4**). These findings complement other studies in HIV treatment settings that use CM and rewards-based interventions to promote antiretroviral therapy adherence and decrease HIV viral load.[101]

Lesbian, Gay, Bisexual, and Transgender Populations

Substance use is more common among men who have sex with men and associated with increased HIV risk behaviors and health disparities. However, there are few high-quality studies to guide how to best implement an approach to care to address tobacco, alcohol, or opioid use among MSM in primary-care based settings.[73] Although a recent review demonstrates support for use of motivational interviewing/motivational enhancement therapy and CBT-based approaches to address alcohol use, future work is needed to address this critical area to generate evidence to guide best practices.[102]

People Transitioning Out of Incarceration

An increasing number of studies have evaluated treatment strategies to address substance use, including alcohol and opioid use, among people transitioning out of incarceration. These approaches include the initiation of pharmacotherapy before release into the community. In post hoc analyses, 1 such study found that, among PLWH, XR naltrexone decreased the time to relapse to heavy drinking.[103] Given the particularly high risk of opioid-related overdose after release from incarceration,[104] there have been a number of studies to address this problem. These studies have largely focused on evaluating use of XR naltrexone before release into the community and demonstrated decreased rates of relapse to opioid use.[105,106]

SUMMARY AND FUTURE CONSIDERATIONS

There are a range of approaches to care, incorporating both medications and behaviorally based interventions, that may be applied to primary care and specialty settings, such as HIV clinics, to address alcohol, opioid, and other substance use. Given the pressing need to address the treatment gap, efforts to design and evaluate interventions that promote implementation of these approaches to care are critical and are underway. Future work should also aim to refine quality metrics for assessing quality of addiction treatment services in primary care-based settings and in coordination with other community-based and addiction specialty settings. Last, the importance of ongoing provider education to the implementation and maintenance of effective approaches to care for patients with substance use disorder is vital.

ACKNOWLEDGMENTS

The editors thank P. Todd Korthuis, Oregon Health and Science University, for providing a critical review of this article. The authors acknowledge Janis Glover for her assistance with conducting the literature review.

REFERENCES

1. Lipari RN, Park-Lee E, Van Horn S. America's need for and receipt of substance use treatment in 2015. The CBHSQ report. Rockville (MD): Substance Abuse and Mental Health Services Administration (US); 2013.
2. Tetrault JM, Petrakis IL. Partnering with psychiatry to close the education gap: an approach to the addiction epidemic. J Gen Intern Med 2017;32(12):1387–9.
3. Saitz R, Daaleman TP. Now is the time to address substance use disorders in primary care. Ann Fam Med 2017;15(4):306–8.
4. Maciosek MV, LaFrance AB, Dehmer SP, et al. Updated priorities among effective clinical preventive services. Ann Fam Med 2017;15(1):14–22.
5. Grant BF, Chou SP, Saha TD, et al. Prevalence of 12-month alcohol use, high-risk drinking, and DSM-IV alcohol use disorder in the United States, 2001-2002 to 2012-2013: results from the national epidemiologic survey on alcohol and related conditions. JAMA Psychiatry 2017;74(9):911–23.
6. Babor TF, Ritson EB, Hodgson RJ. Alcohol-related problems in the primary health care setting: a review of early intervention strategies. Br J Addict 1986; 81(1):23–46.
7. Substance Abuse and Mental Health Services Administration (SAMHSA). Results from the 2013 National survey on drug use and health: summary of national findings. Rockville (MD): Substance Abuse and Mental Health Services Administration; 2014. NSDUH Series H-48, DHHS Publication No. (SMA) 04-4863.
8. U.S. Preventive Services Task Force. Final recommendation statement: alcohol misuse: screening and behavioral counseling interventions in primary care. 2013. Available at: https://www.uspreventiveservicestaskforce.org/Page/Document/RecommendationStatementFinal/alcohol-misuse-screening-and-behavioral-counseling-interventions-in-primary-care. Accessed March 26, 2018.
9. Jonas DE, Garbutt JC, Amick HR, et al. Behavioral counseling after screening for alcohol misuse in primary care: a systematic review and meta-analysis for the U.S. Preventive Services Task Force. Ann Intern Med 2012;157(9):645–54.
10. Bush K, Kivlahan DR, McDonell MB, et al. The AUDIT alcohol consumption questions (AUDIT-C): an effective brief screening test for problem drinking. Ambulatory Care Quality Improvement Project (ACQUIP). Alcohol use disorders identification test. Arch Intern Med 1998;158(16):1789–95.
11. Saitz R. Lost in translation: the perils of implementing alcohol brief intervention when there are gaps in evidence and its interpretation. Addiction 2014;109(7): 1060–2.

12. Moyer VA, Preventive Services Task Force. Screening and behavioral counseling interventions in primary care to reduce alcohol misuse: U.S. preventive services task force recommendation statement. Ann Intern Med 2013;159(3): 210–8.

13. National Institute on Alcohol Abuse and Alcoholism (NIAAA). Helping patients who drink too much: a clinician's guide. U.S. Department of Health & Human Services; 2005. Available at: https://pubs.niaaa.nih.gov/publications/Practitioner/CliniciansGuide2005/guide.pdf. Accessed March 26, 2018.

14. Babor TF, Del Boca F, Bray JW. Screening, brief intervention and referral to treatment: implications of SAMHSA's SBIRT initiative for substance abuse policy and practice. Addiction 2017;112(Suppl 2):110–7.

15. Joseph J, Basu D, Dandapani M, et al. Are nurse-conducted brief interventions (NCBIs) efficacious for hazardous or harmful alcohol use? A systematic review. Int Nurs Rev 2014;61(2):203–10.

16. Sullivan LE, Tetrault JM, Braithwaite RS, et al. A meta-analysis of the efficacy of nonphysician brief interventions for unhealthy alcohol use: implications for the patient-centered medical home. Am J Addict 2011;20(4):343–56.

17. Williams EC, Achtmeyer CE, Young JP, et al. Local implementation of alcohol screening and brief intervention at five veterans health administration primary care clinics: perspectives of clinical and administrative staff. J Subst Abuse Treat 2016;60:27–35.

18. Aldridge A, Dowd W, Bray J. The relative impact of brief treatment versus brief intervention in primary health-care screening programs for substance use disorders. Addiction 2017;112(Suppl 2):54–64.

19. Kim TW, Bernstein J, Cheng DM, et al. Receipt of addiction treatment as a consequence of a brief intervention for drug use in primary care: a randomized trial. Addiction 2017;112(5):818–27.

20. McCambridge J, Rollnick S. Should brief interventions in primary care address alcohol problems more strongly? Addiction 2014;109(7):1054–8.

21. McCambridge J, Saitz R. Rethinking brief interventions for alcohol in general practice. BMJ 2017;356:j116.

22. Williams EC, Lapham GT, Bobb JF, et al. Documented brief intervention not associated with resolution of unhealthy alcohol use one year later among VA patients living with HIV. J Subst Abuse Treat 2017;78:8–14.

23. Bradley KA, Bobb JF, Ludman EJ, et al. Alcohol-Related Nurse Care Management in Primary Care: A Randomized Clinical Trial. JAMA Intern Med 2018; 178(5):613–21.

24. Del Re AC, Gordon AJ, Lembke A, et al. Prescription of topiramate to treat alcohol use disorders in the Veterans Health Administration. Addict Sci Clin Pract 2013;8:12.

25. Harris AH, Kivlahan DR, Bowe T, et al. Pharmacotherapy of alcohol use disorders in the Veterans Health Administration. Psychiatr Serv 2010;61(4):392–8.

26. Harris AH, Oliva E, Bowe T, et al. Pharmacotherapy of alcohol use disorders by the Veterans Health Administration: patterns of receipt and persistence. Psychiatr Serv 2012;63(7):679–85.

27. Marienfeld C, Iheanacho T, Issa M, et al. Long-acting injectable depot naltrexone use in the Veterans' Health Administration: a national study. Addict Behav 2014;39(2):434–8.

28. Petrakis IL, Leslie D, Rosenheck R. Use of naltrexone in the treatment of alcoholism nationally in the Department of Veterans Affairs. Alcohol Clin Exp Res 2003;27(11):1780–4.

29. Anton RF, O'Malley SS, Ciraulo DA, et al. Combined pharmacotherapies and behavioral interventions for alcohol dependence: the COMBINE study: a randomized controlled trial. JAMA 2006;295(17):2003–17.

30. Arbaizar B, Diersen-Sotos T, Gomez-Acebo I, et al. Topiramate in the treatment of alcohol dependence: a meta-analysis. Actas Esp Psiquiatr 2010;38(1):8–12.

31. Johnson BA, Rosenthal N, Capece JA, et al. Topiramate for treating alcohol dependence: a randomized controlled trial. JAMA 2007;298(14):1641–51.

32. Mason BJ, Quello S, Goodell V, et al. Gabapentin treatment for alcohol dependence: a randomized clinical trial. JAMA Intern Med 2014;174(1):70–7.

33. Jonas DE, Amick HR, Feltner C, et al. Pharmacotherapy for adults with alcohol use disorders in outpatient settings: a systematic review and meta-analysis. JAMA 2014;311(18):1889–900.

34. Muench F. The promises and pitfalls of digital technology in its application to alcohol treatment. Alcohol Res 2014;36(1):131–42.

35. Mattick RP, Breen C, Kimber J, et al. Methadone maintenance therapy versus no opioid replacement therapy for opioid dependence. Cochrane Database Syst Rev 2009;(3):CD002209.

36. Mattick RP, Breen C, Kimber J, et al. Buprenorphine maintenance versus placebo or methadone maintenance for opioid dependence. Cochrane Database Syst Rev 2014;(2):CD002207.

37. Korthuis PT, McCarty D, Weimer M, et al. Primary care-based models for the treatment of opioid use disorder: a scoping review. Ann Intern Med 2017;166(4):268–78.

38. Tanum L, Solli KK, Latif ZE, et al. Effectiveness of injectable extended-release naltrexone vs daily buprenorphine-naloxone for opioid dependence: a randomized clinical noninferiority trial. JAMA Psychiatry 2017;74(12):1197–205.

39. Lee JD, Nunes EV Jr, Novo P, et al. Comparative effectiveness of extended-release naltrexone versus buprenorphine-naloxone for opioid relapse prevention (X: BOT): a multicentre, open-label, randomised controlled trial. Lancet 2017; 391(10118):309–18.

40. Macrae J, Hyde P, Slavitt A. HHS launches multi-pronged effort to combat opioid abuse, vol. 2017. HHS Blog; 2015. Available at: https://blog.samhsa.gov/2015/07/27/hhs-launches-multi-pronged-effort-to-combat-opioid-abuse/#.Wrj_3OzwblU. Accessed March 26, 2018.

41. D'Onofrio G, O'Connor PG, Pantalon MV, et al. Emergency department-initiated buprenorphine/naloxone treatment for opioid dependence: a randomized clinical trial. JAMA 2015;313(16):1636–44.

42. Liebschutz JM, Crooks D, Herman D, et al. Buprenorphine treatment for hospitalized, opioid-dependent patients: a randomized clinical trial. JAMA Intern Med 2014;174(8):1369–76.

43. Wakeman SE, Metlay JP, Chang Y, et al. Inpatient addiction consultation for hospitalized patients increases post-discharge abstinence and reduces addiction severity. J Gen Intern Med 2017;32(8):909–16.

44. Englander H, Weimer M, Solotaroff R, et al. Planning and designing the improving addiction care team (IMPACT) for hospitalized adults with substance use disorder. J Hosp Med 2017;12(5):339–42.

45. Kraus ML, Alford DP, Kotz MM, et al. Statement of the American Society Of Addiction Medicine Consensus Panel on the use of buprenorphine in office-based treatment of opioid addiction. J Addict Med 2011;5(4):254–63.

46. Bell JR, Butler B, Lawrance A, et al. Comparing overdose mortality associated with methadone and buprenorphine treatment. Drug Alcohol Depend 2009; 104(1–2):73–7.

47. Fiellin DA, Schottenfeld RS, Cutter CJ, et al. Primary care-based buprenorphine taper vs maintenance therapy for prescription opioid dependence: a randomized clinical trial. JAMA Intern Med 2014;174(12):1947–54.
48. Fiellin DA, Pantalon MV, Chawarski MC, et al. Counseling plus buprenorphine-naloxone maintenance therapy for opioid dependence. N Engl J Med 2006; 355(4):365–74.
49. Tracqui A, Kintz P, Ludes B. Buprenorphine-related deaths among drug addicts in France: a report on 20 fatalities. J Anal Toxicol 1998;22(6):430–4.
50. Haddad MS, Zelenev A, Altice FL. Buprenorphine maintenance treatment retention improves nationally recommended preventive primary care screenings when integrated into urban federally qualified health centers. J Urban Health 2015;92(1):193–213.
51. Stoller KB. A collaborative opioid prescribing (CoOP) model linking opioid treatment programs with office-based buprenorphine providers. Addict Sci Clin Pract 2015;10(Suppl 1):A63.
52. Alford DP, LaBelle CT, Kretsch N, et al. Collaborative care of opioid-addicted patients in primary care using buprenorphine: five-year experience. Arch Intern Med 2011;171(5):425–31.
53. LaBelle CT, Han SC, Bergeron A, et al. Office-based opioid treatment with buprenorphine (OBOT-B): statewide implementation of the Massachusetts collaborative care model in community health centers. J Subst Abuse Treat 2016;60:6–13.
54. Watkins KE, Ober AJ, Lamp K, et al. Collaborative care for opioid and alcohol use disorders in primary care: the SUMMIT randomized clinical trial. JAMA Intern Med 2017;177(10):1480–8.
55. Patient-Centered Primary Care Collaborative. Vermont hub and spokes health homes statewide. Available at: www.pcpcc.org/initiate/vermont-hub-and-spokes-health-homes. Accessed September 22, 2017.
56. Brooklyn JR, Sigmon SC. Vermont hub-and-spoke model of care for opioid use disorder: development, implementation, and impact. J Addict Med 2017;11(4): 286–92.
57. Berger R, Pulido C, Lacro J, et al. Group medication management for buprenorphine/naloxone in opioid-dependent veterans. J Addict Med 2014;8(6):415–20.
58. Suzuki J, Zinser J, Klaiber B, et al. Feasibility of implementing shared medical appointments (SMAs) for office-based opioid treatment with buprenorphine: a pilot study. Subst Abus 2015;36(2):166–9.
59. Sokol R, Albanese C, Chaponis D, et al. Why use group visits for opioid use disorder treatment in primary care? A patient-centered qualitative study. Subst Abus 2018;39(1):52–8.
60. Komaromy M, Duhigg D, Metcalf A, et al. Project ECHO (Extension for Community Healthcare Outcomes): a new model for educating primary care providers about treatment of substance use disorders. Subst Abus 2016;37(1):20–4.
61. Eibl JK, Gauthier G, Pellegrini D, et al. The effectiveness of telemedicine-delivered opioid agonist therapy in a supervised clinical setting. Drug Alcohol Depend 2017;176:133–8.
62. Tofighi B, Grossman E, Bereket S, et al. Text message content preferences to improve buprenorphine maintenance treatment in primary care. J Addict Dis 2016;35(2):92–100.
63. LifeSpring Health Systems. About us: locations. 2016. Available at: www.lifespringhealthsystems.org/about-us/locations. Accessed September 22, 2017.
64. Minozzi S, Cinquini M, Amato L, et al. Anticonvulsants for cocaine dependence. Cochrane Database Syst Rev 2015;(4):CD006754.

65. Minozzi S, Amato L, Pani PP, et al. Dopamine agonists for the treatment of cocaine dependence. Cochrane Database Syst Rev 2015;(5):CD003352.

66. Indave BI, Minozzi S, Pani PP, et al. Antipsychotic medications for cocaine dependence. Cochrane Database Syst Rev 2016;(3):CD006306.

67. Pani PP, Trogu E, Vecchi S, et al. Antidepressants for cocaine dependence and problematic cocaine use. Cochrane Database Syst Rev 2011;(12):CD002950.

68. Pani PP, Trogu E, Vacca R, et al. Disulfiram for the treatment of cocaine dependence. Cochrane Database Syst Rev 2010;(1):CD007024.

69. Fischer B, Blanken P, Da Silveira D, et al. Effectiveness of secondary prevention and treatment interventions for crack-cocaine abuse: a comprehensive narrative overview of English-language studies. Int J Drug Policy 2015;26(4):352–63.

70. Dutra L, Stathopoulou G, Basden SL, et al. A meta-analytic review of psychosocial interventions for substance use disorders. Am J Psychiatry 2008;165(2): 179–87.

71. Kampman KM. The search for medications to treat stimulant dependence. Addict Sci Clin Pract 2008;4(2):28–35.

72. Karila L, Weinstein A, Aubin HJ, et al. Pharmacological approaches to methamphetamine dependence: a focused review. Br J Clin Pharmacol 2010;69(6): 578–92.

73. Coffin PO, Santos GM, Hern J, et al. Extended-release naltrexone for methamphetamine dependence among men who have sex with men: a randomized placebo-controlled trial. Addiction 2018;113(2):268–78.

74. Roll JM. Contingency management: an evidence-based component of methamphetamine use disorder treatments. Addiction 2007;102(Suppl 1):114–20.

75. Roll JM, Petry NM, Stitzer ML, et al. Contingency management for the treatment of methamphetamine use disorders. Am J Psychiatry 2006;163(11):1993–9.

76. Shoptaw S, Huber A, Peck J, et al. Randomized, placebo-controlled trial of sertraline and contingency management for the treatment of methamphetamine dependence. Drug Alcohol Depend 2006;85(1):12–8.

77. Carrico AW, Flentje A, Gruber VA, et al. Community-based harm reduction substance abuse treatment with methamphetamine-using men who have sex with men. J Urban Health 2014;91(3):555–67.

78. Reback CJ, Veniegas R, Shoptaw S. Getting Off: development of a model program for gay and bisexual male methamphetamine users. J Homosex 2014; 61(4):540–53.

79. Office of National AIDS Policy. The national HIV/AIDS strategy: updated to 2020. Washington, DC: The White House; 2015.

80. United Nations Office on Drugs and Crime, International Network of People Who Use Drugs, Joint United Nations Programme on HIV/AIDS, United Nations Development Programme, United Nations Population Fund, World Health Organization, United States Agency for International Development. Implementing comprehensive HIV and HCV programmes with people who inject drugs: practical guidance for collaborative interventions. Vienna (Austria): United Nations Office on Drugs and Crime; 2017.

81. Tetrault JM, Tate JP, McGinnis KA, et al. Hepatic safety and antiretroviral effectiveness in HIV-infected patients receiving naltrexone. Alcohol Clin Exp Res 2012;36(2):318–24.

82. Vagenas P, Di Paola A, Herme M, et al. An evaluation of hepatic enzyme elevations among HIV-infected released prisoners enrolled in two randomized placebo-controlled trials of extended release naltrexone. J Subst Abuse Treat 2014;47(1):35–40.

83. Korthuis PT, Lum PJ, Vergara-Rodriguez P, et al. Feasibility and safety of extended-release naltrexone treatment of opioid and alcohol use disorder in HIV clinics: a pilot/feasibility randomized trial. Addiction 2017;112(6):1036–44.

84. Edelman EJ, Moore B, Holt S, et al. The impact of injectable naltrexone on antiretroviral therapy adherence, HIV viral load, and drinking in HIV-positive heavy drinkers. Paper presented at: Research Society on Alcoholism. Denver, CO, June 26, 2017.

85. Haug NA, Sorensen JL, Gruber VA, et al. HAART adherence strategies for methadone clients who are HIV-positive: a treatment manual for implementing contingency management and medication coaching. Behav Modif 2006;30(6): 752–81.

86. Edelman EJ, Maisto SA, Hansen NB, et al. The Starting Treatment for Ethanol in Primary care Trials (STEP Trials): Protocol for Three Parallel Multi-Site Stepped Care Effectiveness Studies for Unhealthy Alcohol Use in HIV-Positive Patients. Contemp Clin Trials 2017;52:80–90.

87. Edelman EJ, Maisto SA, Hansen NB, et al. Integrated stepped care to address moderate alcohol use among HIV-positive patients with liver disease: Results from a randomized controlled clinical trial. Presented as an oral presentation at INEBRIA, September 15, 2017, New York, New York.

88. Williams EC, Lapham GT, Shortreed SM, et al. Among patients with unhealthy alcohol use, those with HIV are less likely than those without to receive evidence-based alcohol-related care: a national VA study. Drug Alcohol Depend 2017;174:113–20.

89. Chander G, Monroe AK, Crane HM, et al. HIV primary care providers–Screening, knowledge, attitudes and behaviors related to alcohol interventions. Drug Alcohol Depend 2016;161:59–66.

90. Fiellin DA, Weiss L, Botsko M, et al. Drug treatment outcomes among HIV-infected opioid-dependent patients receiving buprenorphine/naloxone. J Acquir Immune Defic Syndr 2011;56(Suppl 1):S33–8.

91. Weiss L, Netherland J, Egan JE, et al. Integration of buprenorphine/naloxone treatment into HIV clinical care: lessons from the BHIVES collaborative. J Acquir Immune Defic Syndr 2011;56(Suppl 1):S68–75.

92. Altice FL, Bruce RD, Lucas GM, et al. HIV treatment outcomes among HIV-infected, opioid-dependent patients receiving buprenorphine/naloxone treatment within HIV clinical care settings: results from a multisite study. J Acquir Immune Defic Syndr 2011;56(Suppl 1):S22–32.

93. Edelman EJ, Chantarat T, Caffrey S, et al. The impact of buprenorphine/naloxone treatment on HIV risk behaviors among HIV-infected, opioid-dependent patients. Drug Alcohol Depend 2014;139:79–85.

94. Tetrault JM, Moore BA, Barry DT, et al. Brief versus extended counseling along with buprenorphine/naloxone for HIV-infected opioid dependent patients. J Subst Abuse Treat 2012;43(4):433–9.

95. Korthuis PT, Tozzi MJ, Nandi V, et al. Improved quality of life for opioid-dependent patients receiving buprenorphine treatment in HIV clinics. J Acquir Immune Defic Syndr 2011;56(Suppl 1):S39–45.

96. Korthuis PT, Fiellin DA, Fu R, et al. Improving adherence to HIV quality of care indicators in persons with opioid dependence: the role of buprenorphine. J Acquir Immune Defic Syndr 2011;56(Suppl 1):S83–90.

97. Drainoni ML, Farrell C, Sorensen-Alawad A, et al. Patient perspectives of an integrated program of medical care and substance use treatment. AIDS Patient Care STDS 2014;28(2):71–81.

98. Walley AY, Palmisano J, Sorensen-Alawad A, et al. Engagement and substance dependence in a primary care-based addiction treatment program for people infected with HIV and people at high-risk for HIV infection. J Subst Abuse Treat 2015;59:59–66.

99. Burch AE, Rash CJ, Petry NM. Cocaine-using substance abuse treatment patients with and without HIV respond well to contingency management treatment. J Subst Abuse Treat 2017;77:21–5.

100. Petry NM, Weinstock J, Alessi SM, et al. Group-based randomized trial of contingencies for health and abstinence in HIV patients. J Consult Clin Psychol 2010;78(1):89–97.

101. Farber S, Tate J, Frank C, et al. A study of financial incentives to reduce plasma HIV RNA among patients in care. AIDS Behav 2013;17(7):2293–300.

102. Wray TB, Grin B, Dorfman L, et al. Systematic review of interventions to reduce problematic alcohol use in men who have sex with men. Drug Alcohol Rev 2016; 35(2):148–57.

103. Springer SA, Di Paola A, Azar MM, et al. Extended-release naltrexone reduces alcohol consumption among released prisoners with HIV disease as they transition to the community. Drug Alcohol Depend 2017;174:158–70.

104. Binswanger IA, Blatchford PJ, Mueller SR, et al. Mortality after prison release: opioid overdose and other causes of death, risk factors, and time trends from 1999 to 2009. Ann Intern Med 2013;159(9):592–600.

105. Lincoln T, Johnson BD, McCarthy P, et al. Extended-release naltrexone for opioid use disorder started during or following incarceration. J Subst Abuse Treat 2018;85:97–100.

106. Lee JD, Friedmann PD, Kinlock TW, et al. Extended-release naltrexone to prevent opioid relapse in criminal justice offenders. N Engl J Med 2016;374(13): 1232–42.

Pharmacotherapy for Alcohol Use Disorder

Stephen R. Holt, MD, MS[a],*, Daniel G. Tobin, MD[b]

KEYWORDS

- Alcohol use disorder • Pharmacotherapy • Addiction • FDA approved • Off-label
- Withdrawal • Personalized medicine

KEY POINTS

- Alcohol use disorder is a devastating disease with profound clinical and economic impact, but pharmacotherapy can be quite effective at reducing alcohol consumption and improving outcomes.
- Despite strong evidence that pharmacotherapy for alcohol use disorder is appropriate for many patients with the disease, it is significantly underused.
- Multiple medications, both approved and not approved by the US Food and Drug Administration, show efficacy in the treatment of alcohol use disorder and are generally well-tolerated.
- Choosing the best medication to treat alcohol use disorder depends on treatment goals, the presence or absence of various comorbidities, medication adherence considerations, and drug availability and cost.

INTRODUCTION

Alcohol use disorder (AUD) is a severe form of problematic drinking characterized by compulsive and uncontrolled alcohol use despite evidence of harm. The fifth edition of the *Diagnostic and Statistical Manual of Mental Disorders* replaced the older diagnoses of alcohol abuse and alcohol dependence with the single diagnosis of AUD, and characterizes AUD as either mild, moderate, or severe, depending on how many of 11 defined criteria a person has experienced in the past year.[1]

According to the 2015 National Survey on Drug Use and Health, more than 16 million people in the United States over the age of 12 suffer from AUD and need treatment.[2] Furthermore, the National Institute on Alcohol Abuse and Alcoholism reports that an estimated 88,000 people die each year from alcohol-related causes, and that

The authors report no commercial or financial conflicts of interest to disclose.
[a] Department of Internal Medicine, Yale University School of Medicine, 1450 Chapel Street, Room P312, New Haven, CT 06511, USA; [b] Department of Internal Medicine, Yale University School of Medicine, 1450 Chapel Street, Room P308, New Haven, CT 06511, USA
* Corresponding author.
E-mail address: stephen.holt@yale.edu

https://doi.org/10.1016/j.mcna.2018.02.008
0025-7125/18/© 2018 Elsevier Inc. All rights reserved.
medical.theclinics.com

alcohol-impaired driving accounted for 31% of driving fatalities in 2014.[3] There is a profound economic impact from AUD as well; 1 study estimated the cost of excessive drinking as nearly $250 billion in 2010.[3,4] Yet despite the high prevalence and destructive nature of AUD to patients, their families, and societies around the world, and the availability of many evidence-based treatments, the vast majority of patients with AUD are left untreated[5–9]

For many patients with AUD, a personalized multidimensional approach that includes both behavioral and pharmacotherapeutic interventions is ideal. Pharmacotherapy represents a potentially effective and yet severely underused treatment option. In 2012, of all privately insured patients with AUD in the United States, only 3% received targeted pharmacotherapy.[10] Likewise, in 2015 only 8.2% of people over the age of 12 who needed treatment for AUD received treatment of any kind, the majority from a source other than a health care provider.[2] Similarly, in the United Kingdom, only 11.7% of 39,980 persons with an incident diagnosis of AUD received any relevant pharmacotherapy in the 12 months after diagnosis.[8] Many reasons have been postulated as to why pharmacotherapies have been so woefully underused, including low patient demand, insurance coverage concerns, perceived lack of effectiveness, the social stigma surrounding addiction disorders, and the lack of training of health providers.[11,12] The forces perpetuating this problem are undoubtedly complex, but effective evidence-based pharmacotherapeutic options do exist.

In this review, we summarize the evidence supporting the use of both US Food and Drug Administration (FDA)-approved and non–FDA-approved medications for the treatment of AUD. Additionally, we offer the prescriber guidance regarding which medications to use in specific circumstances.

MANAGEMENT GOALS

Although achieving complete abstinence from alcohol may be the ultimate treatment target for patients with AUD, it is important to recognize that abstinence may not be the expressed goal of many patients, and that there are several other worthy outcomes. Reducing cravings for alcohol, reducing the quantity of alcohol consumed, or reducing the number of heavy drinking days are all associated with reductions in the morbidity and mortality associated with AUD.[13,14] Likewise, additional objective markers of successful treatment often cited in addiction research literature include reductions in hepatic biomarkers of inflammation (eg, serum gamma-glutamyl transferase), or few visits to the emergency department and fewer hospitalizations.[15,16] Some medications are best used when a reduction in drinking is the focus, whereas others are appropriate only when complete abstinence is the goal (eg, disulfiram).[14] Given their potential benefits (described in detail elsewhere in this article), pharmacotherapy should be considered for all patients who meet criteria for an AUD. Specific approaches to achieving these goals are described herein.

Of note, the majority of AUD pharmacotherapy studies have predominantly recruited male patients, and thus may be less generalizable to women.[17] Many also focused on relatively short-term outcomes, further limiting generalizability. However, our understanding of the clinical management for AUD continues to grow. For example, although most studies have investigated the role of these medications among outpatients in either addiction treatment or primary care settings, some recent studies have explored the role of initiating AUD treatment in the inpatient setting, before discharge from an admission for an alcohol-related issue.[18]

US FOOD AND DRUG ADMINISTRATION–APPROVED MEDICATIONS
Disulfiram

Disulfiram was first approved for the treatment of alcohol dependence in 1948. It is unique among pharmacotherapeutic options for AUD in that its use serves as a deterrent to alcohol consumption, such that the intake of alcohol while taking disulfiram leads to immediate and potentially severe adverse effects. As a deterrent medication, adherence is crucial to disulfiram's efficacy. As such, this medication is best reserved for patients who are either highly motivated, or who have significant external pressure to abstain (eg, law enforcement oversight, residence in a sober house, professional licensure obligations, or accountability to romantic partner, parent).

Disulfiram is an acetaldehyde dehydrogenase inhibitor, inhibiting the metabolism of acetaldehyde to its inert metabolite, acetic acid, when alcohol is consumed. Accumulation of acetaldehyde leads to symptoms typical of the "disulfiram reaction," namely, flushing, headache, nausea and vomiting, diaphoresis, and lightheadedness. In severe cases, the disulfiram reaction can also lead to hemodynamic instability, so it is essential that patients understand the consequences of drinking alcohol while taking disulfiram. When using disulfiram as prescribed, even very small amounts of alcohol are sufficient to precipitate the disulfiram reaction. Patients are thus encouraged to avoid alcohol-based shaving creams, mouth wash, cough syrup, and some sauces for this reason. Abstinence, rather than cutting back on alcohol consumption, must be the explicit goal for patients prescribed disulfiram. Of note, although disulfiram is generally well-tolerated when patients avoid alcohol, severe idiosyncratic reactions such as toxic hepatitis can occur and, thus, careful monitoring is warranted.[19]

The evidence supporting the use of disulfiram for AUD has evolved over the decades. Initial studies often used a double-blind, randomized controlled trial (RCT) strategy for assessing efficacy, and yielded conflicting results.[20] In fact, a 2014 Agency for Healthcare Research and Quality review that included 135 studies of pharmacologic treatment of AUD in ambulatory settings found insufficient evidence to support the use of disulfiram.[21] However, later studies, acknowledging that RCTs are not an appropriate study design for assessing a medication whose mechanism of action depends on the patient not consuming alcohol, have instead used an open-label study design. A 2014 metaanalysis of 22 disulfiram studies found that by excluding the blinded studies and focusing on the 17 open-labeled studies, disulfiram had a substantial abstinence benefit compared with control groups (effect-size g = 0.70; 95% confidence interval, 0.46–0.93).[22] In addition, disulfiram research that has used a community reinforcement approach, in which the provider and patient partner with a family member to support adherence to daily disulfiram, has yielded the most robust outcomes data for this medication.[23,24]

Disulfiram is prescribed as a once daily dose of 250 mg, although some sources recommend a 500 mg/d loading dose for the first 7 days. Aside from the disulfiram reaction, disulfiram is generally well-tolerated with rare side effects that may include hepatitis, neuropathy, and psychosis. At the time this article was written, the average retail price for a 30-day supply of generic disulfiram is approximately $120, but it can be found for less than $40 per month at some pharmacies.[25]

Acamprosate

In contrast with disulfiram, the precise mechanism of action of acamprosate remains uncertain. Historically, acamprosate was thought to exert its effect by restoring equilibrium of the GABA-ergic and glutamatergic neurotransmitter systems, although more recent studies have suggested that it may act instead by affecting calcium metabolism.[26]

Approved by the FDA in 2004, acamprosate is effective for both maintaining abstinence and for reducing heavy drinking days, and may be most effective in patients who are not currently drinking alcohol.[27] In a recent systematic review of AUD treatments, 27 RCTs using acamprosate with 7519 patients showed a number needed to treat of only 12 to prevent return to any drinking, compared with placebo (95% confidence interval, 8–26).[14]

Acamprosate is prescribed in 333 mg tablets, typically dosed at 2 tablets 3 times daily. This thrice-daily dosing may limit adherence in many patients. Side effects of acamprosate include diarrhea in as many as 16% of patients, but it is otherwise usually well-tolerated. This medication is safe to use in patients with moderate liver disease (Child-Pugh class A or B cirrhosis), but should be used with caution in patients with renal dysfunction, which may warrant a dose adjustment. The current average retail price for a month supply of generic acamprosate is approximately $270, but can be found for less than $90 in some retail pharmacies.[28]

Naltrexone

The reward pathways in the brain that reinforce drinking behavior involve both dopamine release within the mesocorticolimbic system and the release of beta-endorphins from the hypothalamus. Naltrexone, a potent opioid antagonist, is believed to work by blocking this endorphin pathway, thereby uncoupling the association between drinking alcohol and experiencing pleasurable effects.

The oral formulation of naltrexone, approved in 1995, consists of a single 50-mg pill administered once daily. Like acamprosate, its efficacy was demonstrated in patients recently abstinent from alcohol.[29] Also similar to acamprosate, a 2014 meta-analysis of 19 RCTs revealed a number needed to treat of only 12 for oral naltrexone compared with placebo for preventing a return to heavy drinking.[14] Oral naltrexone is safe in patients with advanced liver disease (up to Child-Pugh Class B cirrhosis or transaminases less than 5 times the upper limit of normal), but is contraindicated in patients taking opioid medications because its use will precipitate opioid withdrawal and block the intended effects of opioids. Generally, patients should be abstinent from opioids for several days before starting naltrexone (approximately 5 times the half-life of any opioids consumed), and providers may consider confirming abstinence with a urine drug test if uncertainty remains.[29,30] Common side effects include mild nausea, which often resolves in the first several days of taking the medication, and rare hepatotoxicity. Although the package insert for naltrexone lists depression as a potential side effect occurring in 0% to 15% of patients (vs 0%–17% for placebo),[31] studies have not demonstrated a causal relationship or confirmed this association.[32,33]

The extended release injectable formulation of naltrexone, FDA approved in 2006, obviates concerns about medication adherence. Administered as a monthly 380 mg intramuscular gluteal injection, extended release naltrexone is believed to have similar safety and efficacy to the oral formulation, although injection site reactions can occur and may rarely be severe. There are few data directly comparing oral with intramuscular naltrexone, but a recent small study on hospitalized veterans suggests that they may provide comparable results and both are feasible to use when transitioning patients to the outpatient setting.[34] Of note, it is not necessary to pretreat patients with oral naltrexone before starting the intramuscular formulation.[35]

Although the extended release injectable formulation of naltrexone is considerably more expensive than the oral form, studies have shown that its use is cost effective, and, like other FDA-approved medications for AUD, the extended release injectable formulation of naltrexone is covered by most insurance plans.[36] At the time of this writing, a 30-day supply of oral naltrexone has an average retail price of approximately $112 but can be found for as little as approximately $32.[37] In contrast, the retail price for brand name intramuscular naltrexone (marketed as Vivitrol by Alkermes [Dublin, Ireland]) ranges from approximately $1350 to $1700 for a month's supply, although a manufacturer coupon may also be available.[38]

MEDICATIONS NOT APPROVED BY THE US FOOD AND DRUG ADMINISTRATION (OFF-LABEL USE)
Topiramate

The anticonvulsant topiramate has been studied for use in AUD for over 15 years, although it has not been FDA approved for this indication. A recent metaanalysis of 7 studies found that topiramate yielded a small to moderate effect size when compared with placebo in promoting abstinence and reducing heavy drinking days.[16] Similarly, an Agency for Healthcare Research and Quality review found moderate evidence that topiramate decreases the number of drinking days, heavy drinking days, and drinks per day.[21] In addition to its moderate effects on abstinence rates, topiramate has also been shown to improve overall physical health and quality of life, when compared with placebo.[39] Topiramate may exert its effects by virtue of its glutamate blocking properties, as well as by the inhibition of dopamine release.[40] The most common side effects are various paresthesias, taste disturbance, cognitive impairment, weight loss, and diarrhea. It is prescribed as a gradual dose escalation over 4 weeks, starting with 25 mg twice a day for 1 week, and advancing by 25 mg increments each week (ie, 50 mg twice a day for 1 week, then 75 mg twice a day, etcetera) to a goal of 100 mg twice a day.[41] In those with a creatinine clearance of less than 70 mL/min, titration should occur more slowly and the total daily dose should be reduced by 50%. Generic topiramate is quite inexpensive and a 1-month supply of 100 mg tablets taken twice a day can currently be found for less than $13 per month at some retail pharmacies.[42]

Gabapentin

Another anticonvulsant, gabapentin, has been more recently studied in the treatment of AUD with very promising results. A recent 12-week double-blind RCT of 150 patients with AUD compared 600 mg of gabapentin 3 times daily with placebo.[43] The authors found a substantial decrease in the rates of heavy drinking (number needed to treat of 5) and improved rates of abstinence (number needed to treat of 8) compared with placebo, with no significant differences in drug-related adverse events. Gabapentin also has mounting evidence supporting its use in the outpatient management of alcohol withdrawal syndrome.[44,45] In addition to moderate benefit for the treatment of withdrawal symptoms, another review found that sleep quality and mood-related outcomes also improved with gabapentin and the authors suggest that the drug may have long-term benefits if continued beyond the withdrawal period.[46] Although various dosing regimens have been used in the literature, gabapentin is frequently prescribed at a dose of 300 mg 3 times daily and increased by 300 mg/until a target dose of 600 mg 3 time a day is reached. Although generally well-tolerated, side effects may include cognitive impairment, fatigue, and ataxia. Of note, concerns have recently been raised about the abuse potential of gabapentin with increasing numbers of documented accounts of gabapentin overdose, addiction, and diversion.[47] Presently, a 1-month supply of generic gabapentin at the target treatment dose can be purchased for less than $20 at selected pharmacies.[48]

Varenicline

Considering the high prevalence of co-occurring alcohol and tobacco use disorders, recent evidence that varenicline might reduce cravings for both alcohol and nicotine products has garnered substantial interest from researchers. This nicotine receptor partial agonist, known to be the most effective pharmacologic treatment for tobacco use disorder, was found in a 2014 systematic review of 7 RCTs to reduce rates of heavy drinking with a moderate treatment effect size (d = 0.3–0.5).[49] One multisite, 12-week RCT (n = 200) found varenicline-treated alcohol-dependent patients had 37.9% heavy drinking days per week compared with 48.4% heavy-drinking days per week for placebo-treated alcohol-dependent patients (P = .03).[50] No significant differences were found for rates of abstinence. Interestingly, the benefit of varenicline on reducing rates of heavy drinking was independent of baseline smoking status. Nonetheless, varenicline remains a second-tier choice by its modest effect size and less robust data thus far, compared with other options. Side effects can include nausea, vivid dreams, and changes in mood. Currently, varenicline is only available as a trade name product marketed as Chantix by Pfizer; the average retail price of a 30-day supply of varenicline is currently approximately $400, but it is frequently covered by insurance and a manufacturer coupon limiting the out-of-pocket expense is currently available as well.[51]

MEDICATIONS NOT APPROVED BY THE US FOOD AND DRUG ADMINISTRATION (OFF-LABEL USE) WITH WEAK EVIDENCE OF EFFICACY

Several additional medications have emerging data to support use for the treatment of AUD, but have not been sufficiently studied at this point to recommend. For example, the anticonvulsant zonisamide was shown in a recent RCT comparing zonisamide, topiramate, and levetiracetam with placebo to reduce alcohol consumption to a similar degree as topiramate, although zonisamide did not significantly reduce cravings.[52] Pregabalin may also have a role in the treatment of both AUD and alcohol withdrawal, although the data supporting its use are far more limited than that of gabapentin.[53] In 1 notable study, an RCT comparing pregabalin and naltrexone in 71 patients, no differences were seen in drinking outcomes or cravings, but the pregabalin group had fewer symptoms of hostility, anxiety, and psychosis.[54] Yet another agent that may have potential use for the treatment of AUD is ondansetron, a selective serotonin (5-HT3) antagonist approved by the FDA for the treatment of nausea and vomiting. In an intriguing study, a decrease in the number of drinks per day and number of drinking days was noted in patients who developed AUD before the age of 25, although this effect was not seen in patients who were older at the time of diagnosis.[55] The authors suggest that the age discrepancy may represent an underlying biologic predisposition to AUD related to abnormalities in serotonin neurotransmitter function. Subsequent studies have shown that ondansetron may be more effective in patients with particular genotypes of the serotonin transporter gene, suggesting that this drug may be increasingly useful in an evolving era of personalized medicine.[56,57] The muscle relaxant and GABA receptor agonist baclofen has also garnered interest as a possibly effective agent to treat AUD. Numerous case reports and open-label trials suggest that baclofen may be effective, but the results of RCTs have been mixed and somewhat underwhelming.[58,59] Finally, the opioid antagonist nalmefene was recently approved in Europe for the treatment of AUD[60] and has been promoted for use on an as-needed basis,[61] although it is not currently available in the United States. The promotion of nalmefene as an as-needed treatment option for people who have not stopped drinking represents a new approach to AUD pharmacotherapy, although its efficacy has recently been brought into question.[62]

OTHER MEDICATIONS NOT APPROVED BY THE US FOOD AND DRUG ADMINISTRATION (OFF-LABEL USE)

Additional agents have been proposed to treat AUD based on promising early data, but subsequent studies have not supported their use. For example, levetiracetam has not been shown to be particularly effective in multiple RCTs.[63,64] Similarly, the atypical antipsychotic quetiapine seemed to be a promising drug as well, but in a recent RCT there was no significant difference between placebo and quetiapine on a number of measures of alcohol use.[65] Another atypical antipsychotic, aripiprazole, has also yielded disappointing results in a large multisite 12-week RCT.[66] Selective serotonin reuptake inhibitors have been studied as well and seem to be ineffective for the treatment of AUD in patients without coexisting major depression.[67] However, they may be helpful in a subgroup of patients suffering from both disorders.[68] Finally, the NMDA receptor antagonist memantine (used to treat Alzheimer's dementia) has also been found to be largely ineffective.[69,70]

COMBINATION PHARMACOTHERAPY AND FUTURE DIRECTIONS

There are few data on combination approaches and similarly limited guidance on the ideal duration of therapy. Because AUD is a heterogenous disease that seems to involve multiple neurochemical systems in different patients, it is certainly plausible that combination therapy will prove to be more effective than monotherapy. In the COMBINE study, the addition of acamprosate to naltrexone offered no incremental benefit beyond naltrexone used alone.[71] An earlier study found similar results.[72] Likewise, the combination of gabapentin and naltrexone may improve early outcomes compared with the use of naltrexone alone, but in at least 1 RCT this effect was not sustained.[73] In the absence of more definitive data on combination pharmacotherapy, we cannot yet recommend this approach.

As our understanding of various AUD subtypes and genetic polymorphisms evolves, it is likely that a more personalized and targeted approach to treatment will emerge. For example, recent research has investigated the link between responsiveness to specific AUD pharmacotherapies and genetic factors.[74–76] In particular, recent studies have shown that genetic variation in a single nucleotide in exon 1 (Asn40Asp) in the mu-opioid receptor gene (OPRM1) has been identified in numerous retrospective studies as highly correlated with clinical response to naltrexone.[77,78] Understanding the heterogeneity of populations with AUD, and how they influence the efficacy of current pharmacotherapies, may soon lead to more targeted treatment approaches.

It is worth mentioning that the use of pharmacotherapy for AUD lies within the purview of the primary care provider.[79] In the COMBINE study (Combined Pharmacotherapies and Behavioral Interventions for Alcohol Dependence), 1383 alcohol-dependent patients were randomized to either naltrexone, acamprosate, specialist-delivered behavioral therapy, or some combination. All subjects received non–specialist-delivered medical management, intended to be feasible within a primary care setting. Remarkably, the naltrexone alone arm of the study was as effective as the combination of naltrexone and specialist-delivered behavioral therapy with regard to the composite outcome of maintenance of abstinence, reduction in number of heavy drinking days, and reduction in total number of drinks per week.[71]

Table 1
Evidence-based pharmacotherapies for alcohol use disorder

Drug	Dose	Frequency	Comments	Current Retail Cost
Disulfiram[a]	250 mg	Daily	Requires commitment to abstinence; side effects include hepatitis, neuropathy, psychosis, and "disulfiram reaction"	$40–$120 per month
Naltrexone PO[a]	50 mg	Daily	Contraindicated in presence of opioids; side effects include temporary nausea, depressive symptoms, rare hepatotoxicity	$32–$112 per month
Naltrexone IM[a]	380 mg	Monthly	4-mL intergluteal injection; side effects include those above plus injection site reactions	$1350–$1700 per month Manufacturer coupon available
Acamprosate[a]	666 mg	TID	Best evidence for abstinence; diarrhea occurs in 17% of patients	$90–$270 or more per month
Gabapentin	600 mg	TID	Consider with comorbid neuropathy; starting dose 300 mg TID; side effects include fatigue, ataxia, cognitive impairment	$20–$200 or more per month
Topiramate	100 mg	Twice daily	Consider with comorbid seizure disorder; requires 4-wk dose titration; side effects include paresthesias, GI upset, cognitive impairment	$13–$300 per month
Varenicline	1 mg	Twice daily	Consider with comorbid tobacco use; least studied of front-line medications; side effects include nausea, vivid dreams, and mood changes	$380–$455 per month Manufacturer coupon available

Abbreviations: GI, gastrointestinal; IM, intramuscularly; PO, per os; TID, 3 time per day.
[a] Approved by the US Food and Drug Administration.

CHOOSING THE BEST MEDICATION

Given the myriad of options and similar efficacy across drug classes, the decision regarding which medication to use rests on several patient-dependent factors. For example, disulfiram should only be considered when complete abstinence is the treatment goal and the patient is highly motivated to engage in care. Similarly, patients with chronic pain syndromes who require opioids will not be good candidates for naltrexone. Comorbid disease may also limit therapy or guide drug choice; advanced liver or kidney disease, for example, may limit the use of naltrexone, acamprosate, and disulfiram, whereas a coexisting seizure disorder or symptomatic neuropathy may favor the use of anticonvulsive medications such as topiramate or gabapentin. Cost is another very important consideration; in the absence of insurance coverage, the monthly cost of various treatment options ranges from inexpensive (eg, generic topiramate) to exorbitant (brand name Vivitrol [naltrexone]). Drug interactions and dosing regimens must be considered as well; some patients may prefer the sense of control they experience with 3 times daily dosing, whereas others will do much better with a once monthly injection of intramuscular naltrexone without concerns about adherence between visits. A patient-centered and personalized approach is critically important when choosing a medication to treat AUD. **Table 1** provides a summary of relevant factors. A useful resource that offers guidance on selecting FDA-approved medications for AUD and incorporating treatment into clinical practice is worth reviewing; it was updated by The Center for Substance Abuse Treatment in 2013, and is freely available at www.samhsa.gov.[80]

SUMMARY

AUD is a devastating and sometimes fatal chronic disease that profoundly impacts patients, their families, and society. Social stigma, lack of provider training, and financial concerns are among the many barriers that patients face, but effective treatment options do exist and are severely underused. There are now a broad array of safe and effective medication choices available, including both FDA-approved and off-label options. Patient-specific factors must guide treatment decisions, and providers should engage in shared decision making with their patients to clarify goals and potential obstacles to care. The choice of which medication to use can be complex, but by carefully considering medical comorbidities, potential drug interactions, treatment objectives, and drug cost, the best choice is often clear.

ACKNOWLEDGMENTS

The editors thank Ed Day, King's College London, for providing a critical review of this article.

REFERENCES

1. American Psychiatric Association. DSM-5 task force. Diagnostic and statistical manual of mental disorders: DSM-5. 5th edition. Washington, DC: American Psychiatric Association; 2013.
2. Center for Behavioral Health Statistics and Quality. 2015 national survey on drug use and health: detailed tables. Rockville (MD): Substance Abuse and Mental Health Services Administration; 2016.
3. Department of Health and Human Services. National Institute on Alcohol Abuse and Alcoholism. Alcohol Facts and Statistics. 2017. Available at: https://pubs.niaaa.nih.gov/publications/AlcoholFacts&Stats/AlcoholFacts&Stats.pdf. Accessed February 1, 2017.
4. Sacks JJ, Gonzales KR, Bouchery EE, et al. 2010 national and state costs of excessive alcohol consumption. Am J Prev Med 2015;49(5):e73–9.
5. Lim SS, Vos T, Flaxman AD, et al. A comparative risk assessment of burden of disease and injury attributable to 67 risk factors and risk factor clusters in 21 regions, 1990–2010: a systematic analysis for the Global Burden of Disease Study 2010. Lancet 2012;380(9859):2224–60.
6. Saitz R, Freedner N, Palfai TP, et al. The severity of unhealthy alcohol use in hospitalized medical patients. The spectrum is narrow. J Gen Intern Med 2006;21(4): 381–5.

7. Holt S, Tetrault J. Unhealthy alcohol use. Clin Liver Dis 2016;20(3):429–44.

8. Thompson A, Ashcroft DM, Owens L, et al. Drug therapy for alcohol dependence in primary care in the UK: a clinical practice research Datalink study. PLoS One 2017;12(3):e0173272.

9. Mark TL, Kassed CA, Vandivort-Warren R, et al. Alcohol and opioid dependence medications: prescription trends, overall and by physician specialty. Drug Alcohol Depend 2009;99(1–3):345–9.

10. Thomas CP, Hodgkin D, Levit K, et al. Growth in spending on substance use disorder treatment services for the privately insured population. Drug Alcohol Depend 2016;160:143–50.

11. Harris AH, Ellerbe L, Reeder RN, et al. Pharmacotherapy for alcohol dependence: perceived treatment barriers and action strategies among Veterans Health Administration service providers. Psychol Serv 2013;10(4):410–9.

12. Weine ER, Kim NS, Lincoln AK. Understanding lay assessments of alcohol use disorder: need for treatment and associated stigma. Alcohol Alcohol 2016; 51(1):98–105.

13. Plunk AD, Syed-Mohammed H, Cavazos-Rehg P, et al. Alcohol consumption, heavy drinking, and mortality: rethinking the j-shaped curve. Alcohol Clin Exp Res 2014;38(2):471–8.

14. Jonas DE, Amick HR, Feltner C, et al. Pharmacotherapy for adults with alcohol use disorders in outpatient settings: a systematic review and meta-analysis. JAMA 2014;311(18):1889–900.

15. Landy MS, Davey CJ, Quintero D, et al. A systematic review on the effectiveness of brief interventions for alcohol misuse among adults in emergency departments. J Subst Abuse Treat 2016;61:1–12.

16. Blodgett JC, Del Re AC, Maisel NC, et al. A meta-analysis of topiramate's effects for individuals with alcohol use disorders. Alcohol Clin Exp Res 2014;38(6):1481–8.

17. Agabio R, Pani PP, Preti A, et al. Efficacy of medications approved for the treatment of alcohol dependence and alcohol withdrawal syndrome in female patients: a descriptive review. Eur Addict Res 2016;22(1):1–16.

18. Wei J, Defries T, Lozada M, et al. An inpatient treatment and discharge planning protocol for alcohol dependence: efficacy in reducing 30-day readmissions and emergency department visits. J Gen Intern Med 2015;30(3):365–70.

19. Mutschler J, Grosshans M, Soyka M, et al. Current findings and mechanisms of action of disulfiram in the treatment of alcohol dependence. Pharmacopsychiatry 2016;49(04):137–41.

20. Saitz R. Medications for alcohol use disorders. JAMA 2014;312(13):1349.

21. Pharmacotherapy for adults with alcohol-use disorders in outpatient settings executive summary: Agency for Healthcare Research and Quality. 2014. Available at: https://effectivehealthcare.ahrq.gov/topics/alcohol-misuse-drug-therapy/clinician. Accessed March 21, 2018.

22. Skinner MD, Lahmek P, Pham H, et al. Disulfiram efficacy in the treatment of alcohol dependence: a meta-analysis. PLoS One 2014;9(2):e87366.

23. Azrin NH, Sisson RW, Meyers R, et al. Alcoholism treatment by disulfiram and community reinforcement therapy. J Behav Ther Exp Psychiatry 1982;13(2): 105–12.

24. Roozen HG, Boulogne JJ, van Tulder MW, et al. A systematic review of the effectiveness of the community reinforcement approach in alcohol, cocaine and opioid addiction. Drug Alcohol Depend 2004;74(1):1–13.

25. Goodrx.com. Disulfiram. Available at: https://www.goodrx.com/disulfiram?drugname=disulfuram. Accessed August 3, 2017.

26. Spanagel R, Vengeliene V, Jandeleit B, et al. Acamprosate Produces Its Anti-Relapse Effects Via Calcium. Neuropsychopharmacology 2014;39(4):783–91.

27. Maisel NC, Blodgett JC, Wilbourne PL, et al. Meta-analysis of naltrexone and acamprosate for treating alcohol use disorders: when are these medications most helpful? Addiction 2013;108(2):275–93.

28. Goodrx.com. Acamprosate. Available at: https://www.goodrx.com/acamprosate?drug-name=acamprosate. Accessed August 3, 2017.

29. Substance Abuse and Mental Health Services Administration, National Institute on Alcohol Abuse and Alcoholism. Medication for the treatment of alcohol use disorder: a brief guide. 2015. Available at: https://store.samhsa.gov/shin/content//SMA15-4907/SMA15-4907.pdf. Accessed August 3, 2017.

30. Sigmon SC, Bisaga A, Nunes EV, et al. Opioid detoxification and naltrexone induction strategies: recommendations for clinical practice. Am J Drug Alcohol Abuse 2012;38(3):187–99.

31. Revia (naltrexone hydrochloride) Package Insert. Available at: https://www.accessdata.fda.gov/drugsatfda_docs/label/2013/018932s017lbl.pdf. Accessed October 3, 2017.

32. Dean AJ, Saunders JB, Jones RT, et al. Does naltrexone treatment lead to depression? Findings from a randomized controlled trial in subjects with opioid dependence. J Psychiatry Neurosci 2006;31(1):38–45.

33. Mysels DJ, Cheng WY, Nunes EV, et al. The association between naltrexone treatment and symptoms of depression in opioid-dependent patients. Am J Drug Alcohol Abuse 2011;37(1):22–6.

34. Busch AC, Denduluri M, Glass J, et al. Predischarge injectable versus oral naltrexone to improve postdischarge treatment engagement among hospitalized veterans with alcohol use disorder: a randomized pilot proof-of-concept study. Alcohol Clin Exp Res 2017;41(7):1352–60.

35. Alkermes. Vivitrol prescribing information. Waltham (MA): Author; 2013. Available at: https://www.vivitrol.com/content/pdfs/prescribing-information.pdf. Accessed August 3, 2017.

36. Hartung DM, McCarty D, Fu R, et al. Extended-release naltrexone for alcohol and opioid dependence: a meta-analysis of healthcare utilization studies. J Subst Abuse Treat 2014;47(2):113–21.

37. Goodrx.com. Oral naltrexone. Available at: https://www.goodrx.com/naltrexone?drug-name=naltrexone. Accessed March 21, 2018.

38. Goodrx.com. Vivitrol. Available at: https://www.goodrx.com/vivitrol. Accessed March 21, 2018.

39. Johnson BA, Rosenthal N, Capece JA, et al. Improvement of physical health and quality of life of alcohol-dependent individuals with topiramate treatment: US multisite randomized controlled trial. Arch Intern Med 2008;168(11):1188–99.

40. Olmsted CL, Kockler DR. Topiramate for alcohol dependence. Ann Pharmacother 2008;42(10):1475–80.

41. Kranzler HR, Covault J, Feinn R, et al. Topiramate treatment for heavy drinkers: moderation by a GRIK1 polymorphism. Am J Psychiatry 2014;171(4):445–52.

42. Goodrx.com. Topiramate. Available at: https://www.goodrx.com/topiramate?form=tablet&dosage=100mg&quantity=60&days_supply=&label_override=topiramate. Accessed August 3, 2017.

43. Mason BJ, Quello S, Goodell V, et al. Gabapentin treatment for alcohol dependence: a randomized clinical trial. JAMA Intern Med 2014;174(1):70–7.

44. Stock CJ, Carpenter L, Ying J, et al. Gabapentin versus chlordiazepoxide for outpatient alcohol detoxification treatment. Ann Pharmacother 2013;47(7–8): 961–9.

45. Myrick H, Malcolm R, Randall PK, et al. A double-blind trial of gabapentin versus lorazepam in the treatment of alcohol withdrawal. Alcohol Clin Exp Res 2009; 33(9):1582–8.

46. Leung JG, Hall-Flavin D, Nelson S, et al. The role of gabapentin in the management of alcohol withdrawal and dependence. Ann Pharmacother 2015;49(8): 897–906.

47. Smith RV, Havens JR, Walsh SL. Gabapentin misuse, abuse and diversion: a systematic review. Addiction 2016;111(7):1160–74.

48. Goodrx.com. Gabapentin. Available at: https://www.goodrx.com/gabapentin?drug-name=gabapentin&form=capsule&dosage=300mg&quantity=180&days_supply=&label_override=gabapentin. Accessed August 3, 2017.

49. Erwin BL, Slaton RM. Varenicline in the treatment of alcohol use disorders. Ann Pharmacother 2014;48(11):1445–55.

50. Litten RZ, Ryan ML, Fertig JB, et al. A double-blind, placebo-controlled trial assessing the efficacy of varenicline tartrate for alcohol dependence. J Addict Med 2013;7(4):277–86.

51. Goodrx.com. Varenicline. Available at: https://www.goodrx.com/varenicline?drug-name=varenicline. Accessed August 3, 2017.

52. Knapp CM, Ciraulo DA, Sarid-Segal O, et al. Zonisamide, topiramate, and levetiracetam: efficacy and neuropsychological effects in alcohol use disorders. J Clin Psychopharmacol 2015;35(1):34–42.

53. Freynhagen R, Backonja M, Schug S, et al. Pregabalin for the treatment of drug and alcohol withdrawal symptoms: a comprehensive review. CNS Drugs 2016; 30(12):1191–200.

54. Martinotti G, Di Nicola M, Tedeschi D, et al. Pregabalin versus naltrexone in alcohol dependence: a randomised, double-blind, comparison trial. J Psychopharmacol 2010;24(9):1367–74.

55. Johnson BA, Roache JD, Javors MA, et al. Ondansetron for reduction of drinking among biologically predisposed alcoholic patients: a randomized controlled trial. JAMA 2000;284(8):963–71.

56. Johnson BA, Seneviratne C, Wang XQ, et al. Determination of genotype combinations that can predict the outcome of the treatment of alcohol dependence using the 5-HT(3) antagonist ondansetron. Am J Psychiatry 2013;170(9):1020–31.

57. Seneviratne C, Johnson BA. Advances in medications and tailoring treatment for alcohol use disorder. Alcohol Res 2015;37(1):15–28.

58. Ponizovsky AM, Rosca P, Aronovich E, et al. Baclofen as add-on to standard psychosocial treatment for alcohol dependence: a randomized, double-blind, placebo-controlled trial with 1year follow-up. J Subst Abuse Treat 2015;52:24–30.

59. Beraha EM, Salemink E, Goudriaan AE, et al. Efficacy and safety of high-dose baclofen for the treatment of alcohol dependence: a multicentre, randomised, double-blind controlled trial. Eur Neuropsychopharmacol 2016;26(12):1950–9.

60. European Medicines Agency European public assessment report (EPAR) for Selincro. Available at: http://www.ema.europa.eu/ema/index.jsp?curl=pages/medicines/human/medicines/002583/human_med_001620.jsp&mid=WC0b01ac058001d124. Accessed August 4, 2017.

61. van den Brink W, Aubin HJ, Bladstrom A, et al. Efficacy of as-needed nalmefene in alcohol-dependent patients with at least a high drinking risk level: results from

a subgroup analysis of two randomized controlled 6-month studies. Alcohol Alcohol 2013;48(5):570–8.

62. Palpacuer C, Duprez R, Huneau A, et al. Pharmacologically controlled drinking in the treatment of alcohol dependence or alcohol use disorders: a systematic review with direct and network meta-analyses on nalmefene, naltrexone, acamprosate, baclofen and topiramate. Addiction 2018;113(2):220–37.

63. Fertig JB, Ryan ML, Falk DE, et al. A double-blind, placebo-controlled trial assessing the efficacy of levetiracetam extended release in very heavy drinking alcohol-dependent patients. Alcohol Clin Exp Res 2012;36(8):1421–30.

64. Richter C, Effenberger S, Bschor T, et al. Efficacy and safety of levetiracetam for the prevention of alcohol relapse in recently detoxified alcohol-dependent patients: a randomized trial. J Clin Psychopharmacol 2012;32(4):558–62.

65. Litten RZ, Fertig JB, Falk DE, et al. A double-blind, placebo-controlled trial to assess the efficacy of quetiapine fumarate XR in very heavy-drinking alcohol-dependent patients. Alcohol Clin Exp Res 2012;36(3):406–16.

66. Anton RF, Kranzler H, Breder C, et al. A randomized, multicenter, double-blind, placebo-controlled study of the efficacy and safety of aripiprazole for the treatment of alcohol dependence. J Clin Psychopharmacol 2008;28(1):5–12.

67. Torrens M, Fonseca F, Mateu G, et al. Efficacy of antidepressants in substance use disorders with and without comorbid depression. A systematic review and meta-analysis. Drug Alcohol Depend 2005;78(1):1–22.

68. Litten RZ, Wilford BB, Falk DE, et al. Potential medications for the treatment of alcohol use disorder: an evaluation of clinical efficacy and safety. Subst Abus 2016;37(2):286–98.

69. Evans SM, Levin FR, Brooks DJ, et al. A pilot double-blind treatment trial of memantine for alcohol dependence. Alcohol Clin Exp Res 2007;31(5):775–82.

70. Sani G, Serra G, Kotzalidis GD, et al. The role of memantine in the treatment of psychiatric disorders other than the dementias: a review of current preclinical and clinical evidence. CNS Drugs 2012;26(8):663–90.

71. Anton RF, O'Malley SS, Ciraulo DA, et al. Combined pharmacotherapies and behavioral interventions for alcohol dependence: the COMBINE study: a randomized controlled trial. JAMA 2006;295(17):2003–17.

72. Kiefer F, Jahn H, Tarnaske T, et al. Comparing and combining naltrexone and acamprosate in relapse prevention of alcoholism: a double-blind, placebo-controlled study. Arch Gen Psychiatry 2003;60(1):92–9.

73. Anton RF, Myrick H, Wright TM, et al. Gabapentin combined with naltrexone for the treatment of alcohol dependence. Am J Psychiatry 2011;168(7):709–17.

74. Johnson BA. Medication treatment of different types of alcoholism. Am J Psychiatry 2010;167(6):630–9.

75. Choi DS, Nam HW, Karpyak V. PP135—Pharmacometabolomics for individualized treatment of alcoholism: high serum glutamate level is associated with positive response to acamprosate treatment. Clin Ther 2013;35(8):e58.

76. Kuehn BM. Findings on alcohol dependence point to promising avenues for targeted therapies. JAMA 2009;301(16):1643–5.

77. Berrettini W. Alcohol addiction and the mu-opioid receptor. Prog Neuropsychopharmacol Biol Psychiatry 2016;65:228–33.

78. Anton RF, Oroszi G, O'Malley S, et al. An evaluation of mu-opioid receptor (OPRM1) as a predictor of naltrexone response in the treatment of alcohol dependence: results from the Combined Pharmacotherapies and Behavioral Interventions for Alcohol Dependence (COMBINE) study. Arch Gen Psychiatry 2008; 65(2):135–44.

79. O'Malley SS, Rounsaville BJ, Farren C, et al. Initial and maintenance naltrexone treatment for alcohol dependence using primary care vs specialty care: a nested sequence of 3 randomized trials. Arch Intern Med 2003;163(14):1695–704.

80. U.S. Department of Health and Human Services. Substance Abuse and Mental Health Services Administration. Center for Substance Abuse Treatment. Incorporating alcohol pharmacotherapies into medical practice: a treatment improvement protocol. TIP 49. Available at: https://store.samhsa.gov/shin/content// SMA13-4380/SMA13-4380.pdf. Accessed August 4, 2017.

When and How to Treat Possible Cannabis Use Disorder

Annie Lévesque, MD, MSc[a],*, Bernard Le Foll, MD, PhD[b,c,d,e,f]

KEYWORDS

- Cannabis use disorder • Treatment • Psychosocial • Pharmacologic
- Synthetic cannabinoid

KEY POINTS

- Psychosocial interventions are the first-line for the treatment of cannabis use disorder.
- The most effective available treatments are cognitive–behavioral therapy and motivational enhancement therapy, with greater benefits found when combining approaches.
- Adding contingency management to these interventions can provide further benefit.
- There is no pharmacotherapy approved for the treatment of cannabis use disorder.
- Cannabinoid analogues and gabapentin have been tested with preliminarily positive results. Further research is warranted to clarify the potential role of these medications.

INTRODUCTION

Cannabis is the most frequently used illicit drug worldwide.[1] The lifetime probability of developing cannabis use disorder after a first exposure to the substance is approximately 9%.[2,3] Moreover, the likelihood of developing cannabis use disorder increases significantly if an individual starts using cannabis during adolescence.[4] In the United States, 4 million individuals were estimated to fulfill criteria for cannabis use disorder in the past year, representing approximately 1.5% of the American population aged 12 or older in 2015.[5]

Disclosure Statement: The authors have no conflict of interest to declare.
[a] Department of Psychiatry, Mount Sinai West Hospital, 1000 10th Avenue, Suite 8C-02, New York, NY 10019, USA; [b] Translational Addiction Research Laboratory, Centre for Addiction and Mental Health (CAMH), 33 Russell Street, Toronto, Ontario M5S 2S1, Canada; [c] Addiction Division, Addiction Medicine Service, Centre for Addiction and Mental Health, Toronto, Ontario M6J 1H4, Canada; [d] Department of Pharmacology and Toxicology, Institute of Medical Sciences, University of Toronto, Toronto, Ontario M5S 1A8, Canada; [e] Department of Psychiatry, Institute of Medical Sciences, University of Toronto, Toronto, Ontario M5S 1A8, Canada; [f] Department of Family and Community Medicine, Institute of Medical Sciences, University of Toronto, Toronto, Ontario M5S 1A8, Canada
* Corresponding author.
E-mail address: annie.levesque@mountsinai.org

medical.theclinics.com

The plant *Cannabis sativa* contains approximately 60 identified cannabinoid compounds, some of which exert an effect in the human body via interaction with the CB_1 and CB_2 receptors, located predominantly in the central nervous system and in the immune system, respectively.[6,7] The main psychoactive properties of cannabis are attributed to the cannabinoid compound delta-9-tetrahydrocannabinol (THC), a partial agonist of the CB_1 and CB_2 receptors, that has been associated with the high produced by cannabis use and with its effects that lead to the development of addiction.[6,8,9] Recently, there has been a growing interest in cannabidiol, a nonpsychotropic component also present in different strains of cannabis. Cannabidiol has been shown to have antiepileptic properties in well-conducted clinical trials, and preclinical studies suggest it may have possible therapeutic properties, including its ability to decrease THC induced paranoia and euphoria, in addition to exerting a positive impact on anxiety and depression.[6,10–15] It should be noted that, so far, only the antiepileptic effect of cannabidiol has been tested properly in human subjects, and the other properties of cannabidiol remain to be evaluated in rigorous large-scale clinical trials.[15]

Cannabis is often used recreationally for its euphoria-producing effects. Other symptoms and signs of acute cannabis intoxication include increased appetite, tachycardia, tachypnea, high blood pressure, ocular erythema, dry mouth, and altered judgment. Cannabis use has been associated with a number of deleterious health outcomes, including worsening of respiratory problems, worsening of bipolar disorder-associated symptoms, short-term impairment of learning and memory, and higher risks of death from motor vehicle accidents.[16] There is also substantial evidence regarding the association between frequent cannabis use and psychosis, including schizophrenia, although the exact interplay remains controversial.[16] It is possible that exposure to cannabis may precipitate an earlier occurrence of psychotic symptoms in predisposed subjects, as suggested by the transient occurrence of symptoms that resemble those of a psychosis after THC administration in human laboratory studies.[17] However, the fact that the prevalence of schizophrenia has been stable over time while the use of cannabis and the potency of cannabis used has increased does not support a causal relationship between cannabis use and schizophrenia.

A diagnosis of cannabis use disorder as defined by the fifth edition of the *Diagnostic and Statistical Manual of Mental Disorders* (DSM-5) is made when there is a problematic pattern of use leading to significant impairment or distress, as manifested by at least 2 of the symptoms listed in the DSM-5, occurring within a 12-month period.[18] Discontinuation of cannabis use after regular, prolonged use is associated with a withdrawal syndrome that is recognized by the DSM-5, characterized by the emergence of symptoms such as anxiety, dysphoria, sleep disturbance, irritability, and anorexia.[18,19] Although cannabis withdrawal can be distressing, it is not life threatening. Nonetheless, the experience of withdrawal symptoms makes cannabis cessation more challenging and individuals experiencing a higher number of withdrawal symptoms have greater risks of rapid relapse to cannabis use compared with those experiencing fewer symptoms.[20]

Demand for cannabis-related health care services has been increasing in most regions of the world, including North America.[1] This finding may partly be explained by a significant increase over the past decades in the concentration of THC in cannabis as well as by the emergence of synthetic cannabinoid, a group of chemically synthesized highly potent cannabinoid analogues that are often associated with more severe use-related outcomes.[21] Moreover, the recent legalization of marijuana use in numerous US states has contributed to easier access to the substance. Hence, data from the states that have legalized marijuana for recreational use indicate an increase in cannabis use and in cannabis-related emergency room visits and hospitalizations.[22–24]

Despite the high prevalence of cannabis use disorder, awareness regarding effective treatment options remain limited within the medical community. Better knowledge by clinicians regarding the management of cannabis use disorder could likely improve patient outcomes. This article offers an overview of the different effective approaches for the treatment of cannabis use disorder.

GENERAL TREATMENT PRINCIPLES

The intensity of the treatment recommended for a patient using cannabis largely depends on the clinical presentation. Therefore, a proper assessment and screening needs to be performed before establishing an appropriate treatment plan. Although no consensus screening recommendations have been published, authors have suggested the following recommendations. Physicians should question every patient at least once regarding cannabis use. Adolescents, young adults, and patients at high risk for cannabis-related harm (eg, patients with comorbid psychiatric or substance use disorders) should be asked about cannabis use more frequently, for example, at every routine medical visit.[25] When a patient reports using cannabis, the physician should inquire about clinical indicators of problematic cannabis use, including daily or near daily use, poor social functioning, poor functioning at work or school, unsuccessful attempts to reduce use, and concerns from family or friends.[25] When problematic use is suspected, the DSM-5 criteria should be reviewed to establish a diagnosis of cannabis use disorder.

Differentiating between recreational cannabis use and cannabis use disorder is an important step to determine what type of treatment is appropriate. The type of treatment offered also depends on a patient's motivation and desire to quit, and is often related to the level of distress experienced in relation to substance use. For patients using cannabis without fulfilling the criteria for cannabis use disorder, and for patients with cannabis use disorder who have no desire to diminish or discontinue their use, offering counseling as a part of medical visits is appropriate. Counseling can be based on the Lower Risk Cannabis Use Guidelines, a guideline based on a systematic literature review conducted by a group of international experts to identify behaviors that could be modified to decrease adverse health consequences from cannabis use.[26] The main recommendations issued by the group are summarized in **Box 1**.

For patients with a diagnosis of cannabis use disorder who are interested in receiving treatment, it is generally recommended to provide a referral to an addiction physician or to an addiction treatment program. If these options are not available, psychiatrists, psychologists, or counselors with expertise in addiction can also provide valuable specialized care. The treatment of cannabis use disorder is generally performed in an outpatient setting. Inpatient or residential treatments are generally limited to patients with comorbid psychiatric or substance use disorder justifying a higher level of care. It is recommended to establish treatment goals early in the episode of care to inform the appropriate treatment approach. Treatment goals are based on a patient's individual objectives, and may vary greatly, ranging from total abstinence, reducing the amount of cannabis used, to avoiding hazardous use. The use of urine drug screening may be useful in the course of treatment to monitor abstinence in patients aiming to fully discontinue cannabis use, but is of little usefulness in patients aiming to decrease their use, because routine drug screening only provides qualitative results. In patients with regular, heavy cannabis use, the interpretation of cannabis

Box 1
Main recommendations from the lower risk cannabis use guidelines

1. Abstaining from using cannabis to fully prevent cannabis-related health problems.

2. Avoiding initiation of cannabis use before the age of 16 years.

3. Choosing cannabis products with low THC potency or balanced THC-cannabidiol ratio.

4. Abstaining from using synthetic cannabinoid.

5. Favoring nonsmoking methods of consumption.

6. Avoiding deep inhalation practices, which may increase risks of respiratory problems.

7. Avoiding daily or near-daily cannabis use.

8. Abstaining from driving while impaired from cannabis to prevent motor vehicle accidents.

9. Populations at higher risk of cannabis-related adverse effects should refrain from using cannabis, including pregnant women and individuals with a predisposition for, or with a first-degree family history of psychosis or substance use disorder.

10. Avoiding to combine the aforementioned risk behaviors (eg, combining early initiation and high-frequency use could magnify the likelihood of experiencing cannabis-related adverse outcomes).

Abbreviation: THC, delta-9-tetrahydrocannabinol.
Adapted from Fischer B, Russell C, Sabioni P, et al. Lower-risk cannabis use guidelines: a comprehensive update of evidence and recommendations. Am J Public Health 2017;107(8):e4; with permission.

toxicology results can be challenging because qualitative results may remain positive up to 4 weeks after cessation of use. Furthermore, urine drug screening is of little usefulness in patients using synthetic cannabinoid because many of these compounds are not captured by urine drug testing.

Currently, psychosocial interventions are the first line for the treatment of cannabis use disorder, with some specific forms of such interventions having shown effectiveness in reducing cannabis use. A number of pharmacologic approaches have been tested in regard to their impact on cannabis use and on the severity of withdrawal symptoms yielding limited positive outcomes. Although a few medications have shown some promising results warranting further research, no medication is currently approved by the US Food and Drug Administration for the treatment of cannabis use disorder.

PSYCHOSOCIAL INTERVENTIONS

Different psychosocial interventions have been shown to be effective in reducing the frequency of cannabis use and the severity of cannabis use disorder.[27] The most effective approaches are cognitive–behavioral therapy (CBT), motivational enhancement therapy (MET), and a combination of both. Contingency management (CM) is also efficacious when combined with either of these interventions.[27] As a general principle, greater effectiveness is achieved when psychosocial treatments are implemented with higher intensity over longer periods of time (>4 treatment sessions over a period of >1 month).[27] This section presents an overview of the different psychosocial interventions available for the treatment of cannabis use disorder (**Table 1**).

Cognitive–Behavioral Therapy

CBT is a psychotherapeutic approach that focuses on the identification and modification of problematic thoughts and behaviors. It can be delivered in a group or individual

Table 1
Main psychosocial interventions recommended for the treatment of cannabis use and cannabis use disorder

Condition	Intervention	Setting	Outcomes
Cannabis use	Brief counseling Education on safer cannabis use practices based on the LRCUG	Individual; can be delivered by any physician during a regular medical visit	Decrease adverse health consequences from cannabis use
Cannabis use disorder	CBT Identification and modification of problematic thoughts and behaviors	Individual or group setting; generally delivered by a trained addiction professional	Decrease cannabis use[a] Decrease cannabis related-problems
	MET Enhancement of intrinsic motivation to change by exploring and resolving ambivalence	Individual or group setting; generally delivered by a trained addiction professional	Decrease cannabis use[b] Decrease cannabis-related problems Decrease the severity of cannabis use disorder
	CM Providing incentives (vouchers) contingent upon positive treatment outcomes	Used as an augmentation treatment combined with CBT or MET	Enhances the effectiveness of CBT and MET to decrease cannabis use

Abbreviations: CBT, cognitive–behavioral therapy; CM, contingency management; LRCUG, lower risk cannabis use guidelines; MET, motivation enhancement therapy.
[a] The intervention is effective to decrease the number of days of use, to decrease the number of joints per day and to increase past month abstinence.
[b] The intervention is effective to decrease the number of days of use and the number of joints per day.

setting. In the context of substance use disorder, this approach emphasizes coping strategies learning, problem solving, and promoting the substitution of cannabis use by alternative, better adapted behaviors.[28] CBT effectively reduced the frequency of cannabis use among patients with cannabis use disorder.[27,29,30] A 2016 metaanalysis evaluating the effectiveness of different psychosocial interventions for the treatment of cannabis use disorder found that individuals receiving CBT used cannabis on fewer days in the month before assessment compared with those assigned to the inactive control group (mean difference, 10.94; 95% confidence interval [CI], 7.44–14.44; n = 134).[27] Compared with inactive control, CBT was also found effective in increasing abstinence in the month before assessment (risk ratio; 4.81; 95% CI, 1.17–19.70; n = 171), in reducing the number of joints used per day (standardized mean difference [SMD], 4.60; 95% CI, 2.21–7.00; 2 studies [n = 306]) and in decreasing cannabis-related problems (SMD, 7.88; 95% CI, 6.86–8.90; n = 135).[27]

Motivational Enhancement Therapy

MET is a psychotherapeutic approach that promotes the importance of self-efficacy and positive changes. It can be delivered in an individual or group setting. The objective of MET intervention is to enhance intrinsic motivation to change by exploring and resolving ambivalence in a nonjudgmental and empathic environment.[31] The afore-mentioned 2016 metaanalysis found a significant impact of MET on most of the primary outcomes examined (with the exception of past month abstinence), overall supporting the effectiveness of this psychotherapeutic approach for the treatment of cannabis use disorder.[27] MET was found effective in reducing the number of days of cannabis use in the month before assessment among participants treated with MET compared with inactive control (mean difference, 4.45; 95% CI, 1.90–7.00; 4 studies [n = 612]).[27] MET was also found superior to inactive control in reducing cannabis-related problems (SMD, 3.29; 95% CI, 1.85–4.72; 4 studies [n = 612]) and in decreasing the number of joints smoked per day (SMD, 3.14; 95% CI, 2.66–3.61; 4 studies [n = 611]) and the severity of cannabis use disorder (SMD, 4.07; 95% CI, 1.97–6.17; 2 studies [n = 316]).[27] The impact of MET on abstinence from cannabis in the month before assessment was not statistically significant (risk ratio, 1.19; 95% CI, 0.43–3.28; n = 197).[27]

Contingency Management

CM is often combined with other interventions as an augmentation approach for the treatment of substance use disorder. In CM, incentives are provided, often in the form of vouchers contingent upon positive treatment outcomes such as attendance at treatment appointments and abstinence from substance use verified with urine toxicology. A number of studies conducted in different populations of individuals with substance use disorders support the effectiveness of CM in improving retention to treatment and in promoting abstinence.[32,33] Although studies exploring the effectiveness of CM as a standalone treatment for cannabis use disorder are lacking, a number of clinical trials found that augmenting MET, CBT, or the combination of MET and CBT with abstinence-based CM improves the number of abstinent days compared with each of these psychotherapeutic approaches without CM.[27,34]

Alternative Approaches

Although the majority of studies on psychosocial interventions for the treatment of cannabis use disorder examined MET, CBT, or CM, alternative psychosocial approaches have also been tested, yielding weak or negative results. More specifically, evidence on mindfulness-based meditation, drug counseling, social support, and relapse prevention remain insufficient to recommend any of these approaches.[27] Marijuana Anonymous, a mutual help group based on the 12-step principle of Alcohol Anonymous, is widely available; however, its effectiveness has not been rigorously studied.

Combination Therapy

Although CBT and MET approaches were found equally effective for reducing cannabis use when compared with each other, a recent metaanalysis found maximal effectiveness of these interventions when delivered in combination compared with each treatment alone being delivered alone.[27] Furthermore, adding CM to either MET, CBT, or their combination likely further improves effectiveness.[27]

PHARMACOTHERAPY

There is currently no US Food and Drug Administration–approved medication for the treatment of cannabis use disorder, although a few trials have shown promising results. Cannabinoid agonists may be of potential value to decrease symptoms of withdrawal and improve retention to treatment. Some evidence also suggests gabapentin may improve abstinence from cannabis. *N*-Acetylcysteine (NCA) was thought to be a promising approach based on data from an adolescent trial, but the initial positive findings have not been replicated in a recent clinical trial conducted in an adult population.[35,36] Further research is needed to confirm the effectiveness of these treatments. This section reviews the main pharmacotherapies that have shown preliminarily positive results for the treatment of cannabis use disorder.

Cannabinoid Agonists

Delta-9-tetrahydrocannabinol analogues

Dronabinol Dronabinol (Marinol) is a synthetic form of THC that is bioavailable orally. It is currently approved by the US Food and Drug Administration for the treatment of chemotherapy-related nausea and vomiting and for appetite stimulation in patients with advanced human immunodeficiency virus infection.

A few studies support the effectiveness of dronabinol alone or in combination with lofexidine to improve symptoms of cannabis withdrawal.[37–41] A 12-week trial of 156 adults with cannabis use disorder found that dronabinol 20 mg 2 times per day was effective in reducing symptoms of withdrawal and in improving retention to treatment but had no effect on marijuana use and on abstinence at the end of treatment.[39] Two studies also suggested a dose-dependent effect of dronabinol in suppressing withdrawal symptoms with tested doses up to 120 mg/d.[37,40]

Each study reported that the medication was well-tolerated with minimal side effects and an absence of adverse cognitive effects. Possible side effects from dronabinol include palpitations, tachycardia, flushing, vasodilation, euphoria, abnormality in thinking, dizziness, anxiety, and gastrointestinal symptoms.

Nabilone Nabilone (Cesamet) is a synthetic form of delta THC that acts as an agonist of the CB_1 and CB_2 receptors. It is approved for the treatment of nausea and vomiting induced by chemotherapy.

One small study of 11 non–treatment-seeking individuals who smoked cannabis daily found that nabilone significantly decreased relapse and improved withdrawal symptoms of irritability, insomnia, and disrupted food intake.[42] A dose of 8 mg/d was associated with a modest impact on psychomotor task performance. This adverse effect was not found at a dose of 6 mg/d. Adverse effects most frequently reported from nabilone include drowsiness, dizziness, vertigo, euphoria, ataxia, depression, lack of concentration, sleep disorder, xerostomia, and visual disturbance.

Combined delta-9-tetrahydrocannabinol/cannabidiol product

Nabiximols (Sativex) is a medication delivered as a buccal spray that contains THC and cannabidiol in approximately equal proportions. It acts as an agonist at the CB_1 and CB_2 receptors. Although it is not currently available in the United States, it is approved in different countries for the treatment of cancer pain as well as for spasticity and neuropathic pain associated with multiple sclerosis.

One Australian 28-day inpatient study of 51 adults with cannabis use disorder demonstrated the effectiveness of nabiximols administered at a dose up to 86.4 mg of THC and 80 mg of cannabidiol daily to reduce symptoms of withdrawal (including withdrawal- induced irritability, depression, and cravings) and to improve retention to treatment compared with placebo.[43] No symptoms of intoxication were experienced. A Canadian study of 9 patients with cannabis use disorder found that high doses of nabiximols ($\leq$108 mg of THC and $\leq$100 mg of cannabidiol daily) were effective in reducing symptoms of withdrawal during cannabis abstinence, but had no impact on cravings.[44] In both studies, there was no impact of the treatment on cannabis use outcome. More research studies are required to validate its use for cannabis use disorder treatment. It should be noted that, in those trials, the rate of adverse effects did not differ between the medication and placebo. Importantly, symptoms of intoxication were not noted in the groups treated with nabiximols. Side effects most frequently reported with nabiximols include dizziness, drowsiness, fatigue, and nausea.

Gabapentin

Gabapentin is approved for the treatment of seizures and neuralgia. It acts by blocking voltage-dependent calcium channels, which indirectly modulates the inhibitory central nervous system neurotransmitter GABA. A 12-week randomized controlled trial of 50 adults with cannabis use disorder found that 1200 mg of gabapentin daily was effective in reducing cannabis use assessed both via urine drug testing and self-report, as well as in decreasing withdrawal symptoms including craving and improving executive function compared with the placebo group.[45] In this trial, gabapentin was administered 300 mg twice per day and 600 mg at bedtime. Both groups received weekly individual drug counseling. Although these results are promising, more research is needed to support the effectiveness of this medication for the treatment of cannabis use disorder.

The medication was well-tolerated and there was no difference in the proportion of adverse reactions between groups. The most frequent adverse effects reported with gabapentin are dizziness, drowsiness, ataxia, and fatigue.

N-Acetylcysteine

NAC is a derivative of the amino acid cysteine that modulates glutamate transmission. The presumed mechanism underlying NAC's possible efficacy is through the modulation of glutamate in the nucleus acumbens, a part of the brain reward circuitry that plays a significant role in the development of substance use disorders.

A study of 116 adolescents with cannabis use disorder aged between 15 and 21 years old showed that 8 weeks of treatment with NAC at a dose of 2400 mg/d doubled the odds of negative urine drug testing compared with placebo.[35] However, this finding was not replicated in a subsequent study by the same group, where 12 weeks of treatment with NAC at a dose of 2400 mg/d showed no difference in cannabis abstinence compared with placebo amongst 302 adults with cannabis use disorder aged 18 to 50 years old.[36]

Other

Numerous other tested pharmacologic approaches are likely of little value for the treatment of cannabis use disorder. These medications include escitalopram, fluoxetine, bupropion, nefazodone, venlafaxine, valproate, baclofen, modafinil, atomoxetine, buspirone, and naltrexone, all of which failed to demonstrate a significant positive impact on withdrawal or cannabis use outcomes.[38,46–57] In a human laboratory study, mirtazapine was found to improve sleep and food intake during abstinence, but did not impact withdrawal symptoms and relapse.[55] Similarly, a human laboratory study showed that the antipsychotic quetiapine improved sleep quality and food intake, but also increased marijuana craving and self-administration.[58]

Recently, data have emerged on the potential role of cannabidiol as a treatment option for cannabis use disorder given its ability to decrease THC-induced euphoria.[13,14] Although cannabidiol in combination with THC was found to improve symptoms of cannabis withdrawal, one laboratory study of cannabidiol administered alone did not show effectiveness in decreasing cannabis use or the subjective reinforcing effect of cannabis use.[43,44,59] It is unclear whether the impact of combination THC and cannabidiol treatment on reducing withdrawal symptoms can be partly attributed to the cannabidiol component or is instead owing to the effect of THC alone.

Rimonabant, an inverse agonist/antagonist of the CB_1 receptor was found to decrease drug taking behavior and cue-induced reinstatement of drug-seeking behavior in abstinent monkeys and to attenuate the physiologic effect of cannabis intoxication in humans.[60,61] However, it was found to cause adverse psychiatric outcomes such as anxiety and depression and was removed from the market in 2008.[62,63]

AM4113, a CB_1 receptor neutral antagonist has been studied in animal models, showing positive impact on reducing the use of cannabis without the negative psychiatric side effects of rimonabant.[61,64] This may be a promising treatment and further studies would be of interest.

Finally, a number of clinical trials are currently exploring the impact of different medications for the treatment of cannabis use disorder, including clonazepam, quetiapine, lorcaserin, FAAH-inhibitor, nabilone, NAC, cannabidiol, dronabinol in combination with clonidine, dextroamphetamine/amphetamine, and varenicline.

SYNTHETIC CANNABINOIDS

Synthetic cannabinoids are chemically synthesized compounds that are analogues to naturally occurring cannabinoids. They were first developed in laboratories for medical research in the 1960s and started being sold for recreational use around 2008 in the United States, most frequently under the names of "spice" or "K2."[65] Over the past decade, they have gained popularity owing to their accessibility, the unclear legal status regarding their use, and the lack of detection in routine drug screening. An important feature of synthetic cannabinoid is the variability of their composition, with frequent occurrence of new derivative compounds, presumably with the objective of avoiding regulations.[66] The heterogeneity of the synthetic cannabinoid group of compounds makes intoxication symptoms variable and less predictable.

Synthetic cannabinoids and cannabis bind to the same receptors and, therefore, both substances share common features in terms of signs and symptoms of intoxication and withdrawal. However, a number of synthetic cannabinoid compounds can have greater potency and binding affinity to the receptors compared with cannabis.[67,68] Moreover, certain synthetic cannabinoids produce active metabolites that act as full receptor agonists as opposed to the partial agonist activity of THC.[67,68] These pharmacologic properties contribute to the greater severity of synthetic cannabinoids intoxication and withdrawal symptoms compared with regular cannabis.

The majority of cases of intoxication are not life threatening and may present with tachycardia, nausea, vomiting, behavioral perturbation, and anxiety, although some severe symptoms of intoxication have been reported, including new-onset psychosis, kidney injury, rhabdomyolysis, respiratory depression, and seizures.[69–71] A few cases of death have been attributed to direct toxicity from synthetic cannabinoids causing cardiac arrhythmia, seizure, and kidney failure, whereas other cases of death were indirectly due to synthetic cannabinoids, such as hypothermia owing to individuals remaining unconscious outdoor in the winter or suicide.[69]

Management of Acute Intoxication

Mild to moderate symptoms of intoxication are managed in the emergency department until resolution of symptoms (which typically last 4–6 hours), although more severe symptoms may warrant inpatient admission. In the majority of cases, acute intoxication is managed with supportive care and with intravenous fluid repletion.[72]

Benzodiazepines are used as a first line to treat agitation, irritability, psychosis, and seizure.[72] Antipsychotics may also be used to treat agitation and psychotic symptoms.[72] Antiemetic medications can be used to treat hyperemesis, although they are not always effective.[73,74] Poison control centers are available at all times and should be consulted for patients who are critically ill or for whom presentation symptoms are unclear.

Management of Withdrawal

Abrupt discontinuation of synthetic cannabinoid after daily use has been associated with withdrawal symptoms ranging from mild symptoms such as headaches, anxiety, insomnia, nausea, vomiting, loss of appetite, diaphoresis, and craving to severe symptoms including seizure, chest pain, palpitations, and dyspnea.[72] In the absence of instruments designed to assess withdrawal symptoms from synthetic cannabinoids specifically, we suggest that clinicians use the DSM-5 diagnostic criteria for cannabis withdrawal. Similar to the management of acute intoxication, mild to moderate withdrawal symptoms can be managed in an outpatient setting, although severe cases may require inpatient care and continuous monitoring.

Benzodiazepines are used as a first-line treatment for the management of withdrawal symptoms including agitation, anxiety, and seizure.[75,76] Quetiapine has been used with effectiveness to treat withdrawal induced agitation and anxiety after failure of a benzodiazepine trial.[75,76]

Given the recent emergence of synthetic cannabinoids, knowledge regarding best treatment options remain limited and further research is needed to better guide clinical interventions.

FUTURE CONSIDERATIONS AND SUMMARY

Despite the high prevalence of cannabis use disorder, there are few effective treatment options available. MET and CBT are the most effective psychosocial interventions to reduce cannabis use in individuals with cannabis use disorder, with maximal results achieved when combining both approaches.[27] Adding CM in the form of vouchers for negative urine drug test results can provide further benefit in the short term, although little evidence is available regarding long-term benefits.[27] Treatment of greater intensity (>4 sessions over >1 month) is more effective than lower intensity interventions.[27]

Although no pharmacotherapy is approved for the treatment of cannabis use disorder, data suggest that some medications may be of potential value. In line with the concept of using agonist medications to treat other substance use disorders, such as buprenorphine and methadone for opioid use disorder and nicotine replacement and varenicline for nicotine use disorder, there has been a growing interest in the potential role of cannabinoid analogues for the treatment of cannabis use disorder. It has been hypothesized that cannabinoid analogues could improve abstinence by attenuating withdrawal symptoms and by decreasing the pleasurable effect of cannabis. Although studies have consistently demonstrated the ability of cannabinoid analogues to decrease acute cannabis withdrawal symptoms, no impact was found on cannabis use outcomes.[37–44] Hence, the role of cannabinoid medications in the long-term treatment of cannabis use disorder remains to be investigated.

Gabapentin may provide some benefit in decreasing cannabis use and cannabis withdrawal symptoms.[45] There are mixed results regarding the effect of NAC.[35,36] Further research is warranted to clarify the potential role of the aforementioned medications. A number of pharmacotherapies are currently under investigation for the treatment of cannabis use disorder and may lead to the emergence of novel therapeutic options in the future.

Finally, data suggest gender differences in cannabis use and cannabis use disorder. Although men are more likely to initiate cannabis use and to have a lifetime diagnosis of cannabis use disorder, women demonstrate a faster progression from cannabis use to cannabis use disorder.[77,78] Women with cannabis use disorder are also more likely than men to experience withdrawal symptoms, to have low scores on quality of life assessment scales, and to have comorbid mood or anxiety disorders.[2,78–80] These gender differences could potentially lead to the development of gender-specific treatment approaches, such as placing a greater emphasis on withdrawal symptoms and on the treatment of comorbid psychiatric disorders for women. Future studies exploring the impact of gender on response to treatments for cannabis use disorder would be of great interest.

ACKNOWLEDGMENTS

The editors thank Jeanette M. Tetrault, Yale University School of Medicine, for providing a critical review of this article.

REFERENCES

1. United Nations Office on Drugs and Crime. World drug report 2016. Vienna (Austria): 2016. Available at: http://www.unodc.org/wdr2016/. Accessed June, 2017.
2. Lev-Ran S, Le Strat Y, Imtiaz S, et al. Gender differences in prevalence of substance use disorders among individuals with lifetime exposure to substances: results from a large representative sample. Am J Addict 2013;22(1):7–13.
3. Lopez-Quintero C, Perez de los Cobos J, Hasin DS, et al. Probability and predictors of transition from first use to dependence on nicotine, alcohol, cannabis, and cocaine: results of the National Epidemiologic Survey on Alcohol and Related Conditions (NESARC). Drug Alcohol Depend 2011;115(1–2):120–30.
4. Le Strat Y, Dubertret C, Le Foll B. Impact of age at onset of cannabis use on cannabis dependence and driving under the influence in the United States. Accid Anal Prev 2015;76:1–5.
5. SAMHSA. Key substance use and mental health indicators in the United States: results from the 2015 National Survey on Drug Use and Health. 2017. Available at: https://www.samhsa.gov/data/sites/default/files/NSDUH-FFR1-2015/NSDUH-FFR1-2015/NSDUH-FFR1-2015.htm#sudyr04. Accessed June, 2017.
6. Pertwee RG. Ligands that target cannabinoid receptors in the brain: from THC to anandamide and beyond. Addict Biol 2008;13(2):147–59.
7. Mechoulam R, Parker LA. The endocannabinoid system and the brain. Annu Rev Psychol 2013;64:21–47.
8. Solinas M, Goldberg SR, Piomelli D. The endocannabinoid system in brain reward processes. Br J Pharmacol 2008;154(2):369–83.
9. Mechoulam R, Hanus L. A historical overview of chemical research on cannabinoids. Chem Phys Lipids 2000;108(1–2):1–13.
10. Leweke FM, Piomelli D, Pahlisch F, et al. Cannabidiol enhances anandamide signaling and alleviates psychotic symptoms of schizophrenia. Transl Psychiatry 2012;2:e94.
11. Schier AR, Ribeiro NP, Silva AC, et al. Cannabidiol, a Cannabis sativa constituent, as an anxiolytic drug. Rev Bras Psiquiatr 2012;34(Suppl 1):S104–10.

12. Campos AC, Moreira FA, Gomes FV, et al. Multiple mechanisms involved in the large-spectrum therapeutic potential of cannabidiol in psychiatric disorders. Philos Trans R Soc Lond B Biol Sci 2012;367(1607):3364–78.

13. Englund A, Morrison PD, Nottage J, et al. Cannabidiol inhibits THC-elicited paranoid symptoms and hippocampal-dependent memory impairment. J Psychopharmacol 2013;27(1):19–27.

14. Karniol IG, Shirakawa I, Kasinski N, et al. Cannabidiol interferes with the effects of delta 9-tetrahydrocannabinol in man. Eur J Pharmacol 1974;28(1):172–7.

15. Devinsky O, Cross JH, Laux L, et al. Trial of cannabidiol for drug-resistant seizures in the Dravet syndrome. N Engl J Med 2017;376(21):2011–20.

16. National Academies of Sciences, Engineering, and Medicine. The health effects of cannabis and cannabinoids: the current state of evidence and recommendations for research. Washington, DC: The National Academies Press; 2017. p. 486.

17. D'Souza DC, Perry E, MacDougall L, et al. The psychotomimetic effects of intravenous delta-9-tetrahydrocannabinol in healthy individuals: implications for psychosis. Neuropsychopharmacology 2004;29(8):1558–72.

18. American Psychiatric Association. Diagnostic and statistical manual of mental disorders, fifth edition (DSM-5). Arlington (VA): American Psychiatric Association; 2013.

19. Gorelick DA, Levin KH, Copersino ML, et al. Diagnostic criteria for cannabis withdrawal syndrome. Drug Alcohol Depend 2012;123(1–3):141–7.

20. Cornelius JR, Chung T, Martin C, et al. Cannabis withdrawal is common among treatment-seeking adolescents with cannabis dependence and major depression, and is associated with rapid relapse to dependence. Addict Behav 2008; 33(11):1500–5.

21. ElSohly MA, Mehmedic Z, Foster S, et al. Changes in cannabis potency over the last 2 decades (1995-2014): analysis of current data in the United States. Biol Psychiatry 2016;79(7):613–9.

22. Wang GS, Roosevelt G, Heard K. Pediatric marijuana exposures in a medical marijuana state. JAMA Pediatr 2013;167(7):630–3.

23. Kim HS, Anderson JD, Saghafi O, et al. Cyclic vomiting presentations following marijuana liberalization in Colorado. Acad Emerg Med 2015;22(6):694–9.

24. Wen H, Hockenberry JM, Cummings JR. The effect of medical marijuana laws on adolescent and adult use of marijuana, alcohol, and other substances. J Health Econ 2015;42:64–80.

25. Turner SD, Spithoff S, Kahan M. Approach to cannabis use disorder in primary care: focus on youth and other high-risk users. Can Fam Physician 2014;60(9): 801–8.

26. Fischer B, Russell C, Sabioni P, et al. Lower-risk cannabis use guidelines: a comprehensive update of evidence and recommendations. Am J Public Health 2017;107(8):e1–12.

27. Gates PJ, Sabioni P, Copeland J, et al. Psychosocial interventions for cannabis use disorder. Cochrane Database Syst Rev 2016;(5):CD005336.

28. Beck A, Wright F, Newman C, et al. Cognitive therapy of substance abuse. New York: Guilford Press; 1993.

29. Stephens RS, Roffman RA, Curtin L. Comparison of extended versus brief treatments for marijuana use. J Consult Clin Psychol 2000;68(5):898–908.

30. Copeland J, Swift W, Roffman R, et al. A randomized controlled trial of brief cognitive-behavioral interventions for cannabis use disorder. J Subst Abuse Treat 2001;21(2):55–64 [discussion: 5–6].

31. Miller WR, Rollnick S. Motivational interviewing: preparing people for change. New York: The Guilford Press; 2002.
32. Petry NM, Peirce JM, Stitzer ML, et al. Effect of prize-based incentives on outcomes in stimulant abusers in outpatient psychosocial treatment programs: a national drug abuse treatment clinical trials network study. Arch Gen Psychiatry 2005;62(10):1148–56.
33. Peirce JM, Petry NM, Stitzer ML, et al. Effects of lower-cost incentives on stimulant abstinence in methadone maintenance treatment: a National Drug Abuse Treatment Clinical Trials Network study. Arch Gen Psychiatry 2006;63(2):201–8.
34. Stanger C, Budney AJ, Kamon JL, et al. A randomized trial of contingency management for adolescent marijuana abuse and dependence. Drug Alcohol Depend 2009;105(3):240–7.
35. Gray KM, Carpenter MJ, Baker NL, et al. A double-blind randomized controlled trial of N-acetylcysteine in cannabis-dependent adolescents. Am J Psychiatry 2012;169(8):805–12.
36. Gray KM, Sonne SC, McClure EA, et al. A randomized placebo-controlled trial of N-acetylcysteine for cannabis use disorder in adults. Drug Alcohol Depend 2017; 177:249–57.
37. Budney AJ, Vandrey RG, Hughes JR, et al. Oral delta-9-tetrahydrocannabinol suppresses cannabis withdrawal symptoms. Drug Alcohol Depend 2007;86(1): 22–9.
38. Haney M, Hart CL, Vosburg SK, et al. Marijuana withdrawal in humans: effects of oral THC or divalproex. Neuropsychopharmacology 2004;29(1):158–70.
39. Levin FR, Mariani JJ, Brooks DJ, et al. Dronabinol for the treatment of cannabis dependence: a randomized, double-blind, placebo-controlled trial. Drug Alcohol Depend 2011;116(1–3):142–50.
40. Vandrey R, Stitzer ML, Mintzer MZ, et al. The dose effects of short-term dronabinol (oral THC) maintenance in daily cannabis users. Drug Alcohol Depend 2013; 128(1–2):64–70.
41. Haney M, Hart CL, Vosburg SK, et al. Effects of THC and lofexidine in a human laboratory model of marijuana withdrawal and relapse. Psychopharmacology 2008;197(1):157–68.
42. Haney M, Cooper ZD, Bedi G, et al. Nabilone decreases marijuana withdrawal and a laboratory measure of marijuana relapse. Neuropsychopharmacology 2013;38(8):1557–65.
43. Allsop DJ, Copeland J, Lintzeris N, et al. Nabiximols as an agonist replacement therapy during cannabis withdrawal: a randomized clinical trial. JAMA Psychiatry 2014;71(3):281–91.
44. Trigo JM, Lagzdins D, Rehm J, et al. Effects of fixed or self-titrated dosages of Sativex on cannabis withdrawal and cravings. Drug Alcohol Depend 2016;161: 298–306.
45. Mason BJ, Crean R, Goodell V, et al. A proof-of-concept randomized controlled study of gabapentin: effects on cannabis use, withdrawal and executive function deficits in cannabis-dependent adults. Neuropsychopharmacology 2012;37(7): 1689–98.
46. Weinstein AM, Miller H, Bluvstein I, et al. Treatment of cannabis dependence using escitalopram in combination with cognitive-behavior therapy: a double-blind placebo-controlled study. Am J Drug Alcohol Abuse 2014;40(1):16–22.
47. Carpenter KM, McDowell D, Brooks DJ, et al. A preliminary trial: double-blind comparison of nefazodone, bupropion-SR, and placebo in the treatment of cannabis dependence. Am J Addict 2009;18(1):53–64.

48. Levin FR, Mariani J, Brooks DJ, et al. A randomized double-blind, placebo-controlled trial of venlafaxine-extended release for co-occurring cannabis dependence and depressive disorders. Addiction 2013;108(6):1084–94.

49. Cornelius JR, Bukstein OG, Douaihy AB, et al. Double-blind fluoxetine trial in co-morbid MDD-CUD youth and young adults. Drug Alcohol Depend 2010;112(1–2):39–45.

50. Penetar DM, Looby AR, Ryan ET, et al. Bupropion reduces some of the symptoms of marihuana withdrawal in chronic marihuana users: a pilot study. Subst Abuse 2012;6:63–71.

51. Haney M, Ward AS, Comer SD, et al. Bupropion SR worsens mood during marijuana withdrawal in humans. Psychopharmacology 2001;155(2):171–9.

52. Levin FR, McDowell D, Evans SM, et al. Pharmacotherapy for marijuana dependence: a double-blind, placebo-controlled pilot study of divalproex sodium. Am J Addict 2004;13(1):21–32.

53. McRae-Clark AL, Carter RE, Killeen TK, et al. A placebo-controlled trial of buspirone for the treatment of marijuana dependence. Drug Alcohol Depend 2009;105(1–2):132–8.

54. McRae-Clark AL, Carter RE, Killeen TK, et al. A placebo-controlled trial of atomoxetine in marijuana-dependent individuals with attention deficit hyperactivity disorder. Am J Addict 2010;19(6):481–9.

55. Haney M, Hart CL, Vosburg SK, et al. Effects of baclofen and mirtazapine on a laboratory model of marijuana withdrawal and relapse. Psychopharmacology 2010;211(2):233–44.

56. Sugarman DE, Poling J, Sofuoglu M. The safety of modafinil in combination with oral 9-tetrahydrocannabinol in humans. Pharmacol Biochem Behav 2011;98(1):94–100.

57. Haney M, Bisaga A, Foltin RW. Interaction between naltrexone and oral THC in heavy marijuana smokers. Psychopharmacology 2003;166(1):77–85.

58. Cooper ZD, Foltin RW, Hart CL, et al. A human laboratory study investigating the effects of quetiapine on marijuana withdrawal and relapse in daily marijuana smokers. Addict Biol 2013;18(6):993–1002.

59. Haney M, Malcolm RJ, Babalonis S, et al. Oral cannabidiol does not alter the subjective, reinforcing or cardiovascular effects of smoked cannabis. Neuropsychopharmacology 2016;41(8):1974–82.

60. Huestis MA, Boyd SJ, Heishman SJ, et al. Single and multiple doses of rimonabant antagonize acute effects of smoked cannabis in male cannabis users. Psychopharmacology 2007;194(4):505–15.

61. Schindler CW, Redhi GH, Vemuri K, et al. Blockade of nicotine and cannabinoid reinforcement and relapse by a cannabinoid CB1-receptor neutral antagonist AM4113 and inverse agonist rimonabant in squirrel monkeys. Neuropsychopharmacology 2016;41(9):2283–93.

62. Despres JP, Golay A, Sjostrom L. Effects of rimonabant on metabolic risk factors in overweight patients with dyslipidemia. N Engl J Med 2005;353(20):2121–34.

63. Scheen AJ. CB1 receptor blockade and its impact on cardiometabolic risk factors: overview of the RIO programme with rimonabant. J Neuroendocrinol 2008;20(Suppl 1):139–46.

64. Gueye AB, Pryslawsky Y, Trigo JM, et al. The CB1 neutral antagonist AM4113 retains the therapeutic efficacy of the inverse agonist rimonabant for nicotine dependence and weight loss with better psychiatric tolerability. Int J Neuropsychopharmacol 2016;19(12) [pii:pyw068].

65. European Monitoring Centre for Drugs and Drug Addiction. Understanding the 'spice' phenomenon. Luxembourg: Office for Official Publications of the European Communities: EMCDDA; 2009. Available at: http://www.emcdda.europa. eu/system/files/publications/537/Spice-Thematic-paper-final-version.pdf_en.
66. Seely KA, Lapoint J, Moran JH, et al. Spice drugs are more than harmless herbal blends: a review of the pharmacology and toxicology of synthetic cannabinoids. Prog Neuropsychopharmacol Biol Psychiatry 2012;39(2):234–43.
67. Huffman JW, Padgett LW. Recent developments in the medicinal chemistry of cannabimimetic indoles, pyrroles and indenes. Curr Med Chem 2005;12(12): 1395–411.
68. Brents LK, Reichard EE, Zimmerman SM, et al. Phase I hydroxylated metabolites of the K2 synthetic cannabinoid JWH-018 retain in vitro and in vivo cannabinoid 1 receptor affinity and activity. PLoS One 2011;6(7):e21917.
69. Tait RJ, Caldicott D, Mountain D, et al. A systematic review of adverse events arising from the use of synthetic cannabinoids and their associated treatment. Clin Toxicol (Phila) 2016;54(1):1–13.
70. Riederer AM, Campleman SL, Carlson RG, et al. Acute poisonings from synthetic cannabinoids - 50 U.S. toxicology investigators consortium registry sites, 2010-2015. MMWR Morb Mortal Wkly Rep 2016;65(27):692–5.
71. Hoyte CO, Jacob J, Monte AA, et al. A characterization of synthetic cannabinoid exposures reported to the National Poison Data System in 2010. Ann Emerg Med 2012;60(4):435–8.
72. Cooper ZD. Adverse effects of synthetic cannabinoids: management of acute toxicity and withdrawal. Curr Psychiatry Rep 2016;18(5):52.
73. Hermanns-Clausen M, Kneisel S, Szabo B, et al. Acute toxicity due to the confirmed consumption of synthetic cannabinoids: clinical and laboratory findings. Addiction 2013;108(3):534–44.
74. Ukaigwe A, Karmacharya P, Donato A. A gut gone to pot: a case of cannabinoid hyperemesis syndrome due to K2, a synthetic cannabinoid. Case Rep Emerg Med 2014;2014:3.
75. Nacca N, Vatti D, Sullivan R, et al. The synthetic cannabinoid withdrawal syndrome. J Addict Med 2013;7(4):296–8.
76. Macfarlane V, Christie G. Synthetic cannabinoid withdrawal: a new demand on detoxification services. Drug Alcohol Rev 2015;34(2):147–53.
77. Hernandez-Avila CA, Rounsaville BJ, Kranzler HR. Opioid-, cannabis- and alcohol-dependent women show more rapid progression to substance abuse treatment. Drug Alcohol Depend 2004;74(3):265–72.
78. Khan SS, Secades-Villa R, Okuda M, et al. Gender differences in cannabis use disorders: results from the National Epidemiologic Survey of Alcohol and Related Conditions. Drug Alcohol Depend 2013;130(1–3):101–8.
79. Copersino ML, Boyd SJ, Tashkin DP, et al. Sociodemographic characteristics of cannabis smokers and the experience of cannabis withdrawal. Am J Drug Alcohol Abuse 2010;36(6):311–9.
80. Herrmann ES, Weerts EM, Vandrey R. Sex differences in cannabis withdrawal symptoms among treatment-seeking cannabis users. Exp Clin Psychopharmacol 2015;23(6):415–21.

Nontraditional Alcohol and Opioid Agonist Treatment Interventions

Christopher Fairgrieve, MD[a,b], Nadia Fairbairn, MD[b,c],
Jeffrey H. Samet, MD, MA, MPH[d,e], Seonaid Nolan, MD[b,c],*

KEYWORDS

- Managed alcohol • Injectable opioids • Severe opioid use disorder
- Severe alcohol use disorder • Sustained release oral morphine

KEY POINTS

- Alternative treatment interventions for individuals with a severe substance use disorder unsuccessful with standard management have been used in some settings.
- Community-managed alcohol programs combined with low-barrier housing have been used to stabilize some individuals with a severe alcohol use disorder.
- Slow-release oral morphine and injectable opioid agonist treatment can be alternative treatment options for people with severe opioid use disorders unsuccessful with methadone or buprenorphine.

INTRODUCTION

A spectrum of severity exists among individuals with alcohol and/or drug use disorders. Some may repeatedly fail the most aggressive standard treatment regimens. For such individuals, who can experience the worst medical complications and intensive utilization of health services, nonstandard approaches should be considered to mitigate the negative consequences of the use of harmful substances.

Disclosure Statement: All authors have no conflicts of interest to declare.
[a] Department of Family Medicine, University of British Columbia, St. Paul's Hospital, Room 553, 5th Floor Burrard Building, 1081 Burrard Street, Vancouver, British Columbia V6Z 1Y6, Canada; [b] British Columbia Centre on Substance Use, Providence Health Care, St. Paul's Hospital, Room 553, 5th Floor Burrard Building, 1081 Burrard Street, Vancouver, British Columbia V6Z 1Y6, Canada; [c] Department of Medicine, University of British Columbia, St. Paul's Hospital, Room 553, 5th Floor Burrard Building, 1081 Burrard Street, Vancouver, British Columbia V6Z 1Y6, Canada; [d] Clinical Addiction Research and Education Unit, Section of General Internal Medicine, Department of Medicine, Boston University School of Medicine, Boston Medical Center, 801 Massachusetts Avenue, 2nd Floor, Boston, MA 02118, USA; [e] Department of Community Health Sciences, Boston University School of Public Health, 715 Albany Street, Boston, MA 02118, USA
* Corresponding author. St. Paul's Hospital, Room 553, 5th Floor Burrard Building, 1081 Burrard Street, Vancouver, British Columbia V6Z 1Y6, Canada.
E-mail address: seonaidn@gmail.com

These approaches include managed alcohol programs (MAPs), sustained-release oral morphine (SROM) as an opioid agonist treatment, injectable opioid agonist treatment (OAT), and safe injecting facilities. These modalities fall outside the realm of standard medical care, and may not currently be legal in certain locales, but are adopted with some success in other regions. Understanding the current evidence of effectiveness for these nontraditional treatment approaches and the specific populations addressed was the goal of this review.

MANAGED ALCOHOL PROGRAMS

The goal of MAPs is both to eliminate barriers for shelter among individuals with an alcohol use disorder (AUD), which has historically proven challenging, and to provide access to alcohol in a supervised, controlled environment to mitigate the potential harms of ongoing use.[1] AUD is a common comorbidity among individuals who are unstably housed, with estimates approximating between 53% and 73%.[2,3] Such individuals are subject to poor health and social outcomes, including criminal justice system encounters, chronic medical illness, prolonged hospital stays,[4] and high rates of mortality.[5] For many, conventional treatment approaches for the management of an AUD has proven unsuccessful, and consideration of participation in an MAP can offer an effective harm-reduction strategy.

To date, MAPs have been described in several countries, including Canada, Ireland, Norway, and Australia.[6] Eligibility criteria may vary, but participation in an MAP is generally reserved for those who are chronically homeless, have a severe AUD (using criteria from the *Diagnostic and Statistical Manual of Mental Disorders* (DSM) IV or V), have demonstrated evidence of harm to self and community, and for whom abstinence-based programs have failed or been refused.[7] Most MAPs reported in the literature to date have described the use of an MAP in a community-based residential setting,[8] although non–housing-based programs have been reported as well.[9] Community MAPs are generally small, ranging from 8 to 35 participants.[8–10] Although the operational details vary among different programs, MAPs generally provide alcohol in relatively small doses at regular intervals, typically 1 standard drink (SD) per hour administered by a nurse or other staff worker, with total daily amounts ranging from 9 to 16 SD per day.[6]

Several positive outcomes have been reported in 3 Canadian pilot studies on community MAPs.[7,8,11] A reduction in alcohol consumption has been reported in 2 studies: an average decrease in daily alcohol consumption among 10 MAP participants, from 45.6 ± 28.8 SDs (pre-MAP) to 8.3 ± 3.5 SDs (during MAP)[7] (representing a daily decrease of approximately 38 sixteen-ounce pints of beer) and a reduction in alcohol consumption over a 6-month period of MAP participation (n = 18) from an average of 19.1 SDs at MAP initiation to 10.4 SDs 6 months later.[11] In contrast, a small-scale study of 7 participants reported no overall change in alcohol consumption during 9 months.[8] Despite mixed results for the effect of MAP on quantity of alcohol consumption, importantly all 3 studies reported a reduction in self-reported intake of non-beverage alcohol, such as mouthwash or rubbing alcohol.[7,8,11] The potential for underreporting of non-MAP consumption (ie, alcohol obtained independent of an MAP) has appropriately been cited as a study limitation.[8,12]

Other important health outcomes related to participation in an MAP have been evaluated. One study (n = 17) demonstrated an improvement in emergency health service utilization with a reduction in monthly emergency room visits following program enrollment (0.79 ± 1.25 to 0.51 ± 1.17; $P = .004$).[7] Improved engagement with both psychiatric[13] and general medical care has also been demonstrated among MAP participants.[7] Subjective reports from MAP participants noted an improvement in mental health and reduction in psychosocial harms,[8,11] whereas MAP program staff reported less volatility and hostility among participants after program enrollment.[8] Trends of liver enzymes among MAP participants have shown mixed results, with one study demonstrating a reduction,[11] another reporting stability,[7] and a third demonstrating an increase[8] following MAP enrollment.

Other benefits have been reported with MAP participation: a reduction in police reports (1.07 ± 0.66 per month to 0.52 ± 0.68; $P = .018$)[7]; and crime reduction from 4.77 ± 7.83 days to 2.79 ± 2.32 days per 100 days.[12] Community MAPs often provide shelter for those unstably housed. Qualitative studies of these participants have demonstrated an improved sense of community, safety, and quality of life,[14] with the setting itself being capable of both facilitating recovery[15] and acting as an entry point for some individuals requiring end-of-life care.[16] Retention rates in all 3 Canadian MAP studies were high, and ranged between 82% and 100% (with study durations of between 6 months and 2 years).[7,8,11] Of note, however, a 2012 Cochrane Review failed to identify any studies eligible for inclusion and thus was unable to determine the efficacy of MAP,[6] suggesting further research with a focus on the development of relevant measures of MAP success.

Similar MAP programs exist in acute care settings. For example, St. Paul's Hospital located in Vancouver, Canada, has an in-hospital MAP that uses a formalized protocol to guide the continuation of alcohol administration for individuals enrolled in a community MAP, provided no medical contraindication exists to do so. Furthermore, in this setting, newly initiated in-hospital MAP has occasionally been prescribed as a harm-reduction approach to mitigate the potential negative consequences of ongoing alcohol use in an unsupervised fashion (eg, consumption of nonbeverage alcohol, or quantities of alcohol in excess of what would be provided as part of MAP) or lack of access to alcohol all together (eg, leaving hospital against medical advice). Although regular clinical assessments and the use of benzodiazepines remains the standard of care for inpatient alcohol withdrawal syndrome, hospital MAP may offer benefits similar to those described in community MAP settings to select high-risk patients. Such an approach, however, is not without challenges. Particularly problematic is how to effectively manage a community MAP patient who presents to hospital with a medical complication related to alcohol consumption. Although discontinuing MAP in-hospital is a reasonable first step, formulating and engaging such an individual in his or her medical treatment plan can prove problematic. Furthermore, what to do with an individual newly initiated on MAP in-hospital at the time of discharge also can be a challenge because community MAPs are frequently at capacity. To date, provision of an MAP in an acute care setting has exposed numerous ethical and medicolegal concerns, and little is known about the potential benefits of MAP in this setting.

In summary, although not currently available in the United States, community MAPs do exist in several other countries as an attempt to reduce the harms associated with severe AUD among participants who have been unsuccessfully stabilized with conventional pharmacologic or psychosocial treatment options. Many of these programs operate in a setting that concurrently provides MAP participants with access to low-barrier housing. Although beyond the scope of this review, the value of these housing interventions from a public health perspective can be significant and should not be overlooked. To date, several observational studies evaluating community MAPs have demonstrated a reduction in alcohol consumption, a reduction in emergency department presentations and criminal activity, as well as improved health and quality of life among participants. Given the study sample sizes and potential for reporting bias, however, these results should be interpreted with caution. To date, no randomized controlled trials have been undertaken to determine the effectiveness of MAP in either community or acute care settings; individuals most likely to benefit from MAP are unclear. Furthermore, to our knowledge, no economic evaluation of MAPs currently exists. Further research is needed to address these important questions.

OPIOID AGONIST TREATMENT

Use of traditional opioid agonist medications (ie, buprenorphine or methadone) for the treatment of opioid use disorder (OUD) may not be successful, as a consequence of medication adverse effects or repeated unsuccessful treatment attempts. For such individuals, alternative treatment options could be considered to facilitate patient engagement in care and optimize treatment outcomes. These approaches are not currently legal in the United States, although they merit review given the current evidence and the opioid overdose epidemic in the United States.

Slow-Release Oral Morphine

SROM is an alternative treatment option with limited evidence to suggest benefit for the treatment of OUD.[17–21] A 2013 Cochrane Review, which included 3 randomized controlled trials, found no significant difference in treatment retention for SROM when compared with methadone but a higher incidence of adverse events.[19] Since this review, additional studies focused on SROM have been published. A randomized, noninferiority, crossover study demonstrated SROM to be noninferior to methadone (n = 157) for the proportion of heroin-positive urine samples.[17] A randomized controlled trial of participants previously treated with methadone (n = 276) reported SROM to be an effective, well-tolerated treatment option for OUD with a beneficial side-effect profile compared with methadone.[21] The study noted a shorter QTc interval on electrocardiogram, higher treatment satisfaction, and a reduction in mental stress and heroin cravings among participants being prescribed SROM compared with methadone. Similar findings were noted in 2 additional studies.[18,20] Furthermore, among 67 patients who were intolerant to methadone or experienced inadequate withdrawal suppression with its use, 1 multicenter study demonstrated the feasibility and tolerability of transitioning from methadone to SROM with several measurable improvements being subsequently observed (eg, a reduction in opioid withdrawal symptoms, reduced cravings, and fewer psychological problems).[22] The possible explanations for these outcomes were not discussed in detail in the studies included herein and warrant further research.

Despite preliminary research suggesting SROM to be a beneficial alternative treatment option for OUD, no recommendations currently exist in the United States endorsing SROM's use for this purpose, and in fact, such a practice currently remains illegal. In British Columbia, Canada, authors of the Guideline for the Clinical Management of Opioid Addiction do endorse SROM as a treatment option for patients with OUD who have been unsuccessful with or who have contraindications to first-line and second-line treatment options.[23,24] Specific indications and contraindications for SROM treatment according to the guideline can be found in **Table 1**. Furthermore, use of only the once-daily 24-hour formulation of SROM is endorsed by the guideline and the importance of daily witnessed ingestion is emphasized. Additionally, the guideline demonstrates how the provision of SROM can be seamlessly integrated into Canada's existing health care infrastructure, as eligible patients are assessed and evaluated in a clinic setting with daily witnessing of the medication occurring at a pharmacy (as occurs currently with methadone).

Table 1
Indications and contraindications for the use of slow-release oral morphine (SROM) as a treatment option for opioid use disorder (OUD)

Indications	Contraindications
• Adults (≥19 y) with OUD • On methadone while actively using another opioid	• Hypersensitivity to morphine sulfate or any component of the formulation Pregnant or breastfeeding • Significant respiratory depression • Acute or severe bronchial asthma • Known or suspected paralytic ileus • Currently taking monoamine oxidase inhibitors or use within the past 14 d • Severe respiratory compromise or obstructive disease • Severe respiratory distress • Delirium tremens • Acute alcohol intoxication

Adapted from British Columbia Centre on Substance Use (BCCSU). A guideline for the clinical management of opioid use disorder. Available at: http://www.bccsu.ca/wp-content/uploads/2017/06/BC-OUD-Guidelines_June2017.pdf; with permission. Accessed Mar 21, 2018.

Specific details regarding induction and dosing of SROM can be found in Appendix 3 of the guideline.[24] To summarize, a starting dose of 30 to 60 mg of SROM is recommended, with titration occurring every 48 hours according to an individual's withdrawal symptoms. For patients transitioning from methadone to SROM, a conversion factor of 1:4 can be applied (eg, 60 mg methadone = 240 mg SROM). Current literature reports a mean SROM daily dose range between 235 and 791 mg, with the full range of SROM being between 60 and 1200 mg/d. Given the paucity of literature regarding best practice for SROM treatment for OUD and the risk for overdose and diversion, close observation and follow-up with the patient is essential until a stable dose is achieved.

SROM treatment efficacy should be based on several outcomes, including the alleviation of opioid withdrawal symptoms and a reduction or elimination of illicit opioid use and cravings. Monitoring for compliance and/or ongoing use of illicit opiates is particularly challenging, however. The value of quantitative, point-of-care urine drug tests is limited, given SROM and heroin use will give a positive test result, but can provide useful information when the result is negative for opiates (indicating diversion) or positive for fentanyl. Given the challenges associated with ongoing monitoring for heroin use, the potential for diversion and risk for lethality among nontolerant individuals, the guideline recommends indefinite daily witnessed ingestion of SROM (ie, no take-home doses) (see Appendix 4 of the guideline). Only in exceptional circumstances in which a patient has demonstrated high clinical stability or when daily witnessed ingestion presents a significant barrier to treatment can graduated take-home dosing be considered.

Injectable Opioid Agonist Treatment

Injectable opioid agonist therapy is another option for the treatment of OUD when first-line treatment is not effective (eg, buprenorphine, methadone). Individuals with severe OUD who inject opioids but have not benefited from first-line or second-line oral OAT despite repeated treatment attempts are generally the population for which injectable OAT may be considered.

Injectable diacetylmorphine (ie, prescription heroin) is one injectable OAT option currently available for select populations in Denmark, Germany, the Netherlands, Canada, and Switzerland for the treatment of heroin addiction.[25–27] Among individuals with long-term (ie, greater than 2 years) daily heroin use with previous treatment failures in outpatient settings, meta-analyses of clinical trials have demonstrated the efficacy of diacetylmorphine in comparison with methadone for the treatment of an OUD.[28] More specifically, use of injectable diacetylmorphine resulted in a reduction in self-reported illicit heroin use, criminal activity, and involvement in sex work, as well as improved overall health and social functioning.[28–30] These meta-analyses include a 2011 Cochrane Review that examined 8 randomized controlled trials and found that supervised injection of diacetylmorphine, prescribed alone or combined with flexible doses of methadone, was superior to oral methadone alone in retaining treatment-refractory patients (risk ratio 1.44, 95% confidence interval [CI] 1.19–1.75) in treatment while helping reduce the use of illegal or nonmedical drugs.[28] The authors of the Cochrane Review concluded that there is value in coprescribing diacetylmorphine with flexible doses of methadone and that, due to the higher risk of adverse events related to the study medication diacetylmorphine compared with methadone, treatment with diacetylmorphine should be considered for those who have not benefited from oral agonist treatment.[28] Subsequent to the 2011 review, a 2015 systematic review and meta-analysis was conducted on the efficacy of injectable diacetylmorphine.[30] Six randomized controlled trials (conducted in Switzerland, the Netherlands, Spain, Germany, Canada, and England) were identified and included in the analysis (**Table 2**). These 6 trials also were included in the Cochrane Review from 2011; however, the approach in this study differed from that of the Cochrane Review, as only trials in which heroin was prescribed and provided in a supervised setting (as opposed to prescribed, unsupervised, or take-home administration) were included in this review. The outcome confirmed the previous review in finding a greater reduction of illicit heroin use among individuals who received prescribed, supervised injectable diacetylmorphine compared with those who received oral methadone treatment only.[30]

Regarding injectable OAT treatment duration, one study in the United Kingdom found median injectable diacetylmorphine OAT duration to be 6 years.[31] Additionally, in Switzerland it was found that, among injectable diacetylmorphine patients who were retained in treatment long-term (50% after 2.5 years), approximately 62% did eventually transition to less intensive treatment, such as oral OAT.[32] However, a loss of treatment benefit (ie, an increase in street heroin use posttreatment to levels comparable with that of the control group) has been found repeatedly when prescription diacetylmorphine treatment was discontinued at a predetermined end date.[33,34] Thus, the authors of the Treatment Assisted by Diacetylmorphine (TADAM) study in Belgium, in line with World Health Organization recommendations for other OATs, recommend that supervised injection of diacetylmorphine be provided as an open-ended treatment.[33]

The bulk of the literature on injectable OAT to date focuses on injectable diacetylmorphine as opposed to injectable hydromorphone. Although no systematic reviews currently exist evaluating the use of injectable hydromorphone, the SALOME trial (Study to Assess Longer-term Opioid Medication Effectiveness) was a phase 3, double-blind, single-site noninferiority trial conducted in Vancouver, Canada, that compared injectable diacetylmorphine with injectable hydromorphone for the treatment of OUD. The SALOME trial was conducted based on findings from the previous North American Opiate Medication Initiative study[27] (a randomized controlled trial evaluating the feasibility and effectiveness of heroin-assisted treatment compared with methadone) that demonstrated a reduction in illicit heroin use among a small

Table 2
Six randomized trials of supervised injectable heroin (SIH) (plus flexible supplementary doses of oral methadone): key features and outcomes

Main Article	Country	Sample Size; Groups Studied	Time to Follow-up	Cochrane Risk of Bias Using 5 Criteria Recommended by the Cochrane Handbook	Outcomes
Perneger et al	Switzerland	n = 51 SIH (+OM): n = 27 OM, detox, rehab: n = 24	6 mo	Random sequence generation Allocation concealment Incomplete outcome data Selective reporting Blinding (objective outcomes) Blinding (subjective outcomes)	L Retention: SIH: 93% vs OM 92% L Self-reported illicit heroin use: SIH: 22%, OM: 67% (P = .002) U SAE data not reported H H
van den Brink et al	The Netherlands	Injectable trial: n = 174 SIH (+OM): n = 76 OM: n = 98 (also SinhH trial, n = 75)	12 mo	Random sequence generation Allocation concealment Incomplete outcome data Selective reporting Blinding (objective outcomes) Blinding (subjective outcomes)	U Retention: SIH 72% vs OM 85% L Self-reported 40% improvement in at least 1 domain (physical, mental, social): SIH 56% vs OM 31% (P = .002) L SAEs: reported data limited to 11 SAEs (2 definitely or probably and 9 possibly related to injectable heroin)
March et al	Spain	n = 62 SIH (+OM): n = 31 OM: n = 31	9 mo	Random sequence generation Allocation concealment Incomplete outcome data Selective reporting Blinding (objective outcomes) Blinding (subjective outcomes)	U Retention: SIH 74% vs OM 68% L Self-reported illicit heroin use in past 30 d (mean days): SIH = 8.3 vs OM = 16.9 (P = .02) U SAEs: SIH = 7 (2 unrelated and 5 probably or definitely related to study drug) vs OM = 7

(continued on next page)

Table 2
(continued)

Main Article	Country	Sample Size; Groups Studied	Time to Follow-up	Cochrane Risk of Bias Using 5 Criteria Recommended by the Cochrane Handbook	Outcomes
Haasen et al	Germany	n = 1015 SIH (+OM): n = 515 OM: n = 500	12 mo	Random sequence generation Allocation concealment Incomplete outcome data Selective reporting Blinding (objective outcomes) Blinding (subjective outcomes)	L Retention: SIH 67% vs OM 40% L Improvement in drug use (measured by either UDS or self-report): SIH 69%, OM 55% (*P*<.001) U Improvement in physical/mental health: SIH 80%, OM 74% (*P* = .023) U Combined reduced drug use and improved physical/mental health (responder): SIH 57% vs OM 45% (*P*<.001) SAEs: SIH = 177 (58 possibly, probably or definitely related to study drug) vs OM = 15
Oviedo-Joekes et al	Canada	n = 251 SIH (+OM): n = 115 OM: n = 111 (also SIHM + OM, n = 25)	12 mo	Random sequence generation Allocation concealment Incomplete outcome data Selective reporting Blinding (objective outcomes) Blinding (subjective outcomes)	L Retention: SIH 88% vs OM 54% (*P*<.001) L Self-reported reduction in illicit drug use or other illegal activities (improvement of 20% for either domain): SIH = 67%, OM = 48% (*P* = .004) L SAEs: SIH = 51 vs OM = 18
Strang et al	England	n = 127 SIH (+OM): n = 43 OOM: n = 42 (also SIM + OM, n = 42)	6 mo	Random sequence generation Allocation concealment Incomplete outcome data Selective reporting Blinding (objective outcomes) Blinding (subjective outcomes)	L Retention: SIH (or other treatment) 88% vs OOM 69% L Reduction in "street" heroin: 50% or more negative UDS during weeks 14–26 (responder): SIH 66% vs OOM 19% (*P*<.0001) L SAEs: SIH = 7 (2 probably related to study drug) vs OOM = 9

Abbreviations: H, high risk of bias; L, low risk of bias; OM, oral methadone; OOM, optimized oral methadone; SAE, serious adverse event; SIHM, supervised inject-able hydromorphone; SIM, supervised injectable methadone; SinhH, supervised inhalable heroin; U, unclear; UDS, urine drug screen.

From Strang J, Groshkova T, Uchtenhagen A, et al. Heroin on trial: systematic review and meta-analysis of randomised trials of diamorphine-prescribing as treatment for refractory heroin addiction. Br J Psychiatry 2015;207(1):8; with permission.

number of participants (n = 25) being prescribed injectable hydromorphone, instead of diacetylmorphine, for corroboration of self-reported illicit heroin use. Results from the SALOME study (n = 202) demonstrated injectable hydromorphone to be noninferior to diacetylmorphine in reducing illicit opioid use and retaining individuals in treatment.[29] Injectable hydromorphone also was found to have significantly fewer adverse events than diacetylmorphine (rate ratio 0.21, 95% CI 0.06–0.69).[35] These preliminary results suggest that hydromorphone, a licensed analgesic in many jurisdictions, may be a viable alternative for the treatment of refractory OUD, particularly in jurisdictions in which use of diacetylmorphine may not be available or access is difficult.

The British Columbia Centre on Substance Use in Vancouver, Canada, has developed an Injectable Opioid Agonist Treatment for Opioid Use Disorder Guidance Document for injectable OAT as an alternative, high-intensity treatment for severe OUD.[36] The inclusion and exclusion considerations outlined in the guidance document can be found in **Table 3**. Three distinct models of care for injectable OAT are described in the guidance document. The first is a comprehensive and dedicated supervised injectable OAT program that may be a stand-alone facility or located at a hospital or other acute care facility. Participants attend the clinic up to 3 times daily to self-administer injectable OAT under the supervision of qualified health professionals. Patients can be linked with ancillary services housed within the clinic or referred to community services when appropriate. The second model is a supervised injectable OAT program embedded in primary care clinics or harm-reduction programs with linkage to health care professionals and community services. Such a program would operate similar to what has already been described, with patients presenting up to 3 times a daily for their witnessed prescribed medications. The last model described is an emerging pharmacy-based model in which patients receive primary and addiction care at existing clinics, with supervision of injectable OAT provided by appropriately trained pharmacists at select pharmacy locations anywhere from 1 to 3 times daily. This permits a lower intensity of treatment than the comprehensive model and allows for access to injectable OAT in community settings in which a designated clinic may not exist.

As many injectable OAT programs operate in a setting of supervised injection, the potential for additional benefits (beyond opioid-related outcomes) may exist. More specifically, a recent systematic review included 75 articles to examine the effects of supervised injection facilities (SIFs).[37] Briefly, SIF implementation has had a significant impact on fatal overdoses. Beyond no death by overdose having ever been reported at an SIF-designated site, 1 Vancouver-based study also demonstrated a 35% reduction in fatal overdoses in the surrounding area.[38] Beyond this, SIF has been shown to be associated with an improvement on injecting behaviors and consequences, including a reduction in syringe sharing (adjusted odds ratio [aOR] 0.30, 95% CI 0.11–0.82) and syringe reuse (aOR 2.04, 95% CI 1.38–3.01), as well as more regular use of sterile injection materials and requests for education on safer injection practices (aOR 1.47, 95% CI 1.22–1.77).[39–42] Two Vancouver studies also demonstrated SIF to be associated with accessing addiction treatment services, with 18% of SIF users engaging in a detox program, 57% initiating an addiction treatment program, and 23% ceasing injection drug use entirely.[43,44] In the surrounding areas, SIFs have not been shown to be associated with an increase in drug trafficking or crime, but rather a reduction in the daily mean number of people injecting in public, fewer syringes dropped, and less injection-related litter.[45,46] Finally, 4 studies were performed to assess if SIF was a cost-saving system. It was estimated that per year a SIF could prevent 5 to 35 new human immunodeficiency virus (HIV) infections and 3 overdose deaths.[47–50] Over 10 years, this prevention would amount to $14 million

Table 3
Inclusion considerations and precautions for injectable opioid agonist treatment

Inclusion Considerations	Precautions
1. Capacity to consent to and fully understand the goals of treatment	1. Caution should be exercised in prescribing injectable OAT to patients with chronic medical conditions, such as respiratory, hepatic, or renal disease; acute conditions; or a history of recent head injury. Caution is also required for youth and older adults, in whom oral OAT or other forms of treatment may be more appropriate
2. Well-established history of injection drug use with opioids and severe opioid use disorder (DSM-V criteria)	
3. Current opioid injection drug use	
4. Able to attend clinic or pharmacy up to 3 times daily (physically able and reside in proximity)	
5. Able to self-administer (ie, inject via subcutaneous, intravenous, or intramuscular route) medication under supervision	2. The greater inherent risk of overdose with injectable treatments should be individually considered in each case
6. Past experience with appropriately dosed oral agonist treatment in the form of methadone, buprenorphine/naloxone, or slow-release oral morphine, and evidence of regular and ongoing injection opioid use while given these therapies	3. Extreme caution should be exercised in prescribing injectable OAT to patients with existing injection-related infections (eg, septicemia, endocarditis, pneumonia, infective osteomyelitis), and in individuals with coagulation disorders (eg, patients prescribed anticoagulants, severe hepatic disease, deep vein thrombosis); oral treatment options should be preferentially prescribed for such patients
7. Significant risk of medical consequences of injection drug use that would likely benefit from increased health system involvement and engagement in care, or existing significant medical and/or psychiatric comorbidities (eg, HIV positive and antiretroviral nonadherence, severe mental health challenges, history of multiple overdoses)	4. Clinicians should carefully consider drug-drug interactions
8. At least 18 y of age or older	5. Caution should be exercised with pregnant women or women who become pregnant while receiving injectable OAT; this caution should be balanced against the potential harms of denying access to injectable OAT for a pregnant woman who otherwise meets eligibility criteria
9. No coprescribed benzodiazepines and/or other sedatives	
10. Does not fit the criteria for active moderate or severe alcohol use disorder or sedative use disorder	6. Caution should be exercised in prescribing injectable OAT to patients who cannot safely self-administer their medications, due to either inadequate venous access in "low-risk" sites (with consequent injecting in neck or groin veins), or persistently poor injecting technique not remedied by education about intramuscular injection

Abbreviations: DSM-V, Diagnostic and Statistical Manual of Mental Disorders, Fifth Edition; HIV, human immunodeficiency virus; OAT, opioid agonist treatment.

Adapted from British Columbia Centre on Substance Use (BCCSU). Guidance for injectable opioid agonist treatment for opioid use disorder. Available at: http://www.bccsu.ca/wp-content/uploads/2017/10/BC-iOAT-Guidelines-10.2017.pdf; with permission. Accessed Mar 21, 2018.

saved, an increase in 920 years of life, and an avoidance of 1191 new HIV infections and 54 hepatitis C infections.[48]

FUTURE CONSIDERATIONS/SUMMARY

Given that the range of substance use disorders includes individuals who do not benefit from the often-effective medications and psychosocial treatments available, additional strategies to treat and reduce the harms of substances are needed.

Although this review describes 3 such modalities for which evidence exists for effectiveness, the selectivity of participants in these studies, namely individuals with a severe substance use disorder, should be emphasized to ensure promotion of such treatments are recognized to exist beyond the realm of standard medical therapy. Furthermore, it should be highlighted that much of the research presented herein has been conducted in settings outside the United States, where the provision of MAP, SROM, and injectable OAT are regulated and occur in a supportive environment. Despite these treatment approaches being legal in these countries and associated with numerous positive outcomes, many of these programs have been subjected to ongoing scrutiny and criticism. Given the current US opioid epidemic and need to engage the entire spectrum of affected individuals in care, expansion of such newer modalities merits consideration in settings of greatest need with adequate support systems to implement. MAPs are more recent innovations with very early evidence of potential benefit; they merit further examination for the severe end of the AUD spectrum for which standard treatment can seem at times to elude benefit. Although these challenging severely affected individuals can exhaust providers' repeated efforts to address their needs, the proper role of innovative medical care to mitigate harm and consequences of harmful substances merits ongoing study, testing, and description.

ACKNOWLEDGMENTS

The editors thank Nady el-Guebaly, University of Calgary, and Joseph O. Merrill, University of Washington Department of Medicine, for providing a critical review of this article.

REFERENCES

1. Muckle W, Muckle J, Welch V, et al. Managed alcohol as a harm reduction intervention for alcohol addiction in populations at high risk for substance abuse. Cochrane Database Syst Rev 2012;(12):CD006747.
2. Robertson MJ, Zlotnick C, Westerfelt A. Drug use disorders and treatment contact among homeless adults in Alameda County, California. Am J Public Health 1997;87(2):221–8.
3. Fichter M, Quadflieg N. Alcoholism in homeless men in the mid-nineties: results from the Bavarian Public Health Study on homelessness. Eur Arch Psychiatry Clin Neurosci 1999;249(1):34–44.
4. Chin CN, Sullivan K, Wilson SF. A 'snap shot' of the health of homeless people in inner Sydney: St Vincent's Hospital. Aust Health Rev 2011;35(1):52–6.
5. Babidge NC, Buhrich N, Butler T. Mortality among homeless people with schizophrenia in Sydney, Australia: a 10-year follow-up. Acta Psychiatr Scand 2001; 103(2):105–10.
6. Ezard N, Dolan K, Baldry E, et al. Feasibility of a Managed Alcohol Program (MAP) for Sydney's homeless. Canberra: Foundation for Alcohol Research and Education; 2015.
7. Podymow T, Turnbull J, Coyle D, et al. Shelter-based managed alcohol administration to chronically homeless people addicted to alcohol. CMAJ 2006;174(1):45–9.
8. Stockwell T, Pauly B, Chow C, et al. Evaluation of a managed alcohol program in Vancouver, BC: Early findings and reflections on alcohol harm reduction. CARBC Bulletin #9, Victoria, British Columbia: University of Victoria; 2003. Available at: http://www.sunshinecoasthealthcentre.ca/wpcontent/uploads/2014/01/MAPs_EVALUATION_CARBC.pdf. Accessed March 21, 2018.

9. Managed alcohol: housing, health and hospital diversion. Available at: https://www.london.ca/residents/neighbourhoods/Documents/Managed%20Alcohol%20Report.pdf. Accessed March 21, 2018.

10. Wilton P. Shelter "goes wet," opens infirmary to cater to Toronto's homeless. CMAJ 2003;168(7):888.

11. Vallance K, Stockwell T, Pauly B, et al. Do managed alcohol programs change patterns of alcohol consumption and reduce related harm? A pilot study. Harm Reduct J 2016;13(1):13.

12. Pauly B, Stockwell T, Chow C, et al. Towards alcohol harm reduction: preliminary results from an evaluation of a Canadian managed alcohol program. Victoria (Canada): Centre for Addictions Research of British Columbia; 2013.

13. Haney CPT, Muckle WJT. Addressing psychiatric disease in homeless individuals with chronic alcoholism. J Urban Health 2003;80:ii80.

14. Pauly BB, Gray E, Perkin K, et al. Finding safety: a pilot study of managed alcohol program participants' perceptions of housing and quality of life. Harm Reduct J 2016;13(1):15.

15. Evans J, Semogas D, Smalley JG, et al. "This place has given me a reason to care": understanding 'managed alcohol programs' as enabling places in Canada. Health Place 2015;33:118–24.

16. McNeil R, Guirguis-Younger M, Dilley LB, et al. Harm reduction services as a point-of-entry to and source of end-of-life care and support for homeless and marginally housed persons who use alcohol and/or illicit drugs: a qualitative analysis. BMC Public Health 2012;12:312.

17. Beck T, Haasen C, Verthein U, et al. Maintenance treatment for opioid dependence with slow-release oral morphine: a randomized cross-over, non-inferiority study versus methadone. Addiction 2014;109(4):617–26.

18. Falcato L, Beck T, Reimer J, et al. Self-reported cravings for heroin and cocaine during maintenance treatment with slow-release oral morphine compared with methadone: a randomized, crossover clinical trial. J Clin Psychopharmacol 2015;35(2):150–7.

19. Ferri M, Minozzi S, Bo A, et al. Slow-release oral morphine as maintenance therapy for opioid dependence. Cochrane Database Syst Rev 2013;(6):CD009879.

20. Verthein U, Beck T, Haasen C, et al. Mental symptoms and drug use in maintenance treatment with slow-release oral morphine compared to methadone: results of a randomized crossover study. Eur Addict Res 2015;21(2):97–104.

21. Hammig R, Kohler W, Bonorden-Kleij K, et al. Safety and tolerability of slow-release oral morphine versus methadone in the treatment of opioid dependence. J Subst Abuse Treat 2014;47(4):275–81.

22. Kastelic A, Dubajic G, Strbad E. Slow-release oral morphine for maintenance treatment of opioid addicts intolerant to methadone or with inadequate withdrawal suppression. Addiction 2008;103(11):1837–46.

23. Dunlap B, Cifu AS. Clinical management of opioid use disorder. JAMA 2016;316(3):338–9.

24. Wood E, AK, Djurfors C, et al. A guideline for the clinical management of opioid addiction. 2015. Available at: http://www.bccsu.ca/wp-content/uploads/2017/06/BC-OUD-Guidelines_June2017.pdf. Accessed July 20, 2017.

25. Strang J, Groshkova T, Metrevian N. New heroin-assisted treatment: recent evidence and current practices of supervised injectable heroin treatment in Europe and beyond. Available at: http://www.emcdda.europa.eu/system/files/publications/690/Heroin_Insight_335259.pdf. Accessed March 21, 2018.

26. Fischer B, Oviedo-Joekes E, Blanken P, et al. Heroin-assisted Treatment (HAT) a decade later: a brief update on science and politics. J Urban Health 2007;84(4): 552–62.
27. Oviedo-Joekes E, Brissette S, Marsh DC, et al. Diacetylmorphine versus methadone for the treatment of opioid addiction. N Engl J Med 2009; 361(8):777–86.
28. Ferri M, Davoli M, Perucci CA. Heroin maintenance for chronic heroin-dependent individuals. Cochrane Database Syst Rev 2011;(12).
29. Oviedo-Joekes E, Guh D, Brissette S, et al. Hydromorphone compared with diacetylmorphine for long-term opioid dependence: a randomized clinical trial. JAMA Psychiatry 2016;73(5):447–55.
30. Strang J, Groshkova T, Uchtenhagen A, et al. Heroin on trial: systematic review and meta-analysis of randomised trials of diamorphine-prescribing as treatment for refractory heroin addiction. Br J Psychiatry 2015;207(1):5–14.
31. Metrebian N, Carnwath Z, Mott J, et al. Patients receiving a prescription for diamorphine (heroin) in the United Kingdom. Drug Alcohol Rev 2006;25(2): 115–21.
32. Rehm J, Gschwend P, Steffen T, et al. Feasibility, safety, and efficacy of injectable heroin prescription for refractory opioid addicts: a follow-up study. Lancet 2001; 358(9291):1417–20.
33. Demaret I, Quertemont E, Litran G, et al. Loss of treatment benefit when heroin-assisted treatment is stopped after 12 months. J Subst Abuse Treat 2016;69:72–5.
34. van den Brink W, Hendriks VM, Blanken P, et al. Medical prescription of heroin to treatment resistant heroin addicts: two randomised controlled trials. BMJ 2003; 327(7410):310.
35. Oviedo-Joekes E, Brissette S, MacDonald S, et al. Safety profile of injectable hydromorphone and diacetylmorphine for long-term severe opioid use disorder. Drug Alcohol Depend 2017;176:55–62.
36. Injectable opioid agonist treatment for opioid use disorder guidance document. BC Centre on Substance Use. Guidance for injectable opioid agonist treatment for opioid use disorder. Available at: http://www.bccsu.ca/wp-content/uploads/2017/10/BC-iOAT-Guidelines-10.2017.pdf. Accessed March 21, 2018.
37. Potier C, Laprevote V, Dubois-Arber F, et al. Supervised injection services: what has been demonstrated? A systematic literature review. Drug Alcohol Depend 2014;145:48–68.
38. Marshall BD, Milloy MJ, Wood E, et al. Reduction in overdose mortality after the opening of North America's first medically supervised safer injecting facility: a retrospective population-based study. Lancet 2011;377:1429–37.
39. Kerr T, Tyndall M, Li K, et al. Safer injection facility use and syringe sharing in injection drug users. Lancet 2005;366:316–8.
40. Stoltz JA, Wood E, Small W, et al. Changes in injecting practices associated with the use of a medically supervised safer injection facility. J Public Health (Oxf) 2007;29:35–9.
41. Fast D, Small W, Wood E, et al. The perspectives of injection drug users regarding safer injecting education delivered through a supervised injecting facility. Harm Reduct J 2008;5:32.
42. Wood RA, Wood E, Lai C, et al. Nurse delivered safer injection education among a cohort of injection drug users: evidence from the evaluation of Vancouver's supervised injection facility. Int J Drug Policy 2008;19:183–8.
43. Wood E, Tyndall MW, Zhang R, et al. Attendance at supervised injecting facilities and use of detoxification services. N Engl J Med 2006;354:2512–4.

44. DeBeck K, Kerr T, Bird L, et al. Injection drug use cessation and use of North America's first medically supervised safer injecting facility. Drug Alcohol Depend 2011;113:172–6.

45. Wood E, Kerr T, Small W, et al. Changes in public order after the opening of a medically supervised safer injecting facility for illicit injection drug users. CMAJ 2004;171:731–4.

46. Wood E, Tyndall MW, Lai C, et al. Impact of a medically supervised safer injecting facility on drug dealing and other drug-related crime. Subst Abuse Treat Prev Policy 2006;1:13.

47. Andresen MA, Boyd N. A cost-benefit and cost-effectiveness analysis of Vancouver's supervised injection facility. Int J Drug Policy 2010;21:70–6.

48. Bayoumi AM, Zaric GS. The cost-effectiveness of Vancouver's supervised injection facility. CMAJ 2008;179:1143–51.

49. Pinkerton S. Is Vancouver Canada's supervised injection facility cost-saving? Addiction 2010;105:1429–36.

50. Pinkerton SD. How many HIV infections are prevented by Vancouver Canada's supervised injection facility? Int J Drug Policy 2011;22:179–83.

New and Emerging Illicit Psychoactive Substances

Ryan Graddy, MD, Megan E. Buresh, MD, Darius A. Rastegar, MD*

KEYWORDS

- Psychotropic drugs • Novel psychoactive substances • Designer drugs
- Cathinones • Cannabinoids

KEY POINTS

- Globalization and advances in neurochemistry have facilitated the development of novel substances which are often designed to circumvent regulations limiting access to psychoactive drugs.
- Most are in one of 4 broad categories: stimulant, cannabinoid, opioid, or benzodiazepine.
- Some novel stimulants and cannabinoids are potent and users may present with psychosis or seizures.
- Identification of use is hampered by lack of standardized rapid tests to identify these substances and clinicians must rely on history and clinical presentation.
- Treatment of toxicity is generally supportive; naloxone can be used for opioids and flumazenil for benzodiazepine toxicity.

INTRODUCTION

A 28-year-old man is evaluated by emergency medical technicians after a bystander calls 911 for concern about altered mental status. On arrival, the man is slow to respond to questions and has a blank stare. He is brought to the emergency department (ED) where he is lethargic but responds to tactile stimuli. His vital signs and oxygen saturation are within normal limits. On examination, the man has periods of zombielike groaning and moves his arms and legs slowly. Examination is otherwise notable for diffuse diaphoresis, without any focal neurologic deficits. Comprehensive laboratory analysis, including a standard urine immunoassay toxicology test and serum alcohol, is within normal limits without any toxins detected. Seven other patients with similar presentations evaluated in the same hospital on that day also had unremarkable laboratory tests. The patient is placed on an observation unit and his behavior normalizes after approximately 9 hours. On further history obtained later,

Division of Chemical Dependence, Johns Hopkins University School of Medicine, 5200 Eastern Avenue, Suite D5W, Baltimore, MD 21224, USA
* Corresponding author.
E-mail address: drasteg1@jhmi.edu

Med Clin N Am 102 (2018) 697–714
https://doi.org/10.1016/j.mcna.2018.02.010
0025-7125/18/© 2018 Elsevier Inc. All rights reserved.

he reports inhalation of a new substance he purchased recently before the episode. Further analysis identifies a novel synthetic cannabinoid, methyl 2-(1-(4-fluoroben-zyl)-1H-indazole-3-carboxamido)-3-methylbutanoate, in the serum of all 8 patients with similar symptoms.[1]

This case and others illustrate a new and growing phenomenon of individuals presenting with toxicity from psychoactive drugs that have not been seen before. Globalization and advances in neurochemistry have created conditions for the development and dissemination of novel psychoactive substances. Historically, psychoactive drugs have been obtained directly from natural sources (eg, cocaine from coca leaf) or derived from natural sources (eg, heroin derived from morphine in poppy bulbs), but the past few decades have seen the proliferation of drugs that are synthesized de novo without need to access regulated sources or precursors and that, for this reason, are sometimes referred to as designer drugs. Any review of this topic will be limited in that these drugs are new and rapidly evolving. The information on the clinical effects tends to focus on severe presentations and there is limited information on users' typical experience.

Although some of these drugs are brought to North America through traditional smuggling routes from Central and South America, many are marketed through the so-called dark Web (or cryptomarkets) and arrive through the mail.[2] Some arrive through legal channels and are labeled and marketed as not for human consumption or research chemicals to circumvent regulations.

This article provides a brief overview of these drugs, dividing them into 4 broad categories:

1. Stimulants
2. Cannabinoids
3. Opioids
4. Sedatives

Table 1 provides an overview of these substances and **Table 2** provides a summary of the clinical effects, detection, and treatment of exposure.

Stimulants

There are several novel stimulants that have been emerging in the past decades. These can be divided into 4 categories: synthetic cathinones, tryptamines, piperazines, and 2C (2 carbon) phenethylamines.

Synthetic cathinones
Pharmacology Synthetic cathinones are designed to mimic the primary psychoactive substance found in the leaves of the *Catha edulis* plant, colloquially referred to as khat.[3] They are derivatives of phenethylamine and are similar to amphetamines and 3,4-methylenedioxy-N-methylamphetamine (MDMA, or Ecstasy).[4] Cathinones have varying agonist activity on the dopamine, serotonin, and norepinephrine pathways through neurotransmitter reuptake inhibition and stimulation of neurotransmitter release.[5] Contrasting patterns of pathway activation contribute to the clinical effects observed with different compounds: dopamine agonism is associated with psychoactive effects and the addictive potential of cathinones, norepinephrine agonism with sympathomimetic effects, and serotonin agonism with paranoia and hallucinations.[6] The duration of effect is approximately 2 to 4 hours for many synthetic cathinones; 4-methylmethcathinone (mephedrone), the best-studied compound in the class, has a half-life of approximately 2 hours.[3,7]

Table 1
Overview of novel psychoactive substances

NPS Class	Selected Agents	Selected Street Names	Common Routes of Administration	Typical Duration of Effects (h)
Stimulants				
Cathinones	Mephedrone, methylone, MDPV	Bath Salts, Plant Food, research chemicals Meow-Meow, m-CAT, Bubbles, Bounce, Ivory Wave, Vanilla Sky, Energy-1	Nasal insufflation, oral, intravenous	2–4
Tryptamines	AMT, 5-MeO-DiPT	Foxy, Plant Food, research chemicals	Oral, nasal insufflation	6+
Piperazines	BZP, TFMPP	A2, Rapture, Frenzy, Bliss, Charge, herbal Ecstasy, Legal X, and Legal E	Oral	6–8
2C Phenylethylamines	2C-B	Nexus, Afro, Erox, Performax	Oral, nasal insufflation	8
Cannabinoids	Naphthoylindoles (JWH-018, JWH-073 and JWH-398), naphthylmethylindoles, naphthoylpyrroles, naphthylmethylindenes, phenylacetylindoles (ie, benzoylindoles, eg, JWH-250), cyclohexylphenols (eg, CP 47,497) classic cannabinoids (eg, HU-210)	Spice, K2, Scooby Snax, Mojo, Yucatan, Geeked Up, Smacked, Fake Weed, Trippy, Bad Guy, Green Giant, Ice Dragon, AK-47	Smoking, oral, liquid inhalation	2–5
Opioids	Carfentanil, ocfentanil, acetyl fentanyl, furanyl fentanyl, U-47700, AH-7921, and MT-45	Drop Dead, Serial Killer, Gray Death, Pink	Injection, nasal insufflation	2–8
Designer benzodiazepines	Clonazolam, diclazepam, etizolam, flubromazepam, flubromazolam, phenazepam, pyrazolam	Research chemicals	Oral	4–12

Abbreviations: AMT, alpha-methyltryptamine; BZP, N-benzylpiperazine; 2C-B, 4-bromo-2,5-dimethoxyphenethylamine; MDPV, methylenedioxypyrovalerone; 5-MeO-DiPT, 5-Methoxy-N,N-diisopropyltryptamine; JWH, John W. Huffman, an inventor of this class of compounds; NPS, novel psychoactive substances; TFMPP, 1-(3-trifluoromethyl-phenyl) piperazine.

Table 2
Overview of toxicity, testing, and treatment of novel psychoactive substances

NPS Class	Commonly Reported Toxicities	Urine Drug Testing	Treatment of Acute Toxicity
Stimulants			
Cathinones	Agitation, tachycardia, hypertension, restlessness, sweating, hyperthermia, paranoia, visual and auditory hallucinations, delusions, delirium, serotonin syndrome	Standard assay negative or false-positive for PCP	Supportive: benzodiazepines for agitation/anxiety; atypical antipsychotics for refractory agitation/psychosis
Tryptamines	Visual hallucinations, agitation, tachycardia, hyperthermia, delirium, flashbacks	Standard assay negative	Supportive: benzodiazepines for agitation/anxiety; atypical antipsychotics for refractory agitation/psychosis
Piperazines	Seizures, tachycardia, hypertension, hallucinations, insomnia, anxiety, headaches, nausea, tremors, diaphoresis, dizziness, palpitations, dyspnea, paranoia, hyponatremia, delirium, serotonin syndrome	Standard assay negative; BZP may cause false-positive for amphetamine	Supportive: benzodiazepines a mainstay because of high seizure risk
2C phenylethylamines	Hallucinations, tremor, diaphoresis, vision changes, nausea, vomiting, dizziness, seizures, serotonin syndrome, delirium	Standard assay negative	Supportive: benzodiazepines for agitation/anxiety; atypical antipsychotics for refractory agitation/psychosis
Cannabinoids	Agitation, nausea, tachycardia, lethargy, psychosis, seizures	Standard THC assay negative; specific assays for earlier-generation drugs available	Supportive: benzodiazepines for agitation/anxiety; atypical antipsychotics for refractory agitation/psychosis
Opioids	Sedation, respiratory depression	Fentanyl assay may be positive for related agents	Naloxone (2 mg IV/IM or 4 mg IN)
Designer benzodiazepines	Sedation, slurred speech, ataxia	Positive for benzodiazepines	Flumazenil (0.2 mg IV)

Abbreviations: BZP, N-benzylpiperazine; IV, intravenously; IM, intramuscularly; IN, intranasally; PCP, phencyclidine; THC, tetrahydrocannabinol.

Epidemiology Synthetic cathinones are often marketed as Bath Salts because of their white crystalline powder appearance. There are many nicknames for individual compounds; some are listed in **Table 1**. Mephedrone was synthesized in 1929 but does not seem to have been used recreationally until the early 2000s when it reappeared among European dance club populations.[4] Slang terms for this compound include 4-MMC, Meow-Meow, m-CAT, Bubbles, and Bounce. Other synthetic cathinones used widely in the United States include 3,4-methylenedioxymethcathinone (methylone; bk-MDMA) and 3,4-methylenedioxypyrovalerone (MDPV; Ivory Wave, Vanilla Sky, Energy-1).[8,9]

Although synthetic cathinones were previously unregulated, a series of laws in the United Kingdom, United States, and elsewhere placed increasing restrictions on them in the early 2010s. The US Synthetic Drug Abuse Prevention Act of 2012 placed several synthetic cathinones, including mephedrone and MDPV, into the Schedule I category (no accepted medical use and high potential for misuse); subsequent Drug Enforcement Administration (DEA) regulations have expanded the number of synthetic cathinones in this category and no compounds in this class are approved for therapeutic use.[10]

Data on the prevalence of synthetic cathinone use are limited, but consumption seems to be around 1% or less among adults in the developed world.[11–13] Usage seems to be highest among adolescents and adults less than the age of 25 years. In some subpopulations, usage rates are substantially higher; for example, in the dance music scene in the United Kingdom, where rates of use may be higher than 40%, and among some men who have sex with men.[14,15]

Synthetic cathinones are often used with other psychoactive substances; one study found that 89% of mephedrone users also drank alcohol with their initial mephedrone use.[15] Use of other substances often occurs in an attempt to heighten the cathinone effects, alter the comedown, or enhance sexual performance. Common intentionally coadministered substances include heroin, cocaine, cannabis, ketamine, MDMA, methamphetamine, sildenafil, and gamma-hydroxybutyric acid (GHB).[4,6,15] In addition, many coadministered substances are ingested unintentionally, particularly among individuals using so-called party pills.[16]

The most common method of administration for synthetic cathinones is nasal insufflation. However, oral or intravenous use is common and there are reports of rectal, intramuscular, and subcutaneous administration as well.[6] Redosing at intervals of 1 to 2 hours is widespread given the short duration of action.[7]

Clinical effects Synthetic cathinones were initially developed as substitutes for other stimulants and MDMA, and have several shared clinical effects. The most common reason for presentation to EDs and poison control centers after ingestion is agitation.[11] Acute intoxication often presents with other signs and symptoms of sympathetic nervous system activation, including tachycardia, hypertension, restlessness, diaphoresis, and hyperthermia.[15,17,18] Psychiatric effects may include euphoria, paranoia, visual and auditory hallucinations, and delusions.[4,15,19] Serotonin syndrome has been reported in some cases,[19,20] as have seizures[21] and rhabdomyolysis.[22]

Data detailing the health effects of chronic cathinone use are limited; studies of long-term khat users suggest increased rates of psychiatric symptoms, including psychosis, as well as myocardial infarction.[23] Tolerance occurs with repeated use, and many users show behaviors meeting criteria for substance use disorder.[15,24] Withdrawal symptoms from cathinones are similar to those seen in other stimulants, including fatigue, nasal congestion, irritability, depression, anxiety, and insomnia.[15,24]

Causes of death associated with synthetic cathinones include metabolic acidosis, acute kidney injury, acute liver failure, disseminated intravascular coagulation, hyperthermia, arrhythmia, hyponatremia (possibly mediated by vasopressin release related to serotonin reuptake inhibition), and agitated delirium leading to injury.[11,25,26]

Evaluation Evaluation of suspected exposure must rely on the history and clinical presentation. Agitation, delirium, and sympathetic nervous system activation in the setting of unknown ingestion should heighten suspicion for cathinone exposure. Assessment for rhabdomyolysis is important in these scenarios given the apparent increased risk with cathinone ingestion.[22] Because of the frequency of simultaneous use of other psychoactive substances, suspicion for use should be high among individuals with other substance misuse as well.

There are no commercially available drug tests to identify synthetic cathinones.[27,28] Accurate techniques for identification of these compounds depend on liquid chromatography–mass spectrometry (LC-MS) testing but take too long to be clinically useful.[29,30] In some cases, cathinones may cross react with phencyclidine (PCP) enzyme-linked immunoassays (EIA) and result in false-positive results.[31]

Management Treatment of cathinone toxicity is supportive. In a 2011 US study of hospital evaluations for suspected synthetic cathinone toxicity, 49% of patients were treated in the ED and released, 21% admitted to an intensive care unit, 12% admitted to behavioral health or psychiatry, and 12% lost to follow-up.[32] Benzodiazepines are commonly used for management of agitation and seizures, and help with hyperthermia as well.[5] In some cases, cooling therapies are needed for hyperthermia; isotonic fluids for volume depletion, rhabdomyolysis, acute kidney injury, and disseminated intravascular coagulation; and fluid restriction and hypertonic saline to treat severe euvolemic hyponatremia.[11,30,33] Antipsychotics should be avoided in the setting of acute psychosis, because they are known to lower the seizure threshold and can exacerbate the danger of muscle injury and rhabdomyolysis because of the risk of extrapyramidal symptoms and neuroleptic malignant syndrome.[22,34,35] In 1 case, cathinone-induced serotonin syndrome was treated successfully with benzodiazepines and the serotonin antagonist cyproheptadine.[36]

Synthetic tryptamines
Pharmacology Tryptamine is a natural monoamine alkaloid found in plants, animals, fungi, and microbes. Serotonin is a natural derivative of tryptamine, and compounds in this class are typically serotonin receptor agonists.[37] Mushrooms containing psilocin and psilocybin, as well as ayahuasca, a tea containing naturally occurring dimethyltryptamine (DMT), contain tryptamines and are ingested for their hallucinogenic effects.[38,39]

Synthetic tryptamines have been used recreationally since at least the 1960s. Alpha-methyltryptamine (AMT) was initially developed as an antidepressant but was found to have limited medicinal value and intense hallucinogenic properties.[40] 5-Methoxy-N,N-diisopropyltryptamine (5-MeO-DiPT), commonly marketed as Foxy, has been used in the United States since 1999.[41] Both of these tryptamines have been listed as Schedule I substances since 2003.

All synthetic tryptamines are agonists at 5-hydroxytryptamine (5-HT) 2A receptors through serotonin reuptake inhibition, direct receptor agonism, or both.[42] Some tryptamines also interact with norepinephrine receptors, but they typically do not affect the dopaminergic system.[43]

Epidemiology The 2009 to 2013 US National Survey on Drug Use and Health identified psychedelic tryptamines as among the most commonly self-reported novel psychoactive substances used, with rates increasing from 12.9% to 28.8% of all novel psychoactive substances users over this 5-year period.[12] Users tend to be young and male; 1 US study found that 86% of patients seen at ED visits related to use were male, and 86% were less than 21 years of age.[44]

Administration is typically oral or by nasal insufflation, although smoking, injection, and rectal use have been reported.[45] Mixing with other substances for synergy or to avoid adverse effects is common, and concomitant administration of monoamine oxidase inhibitors seems to be widespread in order to potentiate the tryptamine effects.[45]

Clinical effects The onset of effects after oral tryptamine ingestion is typically rapid, within 30 minutes, and can last for 6 hours or more.[46] Visual hallucinations predominate, and many users describe a spiritual experience with euphoria and increased energy. Agitation, tachycardia, and hyperthermia have also been described.[40,41] No obvious tolerance or dependence has been documented with synthetic tryptamines.

Deaths related to synthetic tryptamines have been reported. In one case, a young man walked out into traffic after using N,N-diallyl-5-methoxytryptamine (5-MeO-DALT), and was fatally hit by a car.[37] In another case, fatal neurotoxicity and acute heart failure were attributed to rectal administration of Foxy.[47]

Evaluation and management Evaluation of suspected tryptamine toxicity must rely on clinical evaluation and history. Standard urine EIA drug tests do not detect synthetic tryptamines; individual compounds can be identified through LC-MS testing, but this takes too long to be clinically useful when acute toxicity is suspected.

Treatment of tryptamine toxicity is supportive. In some cases, sedation and intravenous hydration may be required. Benzodiazepines are often used to help with agitation. Activated charcoal may be helpful in the setting of oral ingestion.[45]

Piperazines
Pharmacology Piperazines are a class of compounds with stimulant and hallucinogenic properties with no naturally occurring counterpart. Two major structural groups exist: N-benzylpiperazine (BZP; a single drug) and N-phenylpiperazine [including several drugs, the best documented of which is 1-(3-trifluoromethyl-phenyl) piperazine (TFMPP)].

Piperazines are commonly marketed as alternatives to MDMA. BZP has been listed as a US Schedule I substance since 2002, and TFMPP is currently not assigned a controlled status by the DEA. BZP centrally stimulates dopamine and norepinephrine receptors, whereas TFMPP preferentially agonizes serotonin receptors and inhibits reuptake.[48]

Epidemiology Users of piperazines are predominantly young men[49–51] and use seems common in electronic dance clubs and raves. These drugs are almost exclusively used in combinations with other piperazines or other illicit and legal substances as so-called club drugs or party pills.[49,52]

There are limited data available on the prevalence of piperazine use. Evidence suggests that, in some countries with strict enforcement of laws prohibiting piperazines, rates of use have decreased substantially; in New Zealand, recent use of the piperazine BZP decreased from 15% to 3% following official prohibition in 2008.[53] However, the growth of the dark Web and other online markets for sale of illicit synthetic substances across international borders in recent years has likely contributed to an increase in use in some populations, including those without previous experience. A recent study of new psychoactive substances found in wastewater in major Chinese cities showed BZP (strictly illegal nationwide) detected at 100% of sewage treatment plants evaluated.[54]

Clinical effects Administration of piperazines is typically oral, although intravenous use has been reported.[52] The onset of effects can take up to 2 hours, and last for 6 to 8 hours. BZP ingestion has been associated with euphoria and sympathomimetic effects, described as 10 to 20 times less potent than amphetamine.[55] TFMPP ingestion commonly causes confusion and hallucinations.[51,56] Shared effects of piperazines and those seen with BZP/TFMPP simultaneous ingestion include insomnia, anxiety, headaches, nausea, tremor, diaphoresis, dizziness, palpitations, dyspnea, and paranoia.[49,55,56] Hyponatremia and serotonin syndrome have been described.[57] Seizures have also been associated with piperazine use; in one study of possible BZP-related poisonings at a New Zealand hospital, more than 18% of patients had seizures associated with use.[58] It is important to remember that piperazines are commonly used in party pills as combinations with other piperazines and often including other substances, including MDMA and cocaine.[49,52] Case reports of mortality related to piperazine ingestion have generally involved other drugs, including alcohol, and often result from accidental injuries.[59]

Evaluation and management As with other synthetic stimulants, evaluation of piperazine toxicity is based on history and clinical assessment. Standard urine EIA drug tests do not identify piperazines; however, BZP may trigger false-positives for amphetamines.[52] Treatment of piperazine toxicity is similar to management of synthetic cathinone toxicity, with general supportive measures, benzodiazepines for agitation or seizures, and blood pressure control with close monitoring.[57] Antipsychotic medications are second-line agents for agitation but should be given with caution because of the potential worsening of hyperthermia and cardiac arrhythmias.[48]

Two-carbon phenethylamines
Pharmacology The 2C drugs are a subgroup of phenethylamines, the class of compounds with the same basic structure as catecholamines, amphetamines, and cathinones. The name 2C is derived from the characteristic 2 carbon atoms between a benzene ring and a terminal amine group. Compounds in this class have an affinity for 5-HT2 receptors and occasionally alpha-adrenergic receptors as well, leading to hallucinogenic and sympathomimetic effects.[60] Metabolism occurs through monoamine oxidase, and monoamine oxidase inhibitors may potentiate or heighten the effects of 2C compounds. 2C compounds have been listed as US Schedule I substances since 1994. Although this class of substance has been in use for several decades, novel compounds continue to emerge.[61]

Epidemiology Users of 2C drugs are typically young men; raves and dance parties are common settings of use.[62] A nationally representative US survey found that self-reported lifetime use of psychedelic phenethylamines (of which the most commonly used compounds were from the 2C series) increased from 9.7% to 31.9% among individuals who had used any novel psychoactive substances from 2009 to 2013.[12] Lifetime prevalence of 2C series compounds in US adults was estimated at 0.2% in 2013.

2C compounds are commonly used in combination with other substances; one survey of recent users in Spain found that 69% had mixed MDMA with a 2C compound, and significant numbers also used alcohol and marijuana.[63] Administration is most commonly oral or by nasal insufflation.[58]

Clinical effects The onset of effects for 2C substances is rapid. The most widely studied compound in the 2C class, 4-bromo-2,5-dimethoxyphenethylamine (2C-B), produces effects approximately 30 minutes after oral ingestion, peaks around 2 hours, and lasts up to 8 hours.[64] Reported desirable effects include changes in tactile, auditory, and visual perception; euphoria; and hallucinations. Negative effects include trembling, sweating, difficulty seeing straight, nausea, vomiting, and dizziness.[65,66] The subjective experience of users seems similar to that of ayahuasca[39] (a hallucinogenic traditional brew used ritually in the northwest Amazon containing a 5-HT_{2A} agonist), salvia, and LSD (lysergic acid diethylamide). Seizures, serotonin syndrome, and agitated delirium have all been observed in the setting of use, and deaths have been reported.[66–68]

Evaluation and management As with the synthetic cathinones and other novel psychoactive substances, evaluation of suspected toxicity must rely on history and clinical assessment; standard urine EIA drug testing does not identify 2C compounds and LC-MS testing can be used for definitive detection. Timely diagnosis requires a high level of clinical suspicion in the appropriate setting. Treatment involves supportive care and may require rapid sedation, fluid resuscitation, and reduction of hyperthermia. Benzodiazepines are preferred agents for sedation given their antiepileptic activity; antipsychotics have also been used effectively.[59,69]

Synthetic Cannabinoids

Pharmacology

First developed in research laboratories in the 1960s to study the endocannabinoid system, synthetic cannabinoids emerged as drugs of illicit use in 2008.[69] These substances are structurally very different from Δ^9-tetrahydrocannabinol (Δ^9-THC), the cannabinoid found in marijuana. Synthetic cannabinoids are potent, full agonists of the cannabinoid type-1 (CB-1) receptors found in the central nervous system (CNS), lungs, liver, and kidneys,[70] and weaker agonists of CB-2 receptors found in immune system and at low levels in CNS.[71] They are 2 to 100 times more potent agonists of the CB-1 receptor than THC, which is only a partial agonist of CB-1.[72] Binding of CB-1 induces the classic cannabinoid tetrad of hypothermia, analgesia, cataplexy, and locomotor suppression[72] with psychoactive effects achieved via modulation of glutamate and GABA (gamma-aminobutyric acid) neurotransmitters.[2] Chronic activation of CB-2 in mice leads to dysregulation of 5-HT_{2A} receptors and has been associated with anxiety and psychosis, which are common side effects of synthetic cannabinoids not seen with THC.[73] The greater toxicity of synthetic cannabinoids compared with marijuana is thought to be caused by their greater agonist potency for CB-1 as well as lack of cannabidiol, terpenes, and other constituents of cannabis that may balance some effects.[71] They have multiple downstream metabolites that retain high affinity at CB-1 and CB-2, further potentiating their effects.[71,73]

Epidemiology

Often referred to as Spice and K2, synthetic cannabinoids are sold under hundreds of names; **Table 1** lists some of these.[2] They are dissolved in solvent and sprayed onto inert plant material, which is saturated and dried, leaving highly variable amounts of the substance.[69] They are marketed to consumers as safe and legal alternatives to marijuana, but are in fact much more potent.[69] They are sold in gas stations, convenience stores, marijuana paraphernalia stores, and over the Internet in addition to traditional black market dealers.[69] They are often labeled "Not for human consumption" to avoid government regulations. Synthetic cannabinoids are most commonly smoked or ingested,[74] but can also be administered by liquid inhalation and smoking liquid via refillable vaporizers.[75] As of July 2016, the DEA had banned 25 synthetic cannabinoids; however, laboratories quickly synthesize compounds with minor structural adjustments to evade scheduling laws.[69,76]

Synthetic cannabinoids increased in popularity as so-called legal highs, often viewed as safe and legal alternatives to marijuana.[70] Use is most common among young men and associated with cannabis, alcohol, and other illicit drugs.[72,77,78] It is also popular among military personnel and athletes seeking to avoid detection through drug tests.[72] In a survey of US high school students, use peaked at 11.9% in 2011 and has declined steadily since the 2012 DEA ban, to 4.8% in 2015, likely because of increased awareness of risk.[77,79] Despite the decline in reported use, clusters of synthetic cannabinoid intoxication (sometimes referred to as zombie outbreaks) seem to be increasing and have been reported in many US cities,[1,76,80,81] a likely result of the higher potency of later-generation compounds.

Clinical effects

Acute intoxication with synthetic cannabinoids produces cannabis-like effects that are more severe than those of marijuana.[70,82] Users are 30 times more likely to seek emergency services than marijuana users[83] and have higher rates of psychosis, agitation, and aggression.[84] Effects are seen within 10 minutes of smoking and peak at an average of 2 to 5 hours; most effects resolve in less than 24 hours,[70] although they may persist for days in severe cases.[85] In a systematic review of published cases, the most common effects were tachycardia (37%–77%), nausea (13%–94%), agitation (19%–32%), and lethargy (19%–32%).[86] Although most cases are mild, severe toxicity has been reported and includes seizures,[87] acute kidney injury,[88] rhabdomyolysis,[89] and ischemic stroke.[90] Adverse cardiac effects include myocardial ischemia,[91] bradycardia,[92] heart block,[93] and corrected QT prolongation.[94] Mortalities are 0.5% to 1% among US poison control calls.[73]

Little is known about the chronic effects of synthetic cannabinoid use in humans. Animal studies suggest that chronic exposure during adolescence can lead to behavioral deficits and increased anxiety as adults,[70] as well as increased vulnerability to substance use disorder and depression.[94] The withdrawal syndrome is marked by agitation, irritability, anxiety, mood swings, and tachycardia, and is more severe than withdrawal from marijuana.[95–97]

Evaluation

Evaluation of suspected exposure depends on history and clinical presentation. Synthetic cannabinoids are not detected in standard urine drug tests for THC metabolites. Although commercial testing for older synthetic cannabinoids is available, these tests do not detect most newer compounds.[98,99] LC-MS can detect a wider spectrum of synthetic cannabinoids, but it is too slow to be clinically useful and is limited by lack of reference samples. Exposure should be suspected in substance users who report marijuana use but present with more extreme psychosis and agitation.

Management

There is no reversal agent for synthetic cannabinoids and care for acute toxicity is supportive. Intravenous fluids should be given to prevent acute kidney injury and rhabdomyolysis. Benzodiazepines are first-line agents for management of anxiety and agitation. Atypical antipsychotics such as quetiapine may be used as second-line treatment of severe agitation and psychosis; however, caution should be used with medications that decrease seizure threshold because synthetic cannabinoids are associated with seizures.[83] Withdrawal may require inpatient treatment and can also be managed with benzodiazepines and antipsychotics.[97]

Opioids

Pharmacology

The past decade has seen an increase in the distribution and use of illicitly manufactured fentanyl and fentanyl-related compounds, including carfentanil, ocfentanil, acetyl fentanyl, and furanyl fentanyl.[100] There are several other synthetic opioids that have been reported, including U-47700, AH-7921, and MT-45.[101] The pharmacologic effects are similar to those of other opioids and the potency varies depending on the substance. Some are highly potent; compared with morphine, acetyl fentanyl is 16 times more potent, fentanyl and furanyl fentanyl are 50 to 100 times more potent, ocfentanil is 200 times more potent,[102] and carfentanil is 10,000 times more potent.[103] The potency of U-47700 is about 7.5 times that of morphine.[101]

Epidemiology

Fentanyl-related compounds are often sold as heroin (or mixed with heroin) or in the form of counterfeit pills, which resemble oxycodone, Xanax, or Norco.[100] Most of the epidemiologic data come from law enforcement seizures. In 2016, the DEA reported that the most commonly seized synthetic opioids were fentanyl, followed by furanyl fentanyl, acetyl fentanyl, and U-47700.[104]

Clinical effects

There are limited data on the clinical effects of these substances, but they seem to be similar to those of other opioids: euphoria, analgesia, and respiratory depression.[101] The main difference is the potency, which may lead to an increased risk of overdose, particularly when individuals are not aware of what they are using, because they are often sold as heroin.

Evaluation

Opioid exposure should be suspected in anyone presenting with the typical signs and symptoms: decreased level of consciousness, respiratory depression, and miosis. These substances are not detected in standard urine drug screens. Fentanyl can be detected by a separate EIA drug test and many of the fentanyl-related compounds cross react with this test, but they cannot be distinguished from fentanyl through this method.[101] They can be identified through LC-MS testing, but this takes more time and most laboratories do not have the reference materials needed to do this; these may become available in the future.

Management

The standard treatment of intoxication or overdose with these agents is the opioid antagonist naloxone, given intravenously (IV), intramuscularly (IM), or intranasally (IN). The usual dose for treatment of opioid overdose is 0.4 mg IV/IM; however, it has been reported that overdoses with the more potent agents often require higher doses of naloxone and it is recommended that 2 mg IV/IM or 4 mg IN be used.[101] Among patients who have an opioid use disorder, the most effective treatment is opioid agonist therapy with buprenorphine or methadone; the opioid antagonist naltrexone is another option.

Sedatives

Pharmacology

There are several so-called designer benzodiazepines that have become available in illicit drug markets in recent years. Some of these are available by prescription in other countries; others are classified as research chemicals. **Table 1** provides a list of some of these drugs.

Epidemiology
There is very little information on the epidemiology of use of these drugs. The DEA "Emerging Threat Report" from the first quarter of 2017 identified 7 instances of etizolam contributing to drug seizures, which is significantly lower that of many other novel psychoactive substances.[105] In an analysis of blood samples from drugged drivers and suspected drug offenders in Norway, designer benzodiazepines were detected in 0.3% of cases.[106]

Clinical effects
There is very little information on the clinical effects of these drugs. It would be expected that they would have many of the same effects of other benzodiazepines, but there may be differences in relative anxiolytic or hypnotic effects, as well as onset and duration of action.

Evaluation and management
Benzodiazepine toxicity should be suspected in anyone presenting with a decreased level of consciousness or confusion and concern for ingestion. Designer benzodiazepines may be detected in standard EIA drug tests but cannot be differentiated from other benzodiazepines.[107]

The standard treatment of benzodiazepine toxicity is supportive measures, including intravenous fluids and ventilator support, if needed. A benzodiazepine antagonist, flumazenil, can be given IV in serious cases. There are limited data on its use for designer benzodiazepine overdose, but it has been reported to be effective in some case reports.[108]

FUTURE CONSIDERATIONS/SUMMARY

Novel psychoactive substances are a growing problem and require ongoing vigilance to deal with the adverse consequences of use. Clinicians need to be aware of the substances being used in their community; the National Institute of Drug Abuse (NIDA) publishes a periodic update on emerging trends that is available online (https://www.drugabuse.gov/drugs-abuse/emerging-trends-alerts). Clinicians also need to question patients about use of these substances, particularly among young people who use other drugs and those presenting with agitation, seizures, or other possible complications. Rapid tests are needed to identify these drugs and to aid in the evaluation and treatment of acutely ill patients. Counseling users on the realistic risks of these substances is likely the best initial approach; more research is needed on effective management strategies.

ACKNOWLEDGMENTS

The authors wish to thank Paul Christopher, Brown University, for providing a critical review of this article.

REFERENCES

1. Adams AJ, Banister SD, Irizarry L, et al. "Zombie" outbreak caused by the synthetic cannabinoid AMB-FUBINACA in New York. N Engl J Med 2017;376(3):235–42.
2. Kemp AM, Clark MS, Dobbs T, et al. Top 10 facts you need to know about synthetic cannabinoids: not so nice spice. Am J Med 2016;129:240–4.
3. Valente MJ, Guedes De Pinho P, De Lourdes Bastos M, et al. Khat and synthetic cathinones: a review. Arch Toxicol 2014;88:15–45.

4. Papaseit E, Molto J, Muga R, et al. Clinical pharmacology of the synthetic cathinone mephedrone. Curr Top Behav Neurosci 2017;32:313–32.
5. Schifano F, Orsolini L, Duccio Papanti G, et al. Novel psychoactive substances of interest for psychiatry. World Psychiatry 2015;14:15–26.
6. Zawilska JB. Mephedrone and other cathinones. Curr Opin Psychiatry 2014;27:256–62.
7. Capriola M. Synthetic cathinone abuse. Clin Pharmacol Adv Appl 2013;5:109–15.
8. 3,4-Methylenedioxypyrovalerone (MDPV). (2013). [online] Drug Enforcement Administration Office of Diversion Control. Available at: https://www.deadiversion.usdoj.gov/drug_chem_info/mdpv.pdf. Accessed July 18, 2017.
9. 3,4-Methylenedioxymethcathinone (Methylone). (2013). [online] Drug Enforcement Administration Office of Diversion Control. Available at: https://www.deadiversion.usdoj.gov/drug_chem_info/methylone.pdf. Accessed July 18, 2017.
10. 112th Congress. Synthetic Drug Control Act of 2012, S3190. Senate, Washington, DC, May 16, 2012.
11. Karila L, Megarbane B, Cottencin O, et al. Synthetic cathinones: a new public health problem. Curr Neuropharmacol 2015;13:12–20.
12. Palamar JJ, Martins SS, Su MK, et al. Self-reported use of novel psychoactive substances in a US nationally representative survey: prevalence, correlates, and a call for new survey methods to prevent underreporting. Drug Alcohol Depend 2015;156:112–9.
13. Patrick ME, O'Malley PM, Kloska DD, et al. Novel psychoactive substance use by US adolescents: characteristics associated with use of synthetic cannabinoids and synthetic cathinones. Drug Alcohol Rev 2016;35(5):586–90.
14. Winstock AR, Mitcheson LR, Deluca P, et al. Mephedrone, new kid for the chop? Addiction 2011;106:154–61.
15. Winstock A, Mitcheson L, Ramsey J, et al. Mephedrone: use, subjective effects and health risks. Addiction 2011;106:1991–6.
16. Palamar JJ, Salamone A, Vincenti M, et al. Detection of "bath salts" and other novel psychoactive substances in hair samples of ecstasy/MDMA/"Molly" users. Drug Alcohol Depend 2016;161:200–5.
17. Dargan PI, Sedefov R, Wood DM. The pharmacology and toxicology of the synthetic cathinone mephedrone (4-methylmethcathinone). Drug Test Anal 2011;3:454–63.
18. Papaseit E, Pérez-Mañá C, Mateus J-A, et al. Human pharmacology of mephedrone in comparison with MDMA. Neuropsychopharmacology 2016;41:2704–13.
19. Joksovic P, Mellos N, van Wattum PJ, et al. "Bath salts"–induced psychosis and serotonin toxicity. J Clin Psychiatry 2012;73:1125.
20. Miotto K, Striebel J, Cho AK, et al. Clinical and pharmacological aspects of bath salt use: a review of the literature and case reports. Drug Alcohol Depend 2013;132:1–12.
21. Wood DM, Greene SL, Dargan PI. Clinical pattern of toxicity associated with the novel synthetic cathinone mephedrone. Emerg Med J 2011;28:280–2.
22. O'Connor AD, Padilla-Jones A, Gerkin RD, et al. Prevalence of rhabdomyolysis in sympathomimetic toxicity: a comparison of stimulants. J Med Toxicol 2015;11(2):195–200.
23. Al-Habori M. The potential adverse effects of habitual use of *Catha edulis* (khat). Expert Opin Drug Saf 2005;4(6):1145–54.

24. Carhart-Harris RL, King LA, Nutt DJ. A web-based survey on mephedrone. Drug Alcohol Depend 2011;118:19–22.

25. Karila L, Billieux J, Benyamina A, et al. The effects and risks associated to mephedrone and methylone in humans: a review of the preliminary evidences. Brain Res Bull 2016;126:61–7.

26. Banks ML, Worst TJ, Rusyniak DE, et al. Synthetic cathinones ("Bath salts"). J Emerg Med 2014;46:632–42.

27. Ellefsen KN, Anizan S, Castaneto MS, et al. Validation of the only commercially available immunoassay for synthetic cathinones in urine: Randox Drugs of Abuse V Biochip Array Technology. Drug Test Anal 2015;6:728–38.

28. Moeller KE, Kissack JC, Atayee RS, et al. Clinical interpretation of urine drug tests: what clinicians need to know about urine drug screens. Mayo Clin Proc 2016;92:774–96.

29. Concheiro M, Anizan S, Ellefsen K, et al. Simultaneous quantification of 28 synthetic cathinones and metabolites in urine by liquid chromatography-high resolution mass spectrometry. Anal Bioanal Chem 2013;405:9437–48.

30. Swortwood MJ, Boland DM, Decaprio AP. Determination of 32 cathinone derivatives and other designer drugs in serum by comprehensive LC-QQQ-MS/MS analysis. Anal Bioanal Chem 2013;405:1383–97.

31. Penders TM, Gestring RE, Vilensky DA, et al. Intoxication delirium following use of synthetic cathinone derivatives. Am J Drug Alcohol Abuse 2012;38:616–7.

32. Spiller HA, Ryan ML, Weston RG, et al. Clinical experience with and analytical confirmation of "bath salts" and "legal highs" (synthetic cathinones) in the United States. Clin Toxicol 2011;49:499–505.

33. Boulanger-Gobeil C, St-Onge M, Laliberté M, et al. Seizures and hyponatremia related to ethcathinone and methylone poisoning. J Med Toxicol 2012;8:59–61.

34. Jerry J, Collins G, Streem D. Synthetic legal intoxicating drugs: the emerging "incense" and "bath salt" phenomenon. Cleve Clin J Med 2012;79:258–64.

35. Kersten BP, McLaughlin ME. Toxicology and management of novel psychoactive drugs. J Pharm Pract 2015;28:50–65.

36. Mugele J, Nañagas KA, Tormoehlen LM. Serotonin syndrome associated with MDPV use: a case report. Ann Emerg Med 2012;60:100–2.

37. Corkery JM, Durkin E, Elliott S, et al. The recreational tryptamine 5-MeO-DALT (N,N-diallyl-5-methoxytryptamine): a brief review. Prog Neuropsychopharmacol Biol Psychiatry 2012;39:259–62.

38. Tittarelli R, Mannocchi G, Pantano F, et al. Recreational use, analysis and toxicity of tryptamines. Curr Neuropharmacol 2015;13:26–46.

39. dos Santos RG, Bouso JC, Hallak JEC. Ayahuasca, dimethyltryptamine, and psychosis: a systematic review of human studies. Ther Adv Psychopharmacol 2017;7:141–57.

40. Boland DM, Andollo W, Hime GW, et al. Fatality due to acute alpha-methyltryptamine intoxication. J Anal Toxicol 2005;29:394–7.

41. Drug Enforcement Administration Office of Diversion Control. 3,4-Methylenedioxypyrovalerone (MDPV). (2013). [online] Drug Enforcement Administration Office of Diversion Control. Available at: https://www.deadiversion.usdoj.gov/drug_chem_info/methylone.pdf. Accessed July 18, 2017.

42. Scherbaum N, Schifano F, Bonnet U. New psychoactive substances (NPS) - a challenge for the addiction treatment services. Pharmacopsychiatry 2017;50(3):116–22.

43. Rickli A, Moning OD, Hoener MC, et al. Receptor interaction profiles of novel psychoactive tryptamines compared with classic hallucinogens. Eur Neuropsychopharmacol 2016;26(8):1327–37.

44. Maxwell JC. Psychoactive substances—some new, some old: a scan of the situation in the U.S. Drug Alcohol Depend 2014;134:71–7.

45. Araujo AM, Carvalho F, Bastos Mde L, et al. The hallucinogenic world of tryptamines: an updated review. Arch Toxicol 2015;89:1151–73.

46. Meyer MR. New psychoactive substances: an overview on recent publications on their toxicodynamics and toxicokinetics. Arch Toxicol 2016;90:2421–44.

47. Tanaka E, Kamata T, Katagi M. A fatal poisoning with 5-methoxy-N,N-diisopropyltryptamine, foxy. Forensic Sci Int 2006;163:152–4.

48. Schep LJ, Slaughter RJ, Vale JA, et al. The clinical toxicology of the designer "party pills" benzylpiperazine and trifluoromethylphenylpiperazine. Clin Toxicol 2011;49:131–41.

49. Wilkins C, Sweetsur P, Girling M. Patterns of benzylpiperazine/trifluoromethylphenylpiperazine party pill use and adverse effects in a population sample in New Zealand. Drug Alcohol Rev 2008;27:633–9.

50. Drug Enforcement Administration Office of Diversion Control. N-benzylpiperazine. Available at: https://www.deadiversion.usdoj.gov/drug_chem_info/bzp.pdf. Accessed July 18, 2017.

51. 1-[3-(Trifluoro-methyl)-phenyl]piperazine. (2013). [online] Drug Enforcement Administration Office of Diversion Control. Available at: https://www.deadiversion.usdoj.gov/drug_chem_info/tfmpp.pdf. Accessed July 18, 2017.

52. Arbo M, Bastos M, Carmo H. Piperazine compounds as drugs of abuse. Drug Alcohol Depend 2012;122(3):174–85.

53. Wilkins C, Sweetsur P. The impact of the prohibition of benzylpiperazine (BZP) 'legal highs' on the prevalence of BZP, new legal highs and other drug use in New Zealand. Drug Alcohol Depend 2013;127(1–3):72–80.

54. Gao T, Du P, Xu Z, et al. Occurrence of new psychoactive substances in wastewater of major Chinese cities. Sci Total Environ 2017;575:963–9.

55. Lin JC, Jan RK, Kydd R, et al. Subjective effects in humans following administration of party pill drugs BZP and TFMPP alone and in combination. Drug Test Anal 2011;3:582–5.

56. Musselman ME, Hampton JP. "Not for human consumption": a review of emerging designer drugs. Pharmacotherapy 2014;34:745–57.

57. Gee P, Richardson S, Woltersdorf W, et al. Toxic effects of BZP-based herbal party pills in humans: a prospective study in Christchurch, New Zealand. N Z Med J 2005;118:35–44.

58. Gee P, Gilbert M, Richardson S, et al. Toxicity from the recreational use of 1-benzylpiperazine. Clin Toxicol 2008;46:802–7.

59. Elliott S, Smith C. Investigation of the first deaths in the United Kingdom involving the detection and quantitation of the piperazines BZP and 3-TFMPP. J Anal Toxicol 2008;32:172–7.

60. Dean BV, Stellpflug SJ, Burnett AM, et al. 2C or not 2C: phenethylamine designer drug review. J Med Toxicol 2013;9:172–8.

61. Nikolau P, Papoutsis I, Stefanidou M, et al. 2C-I-NBOMe, an "N-bomb" that kills with "smiles". Drug Chem Toxicol 2015;38(1):113–9.

62. Nelson ME, Bryant SM, Aks SE. Emerging drugs of abuse. Emerg Med Clin North Am 2014;32:1–28.

63. Caudevilla-Gálligo F, Riba J, Ventura M, et al. 4-Bromo-2,5-dimethoxyphenethyl-amine (2C-B): presence in the recreational drug market in Spain, pattern of use and subjective effects. J Psychopharmacol 2012;7:1026–35.

64. 4-Bromo-2,5-Dimethoxyphenethylamine. (2013). [online] Drug Enforcement Administration Office of Diversion Control. Available at: https://www.deadiversion.usdoj.gov/drug_chem_info/bromo_dmp.pdf. Accessed July 18, 2017.

65. Sanders B, Lankenau SE, Bloom JJ, et al. "Research chemicals": tryptamine and phenethylamine use among high-risk youth. Subst Use Misuse 2008;43:389–402.

66. Hill SL, Thomas SHL. Clinical toxicology of newer recreational drugs. Clin Toxicol 2011;49:705–19.

67. Curtis B, Kemp P, Choi C, et al. Postmortem identification and quantitation of 2,5-dimethoxy-4-n-propylthiophenethylamine using GC-MSD and GC-NPD. J Anal Toxicol 2003;27:493–8.

68. Bosak A, Lovecchio F, Levine M. Recurrent seizures and serotonin syndrome following "2C-I" ingestion. J Med Toxicol 2013;9:196–8.

69. Auwarter V, Dresen S, Weinmann W, et al. 'Spice' and other herbal blends: harmless incense of cannabinoid designer drugs? J Mass Spectrom 2009;44:832–7.

70. White CM. The pharmacologic and clinical effects of illicit synthetic cannabinoids. J Clin Pharmacol 2017;57:297–304.

71. Castaneto MS, Gorelick DA, Desrosiers NA, et al. Synthetic cannabinoids: epidemiology, pharmacodynamics, and clinical implications. Drug Alcohol Depend 2014;144:12–41.

72. Fantegrossi WE, Moran JH, Radominska-Pandyab A, et al. Distinct pharmacology and metabolism of K2 synthetic cannabinoids compared to Δ9-THC: mechanism underlying greater toxicity? Life Sci 2014;97:45–54.

73. Tai S, Fantegrossi WE. Pharmacological and toxicological effects of synthetic cannabinoids and their metabolites. Curr Top Behav Neurosci 2017;32:249–62.

74. Law R, Schier J, Martin C, et al. Centers for Disease Control (CDC). Notes from the field: increase in reported adverse health effects related to synthetic cannabinoid Use - United States, January-May 2015. MMWR Morb Mortal Wkly Rep 2015;64:618–9.

75. Springer YP, Gerona R, Scheunemann E, et al. Increase in adverse reactions associated with use of synthetic cannabinoids - Anchorage, Alaska, 2015-2016. MMWR Morb Mortal Wkly Rep 2016;65:1108–11.

76. DEA, Controlled Substances Act, 1308.11 Schedule I. Available at: https://www.deadiversion.usdoj.gov/21cfr/cfr/1308/1308_11.htm. Accessed July 31, 2017.

77. Palamar JJ, Acosta P. Synthetic cannabinoid use in a nationally representative sample of US high school seniors. Drug Alcohol Depend 2015;149:194–202.

78. Caviness CM, Tzilos G, Anderson BJ, et al. Synthetic cannabinoids: use and predictors in a community sample of young adults. Subst Abus 2015;36:368–73.

79. Keyes KM, Rutherford C, Hamilton A, et al. Age, period, and cohort effects in synthetic cannabinoid use among US adolescents, 2011-2015. Drug Alcohol Depend 2016;166:159–67.

80. Monte AA, Bronstein AC, Cao DJ, et al. An outbreak of exposure to a novel synthetic cannabinoid. N Engl J Med 2014;370:389.

81. Kasper AM, Ridpath AD, Arnold JK, et al. Severe illness associated with reported use of synthetic cannabinoids - Mississippi, April 2015. MMWR Morb Mortal Wkly Rep 2015;64(39):1121–2.

82. Gunderson EW, Haughey HM, Ait-Daoud N, et al. "Spice" and "K2" herbal highs: a case series and systematic review of the clinical effects and biopsychosocial implications of synthetic cannabinoid use in humans. Am J Addict 2012;21: 320–6.

83. Winstock A, Lynskey M, Borschmann R, et al. Risk of emergency medical treatment following consumption of cannabis or synthetic cannabinoids in a large global sample. J Psychopharmacol 2015;29:698–703.

84. Bassir Nia A, Medrano B, Perkel C, et al. Psychiatric comorbidity associated with synthetic cannabinoid use compared to cannabis. J Psychopharmacol 2016;30:1321–30.

85. Hermanns-Clausen M, Kneisel S, Szabo B, et al. Acute toxicity due to the confirmed consumption of synthetic cannabinoids: clinical and laboratory findings. Addiction 2013;108:534–44.

86. Tait RJ, Caldicott D, Mountain D, et al. A systematic review of adverse events arising from the use of synthetic cannabinoids and their associated treatment. Clin Toxicol (Phila) 2016;54:1–13.

87. Courts J, Maskill V, Gray A, et al. Signs and symptoms associated with synthetic cannabinoid toxicity: systematic review. Australas Psychiatry 2015;24: 598–601.

88. Zarifi C, Vyas S. Spice-y kidney failure: a case report and systematic review of acute kidney injury attributable to the use of synthetic cannabis. Perm J 2017; 21. https://doi.org/10.7812/TPP/16-160.

89. Adedinsewo DA, Odewole O, Todd T. Acute rhabdomyolysis following synthetic cannabinoid ingestion. N Am J Med Sci 2016;8:256–8.

90. Bernson-Leung ME, Leung LY, Kumar S. Synthetic cannabis and acute ischemic stroke. J Stroke Cerebrovasc Dis 2014;23:1239–41.

91. Mir A, Obafemi A, Young A, et al. Myocardial infarction associated with use of the synthetic cannabinoid K2. Pediatrics 2011;128:e1622–7.

92. Andonian DO, Seaman SR, Josephson EB. Profound hypotension and bradycardia in the setting of synthetic cannabinoid intoxication - A case series. Am J Emerg Med 2017;35:940.e5-6.

93. Von Der Haar J, Talebi S, Ghobadi F, et al. Synthetic cannabinoids and their effects on the cardiovascular system. J Emerg Med 2016;50:258–62.

94. Seely KA, Lapoint J, Moran JH, et al. Spice drugs are more than harmless herbal blends: a review of the pharmacology and toxicology of synthetic cannabinoids. Prog Neuropsychopharmacol Biol Psychiatry 2012;39:234–43.

95. Nacca N, Vatti D, Sullivan R, et al. The synthetic cannabinoid withdrawal syndrome. J Addict Med 2013;7:296–8.

96. Zimmermann US, Winkelmann PR, Pilhatsch M, et al. Withdrawal phenomena and dependence syndrome after the consumption of "spice gold". Dtsch Arztebl Int 2009;106:464–7.

97. Macfarlane V, Christie G. Synthetic cannabinoid withdrawal: a new demand on detoxification services. Drug Alcohol Rev 2015;34:147–53.

98. Franz F, Angerer V, Jechle H, et al. Immunoassay screening in urine for synthetic cannabinoids - an evaluation of the diagnostic efficiency. Clin Chem Lab Med 2017;55(9):1375–84.

99. Namera A, Kawamura M, Nakamoto A, et al. Comprehensive review of the detection methods for synthetic cannabinoids and cathinones. Forensic Toxicol 2015;33:175–94.

100. Centers for Disease Control and Prevention. Influx of fentanyl-laced counterfeit pill and toxic fentanyl-related compounds further increases risk of fentanyl-related overdose and fatalities. Atlanta (GA): CDC HAN; 2016. p. 00395. Available at: https://emergency.cdc.gov/han/han00395.asp.

101. Prekupec MP, Mansky PA, Baumann MH. Misuse of novel synthetic opioids: a deadly new trend. J Addict Med 2017;11(4):256–65.

102. Dussy FE, Hangartner S, Hamberg C, et al. An acute ocfentanil fatality: a case report with postmortem concentrations. J Anal Toxicol 2016;40:761–6.

103. George AV, Lu JJ, Pisaon MV, et al. Carfentanil–an ultra potent opioid. Am J Emerg Med 2010;28:530–2.

104. Emerging threat report: Annual 2016. (2017). [online] Drug Enforcement Administration. Available at: https://ndews.umd.edu/sites/ndews.umd.edu/files/emerging-threat-report-2016-annual.pdf. Accessed June 4, 2017.

105. Drug Enforcement Administration. Emerging threat report: first quarter 2017.

106. Høiseth G, Skogstad S, Karinen R. Blood concentrations of new designer benzodiazepines in forensic cases. Forensic Sci Int 2016;268:35–8.

107. O'Connor LC, Torrance HJ, McKeown DA. ELISA detection of phenazepam, etizolam, pyrazolam, flubormazepam, diclazepam, and delorazepam in blood using Immunalysis benzodiazepine kit. J Anal Toxicol 2016;40:159–61.

108. O'Connell CW, Sadler CA, Tolia VM, et al. Overdose of etizolam: the abuse and risk of a benzodiazepine analog. Ann Emerg Med 2015;65:465–6.

The Role of Technology-Based Interventions for Substance Use Disorders in Primary Care: A Review of the Literature

Babak Tofighi, MD, MSc[a,b],*, Ana Abrantes, PhD[c,d],
Michael D. Stein, MD[e]

KEYWORDS

- Technology • Addiction • Mobile • Substance-related disorders

KEY POINTS

- The burden of alcohol and drug use disorders (substance use disorders [SUDs]) has intensified efforts to expand access to cost-effective psychosocial interventions and pharmacotherapies.
- This article provides an overview of technology-based interventions (eg, computer-based and Web-based interventions, text messaging, interactive voice recognition, smartphone apps, and emerging technologies) that are extending the reach of effective addiction treatments both in substance use treatment and primary care settings.
- This article discusses the efficacy of existing technology-based interventions for SUDs, prospects for emerging technologies, and special considerations when integrating technologies in primary care (eg, privacy and regulatory protocols) to enhance the management of SUDs.

INTRODUCTION

The burden of alcohol and substance use disorders (SUDs) is significant. For example, costs associated with opioid use disorder in 2013 were estimated at $78.5 billion and opioid-related overdose deaths have increased by 200% in the last 15 years.[1] Excessive

Disclosure: B. Tofighi is supported by an NIH Mentored Patient-oriented Research Career Development Award (NIDA K23DA042140 - 01A1).
[a] Department of Population Health, New York University School of Medicine, 227 East 30th Street 7th Floor, New York, NY 10016, USA; [b] Division of General Internal Medicine, New York University School of Medicine, New York, NY 10016, USA; [c] Butler Hospital, Department of Psychiatry and Human Behavior, Behavioral Medicine and Addictions Research, Butler, PA, USA; [d] Department of Psychiatry and Human Behavior, Alpert Medical School of Brown University, Providence, RI, USA; [e] Department of Health Law, Policy, and Medicine, Boston University, Boston, MA 02118, USA
* Corresponding author. 227 East 30th Street 7th Floor, New York, NY, 10016.
E-mail address: babak.tofighi@nyumc.org

alcohol use remains a leading modifiable cause of death and cost an estimated $250 billion in 2010.[2,3] However, nearly 50 years after the introduction of pharmacotherapies for SUDs, fewer than 10% of individuals with SUD are linked to treatment.[4]

Primary care settings are optimally positioned to reduce the burden of SUDs by providing a patient-centered care model for addiction treatment and related comorbidities (prescribing pharmacotherapies, patient education, and access to specialty care).[5,6] Costs of expanding addiction treatment to office-based settings are offset by reductions in emergency department visits and hospitalizations, and improved addiction and medical outcomes.[6,7] However, effective management of SUDs is seldom delivered in primary care. Patient-level barriers to office-based management of SUDs include cost, insurance limitations, stigma, and transportation.[8,9] Among physicians trained in SUD care, lack of adequate administrative and clinical support impede the delivery of effective medication-assisted therapies and psychosocial interventions targeting SUDs.[10,11]

The integration of innovative technology-based interventions (eg, computer-based and Web-based interventions, text messaging, interactive voice recognition, smartphone apps, and emerging technologies) in primary care has the potential to address gaps in care for individuals with SUDs (**Table 1**).[12–14] This pairing of effective

Table 1
Published data on technology-based interventions for substance use disorders

Reference	Device	Target Substances	Target Behaviors or Behavior Change Model	Contact Information
Carroll, et al,[34] 2008	Internet/Web	Alcohol, cocaine, opioid, cannabis	CBT	http://www.cbt4cbt.com/
Marsch et al,[36] 2014	Internet/Web	Opioids	CRA, CBT	http://www.c4tbh.org/
Postel et al,[37] 2010	Internet/Web	Alcohol	CBT, biopsychosocial model	www.lookatyourdrinking.com
Campbell, et al,[38] 2014	Internet/Web	Alcohol, cocaine, cannabis, opiates, stimulants	CRA	http://sudtech.org/
Stoner et al,[43] 2015	Text message	Alcohol	Adherence to oral naltrexone	sastoner@uw.edu
Dulin et al,[56] 2013	Smartphone app	Alcohol		http://stepaway.biz/
Gustafson et al,[23] 2014	Smartphone app	Alcohol	Self-determination theory, cognitive-behavioral relapse prevention	https://chess.wisc.edu
Kay-Lambkin et al,[82] 2011	Internet/Web	Alcohol	Depression	http://www.shadetreatment.com/

Abbreviations: CBT, cognitive behavior therapy; CRA, community reinforcement approach.

technology-based interventions (TBIs) with primary care has already shown improvements in appointment adherence, diabetes self-management, smoking cessation, and human immunodeficiency virus (HIV) care.[15-17] Importantly, TBIs readily enhance between-visit patient engagement with their care by easing patient-physician communication, point of service data gathering, and adherence management, and offering the delivery of evidence-based psychosocial interventions with high fidelity.[12,13,16,18]

Advances in emerging technologies have also accelerated the development and delivery of effective TBIs targeting SUDs in specialty addiction treatment settings.[12,13,18,19] Patient surveys in primary care signal high acceptability and uptake of TBIs to enhance the management of SUDs.[20,21] Although primary care often constitutes the mainstay of medical care for populations with SUDs,[22] efforts to expand TBIs in primary care for the treatment of SUDs have yet to be fully realized. Adoption of evidence-based interventions targeting SUDs in primary care may produce positive outcomes comparable with those observed in specialty addiction treatment settings.[14,19,23,24]

This article describes the rapidly evolving nature of TBIs targeting alcohol and illicit substance use in community and outpatient addiction treatment settings and implications for integrating TBIs in primary care to reduce the burden of SUDs. It primarily focuses on computer-based and Web-based interventions, text messaging, interactive voice recognition, and smartphone applications supported by randomized controlled trials and evidence-based behavior change models (eg, cognitive behavior therapy [CBT], community reinforcement approach [CRA], therapeutic education system).[18]

Computer and Web-Based Interventions

Recent reviews and meta-analyses suggest that computer-based and Web-based interventions are a cost-effective approach to expand the reach of evidence-based psychotherapeutic interventions, reduce the burden of SUDs in community and specialty addiction treatment settings, and show clinical outcomes (improved cognitive functioning, retention of behavior change techniques, treatment engagement, and abstinence) comparable with studies evaluating the impact of individual counseling.[13,25,26] Web-based interventions are available to patients remotely through any Internet browser and may consist of a home page linking participants to addiction treatment services, self-selected modules, and peer discussion forums. In a meta-analysis by Riper and colleagues,[27] Web-based interventions used by participants in community settings (eg, home, employment) targeting alcohol use showed a small but significant effect (g = 0.20; 95% confidence interval [CI], 0.13–0.27; $P<.001$).

The effect of Web-based interventions is potentiated when delivered in multiple sessions at home or in specialty addiction treatment settings.[28,29] Findings in a systematic review by Riper and colleagues[28] reported higher effect sizes in multisession modularized Web-based interventions (g = 0.61, 95% CI 0.33–0.90) targeting alcohol use in community settings (eg, home, library, work) compared with single-session personalized feedback programs (g = 0.27, 95% CI 0.11–0.43, $P = .04$). Kay-Lambkin and colleagues[30] described equivalent treatment outcomes among participants recruited from primary care and mental health settings with major depressive disorder and problematic alcohol use (>4 drinks per day for men or >2 drinks per day for women) or at least weekly marijuana use randomized to a computer-based motivational interviewing (MI)/CBT intervention (SHADE [self-help for alcohol and other drug use and depression] therapy) versus therapist-delivered MI/CBT sessions. Bickel and colleagues[31] also reported comparable weeks of continuous opioid and cocaine abstinence and significantly greater weeks of abstinence among patients enrolled in buprenorphine maintenance treatment in a university-based research clinic receiving a computer-assisted intervention grounded in the CRA combined with contingency management versus standard treatment (CRA-based in-person counseling plus contingency management). CRA reinforces the client's motivation and coping strategies to reduce substance use and integrate social, recreational, and vocational reinforcers to avoid substance use.[32] CM is based on operant conditioning and offers a system of incentives to enhance patient motivation for abstinence.[33] Carroll and colleagues[34] reported that individuals recruited from a community-based outpatient addiction treatment program who met Diagnostic and Statistical Manual of Mental Disorders, Fourth Edition criteria for alcohol, cocaine, opioid, or marijuana dependence randomized to a CBT-based computer intervention (CBT4CBT) showed similar rates of treatment retention compared with standard treatment; further, participants assigned to the CBT4CBT program provided significantly more negative urine drug screen tests and longer continuous durations of abstinence.[35]

Subsequent studies assessed the impact of substituting portions of in-person counseling with Web-based interventions to reduce the burden on health care personnel while ensuring improved therapeutic support and clinical outcomes. Marsch and colleagues[36] evaluated the effectiveness of the Therapeutic Education System (TES), a Web-based psychosocial intervention constituted of modules grounded in the CRA and CBT models among methadone maintenance treatment patients (N = 160) randomized to standard treatment or TES partially substituting for in-person counseling. Findings showed significantly higher rates of abstinence among participants receiving the TES (48%) compared with standard treatment (37%) across all study weeks ($P<.05$). Notably, participants exposed to the TES system showed less dropout compared with patients receiving only clinician-delivered treatment (log-rank $P = .017$) and were exposed to a higher "dose" of the psychosocial intervention.[36] Postal and colleagues[37] assessed the effectiveness of the Alcohol de Baas intervention, a Web-based platform integrating CBT to reduce alcohol use and problem drinking behavior, and improve health status. Participants were recruited from the community and showed significantly improved health status and abstinence, reduced problem drinking, and higher readiness to initiate alcohol treatment compared with the control group. At 6 and 9 months, weekly consumption was less than baseline and participants showed significant improvements in depression, anxiety, and stress scores.[38]

Campbell and colleagues[39] evaluated the effectiveness of the TES, consisting of 62 interactive multimedia modules (eg, basic cognitive-behavioral relapse prevention skills; improving psychosocial functioning; and prevention of HIV, hepatitis, and sexually transmitted infections) requiring approximately 30 minutes each to complete. Interactive modules substituted for 2 hours of standard clinician-led group therapy sessions per week. Incentives were earned by participants for negative urine or alcohol breathalyzer screens and TES module completion, and redeemed using the TES platform to reduce high dropout and relapse rates in the early stages of treatment. Nearly half of the draws consisted of supportive content (eg, "Good job"), and the remaining draws rewarded participants with prizes worth $1, $20, or $80 to $100 in decreasing probability. Participants in the TES group had a significantly greater abstinence rate (odds ratio, 1.62; 95% CI, 1.12, 2.35), and improved retention in treatment (log-rank $P = .017$).[39]

Findings from these trials show the effectiveness of Web-based TES interventions targeting SUDs while overcoming administrative and clinical barriers limiting the reach of evidence-based psychotherapeutic interventions in diverse specialty addiction treatment settings.[39] The applicability of similar Web-based TES interventions across traditional primary care settings remains promising and requires further implementation studies to inform TES integration into service delivery.

Text Message–Based Interventions

Less technologically complex compared with computer-based, Internet-based, or smartphone-based interventions, text messaging (TM) remains a cost-effective platform for improving chronic disease management in primary care (eg, smoking cessation, appointment adherence, and adherence to antiretroviral therapies).[19,40,41] It is the most popular mobile phone feature nationally among patients in addiction treatment and in primary care.[12,42] TM may deliver multimedia content (eg, images, videos, audio) and incorporate behavior change approaches, including CBT, and motivational interventions, with high fidelity.[12]

Recent systematic reviews have described the feasibility and preliminary efficacy of TM interventions to reduce the burden of alcohol and illicit substance use in primary care and university-based research clinic settings. Studies indicate improved retention in treatment; medication adherence; and reduced alcohol, methamphetamine, and opioid use.[12,18,35,36] Stoner and colleagues[43] randomized participants with alcohol use disorder to a text-based tool providing medication reminders for oral naltrexone, adherence support, and prompts eliciting potential side effects, cravings, and alcohol use versus the control condition (i.e., receipt of a prepaid phone and prompts for alcohol use and related side effects). Although adherence to naltrexone did not predict drinking outcomes, the intervention group reported significantly longer periods of adherence to naltrexone (mean = 19 days; 95% CI, 0.0–44.0) than those in the control group (mean = 3 days; 95% CI, 0.0–8.1) during the first month of treatment (P = .04).

Researchers have also leveraged TM to enhance appointment adherence,[44] self-efficacy, relapse prevention, social support, and linkage with peer support groups.[45] Gonzales and colleagues[46] described significantly improved participation in extracurricular recovery activities, rates of abstinence, and reduced substance use problem severity among young adults (aged 12–24 years) recruited from outpatient and residential treatment programs randomized to TM-based self-monitoring prompts, educational content, and information regarding social support resources. TM tools may also enhance access to health care providers in real time to reduce the risk of relapse or other adverse events. Lucht and colleagues[47] randomized participants completing inpatient detoxification for alcohol and scheduled to follow-up in outpatient addiction treatment with a TM intervention offering as-needed counselor telephone support and showed significantly improved rates of low-risk alcohol use, treatment retention, and later episodes of relapse compared with standard care.

TM interventions have also addressed clinical barriers to managing SUDs in primary care, including the management of comorbidities prevalent in patients with SUDs (ie, HIV, depression).[48,49] Agyapong and colleagues[48] randomized dual-diagnosis participants with alcohol use and major depressive disorder to a twice-daily supportive TM tool in combination with primary care. TM content was designed to reduce cravings, stress, relapse, and nonadherence to medications, and to provide general support. Although there were no significant improvements in depression symptoms, participants randomized to the TM tool showed increased days to first drink.

Interactive Voice Recognition

Outpatient management of SUDs requires close monitoring of daily substance use, medication adherence, cravings, and adverse events. Similar to TM, Interactive voice response (IVR) offers a seamless approach to enhance between-visit patient engagement with care. IVR technology uses a telephone-delivered system of recorded scripts to persons seeking substance use treatment. IVR automatizes scheduled phone calls to elicit participant responses in real time using telephone keypad responses or voice recognition, which is preferable for certain patient subgroups that are less comfortable with TM or with limited literacy skills.[50] More dynamic IVR systems include automatic logical skipping or branching sequences to offer more user-centered feedback. Notably, some patients report increased comfort reporting sensitive information to the IVR system than to their clinician.[51] IVR has also shown an impact on chronic illness management outcomes (blood pressure and glycemic control),[51] but the clinical efficacy of IVR in reducing substance use (other than cigarette use)[52] remains unclear.[53–55]

Smartphone Applications

The near ubiquity of mobile phones and increasing popularity of smartphone ownership has hastened the development and study of mobile phone–based health interventions to reduce the burden of SUDs. Smartphone applications offer a diverse range of functions with advanced software capabilities to enhance chronic illness management. The effectiveness of smartphone applications has been supported in recent trials among participants with alcohol use disorder in specialty addiction treatment settings. Dulin and colleagues[56] conducted a pilot randomized controlled trial to evaluate the clinical impact of a stand-alone, self-administered smartphone-delivered intervention for participants recruited from the community with alcohol use disorder (ie, drinking a minimum of ≥ 14 drinks for women or ≥ 21 drinks for men per week over a consecutive 30-day period and ≥ 2 heavy drinking days consisting of 4 or more drinks for women and 5 or more drinks for men in the same 30-day period) who were not enrolled in specialty addiction treatment. The intervention modules enhanced patient awareness of their drinking problems, assessment of daily alcohol use, triggers, personalized weekly feedback reports, and reinforcement of users' social support networks. These features were coupled with offering users coping strategies to reduce cravings and psychological distress to reduce the risk of drinking. The intervention reduced the number of hazardous drinking days and numbers of drinks per day. These preliminary findings suggest clinical benefit for stand-alone evidence-based interventions for individuals unable to access specialty treatment and require further study for potential adoption in primary care.

More recently, Gustafson and colleagues[23] examined the effectiveness of A-CHESS (Alcohol – Comprehensive Health Enhancement Support System) among participants transitioning from residential alcohol treatment to outpatient treatment. A-CHESS is based on self-determination theory[57] and cognitive-behavioral relapse prevention[58] to enhance perceived competence, social relatedness, and motivation to reduce alcohol use. This multifeatured smartphone intervention offers self-assessments, discussion groups, counselor support, links to online resources on addiction management, GPS (global positioning system) tracking to prompt patients if they approach a high-risk location that may lead to relapse, and personalized therapeutic goals. Patients randomized to A-CHESS showed significantly fewer risky drinking days (mean difference, 1.37; 95% CI, 0.46–2.27; $P = .003$), and increased abstinence in the previous 30 days at months 8 and 12 ($P = .04$ and .02), compared with patients receiving treatment as usual, and sustained engagement with the application.[23]

Online Forums and Social Media

Online platforms (eg, discussion/chat rooms, e-mail threads, social media) offer anonymous and socially supportive communication that reinforces self-management, self-esteem, and assistance linking with treatment.[59] Twelve-step–based online sites remain the most popular among participants with SUDs. In addition, an increasing number of sites offer alternatives to the 12-step approach (eg, Women For Sobriety, Rational Recovery Center, SMART [Self-Management and Recovery Training] recovery, Rational Emotive Behavior Therapy). The popularity, quality of information, and clinical impact of such online forums as yet remains unclear.[20] However, given the effectiveness of in-person peer support as an adjunct to primary care–based approaches to managing SUDs,[60] similar online forums based on the 12-step or SMART recovery model have the potential to also enhance clinician-delivered interventions in primary care for SUDs. There are also hundreds of commercial online sites and social media pages promising access to therapists, peer support networks, and motivational and informational content. Sites accredited by the Joint Commission on Accreditation of Healthcare Organizations (eg, soberrecovery.com) may assist some patients in accessing potentially beneficial content (**Table 2**). Recent National Institutes of Health funding of research that leverages social media and online forums promises to reveal important insights into these diversifying platforms facilitating recovery.[61]

Emerging Technologies

In addition to the TBIs reviewed earlier, there are also several emerging technologies that are likely to have an impact on SUD treatment in the years ahead. Technological advances have been rapid over the last decade, resulting in smaller, faster devices with increased computing power. In addition, wireless communication between devices can allow real-time information gathering and transfer between patients and providers. Further, relevant data that extend beyond alcohol and drug use (eg, heart rate, tone of voice) can be processed with machine learning approaches that can ultimately lead to the ability to predict patient behaviors. These novel technological approaches coupled with existing theoretically informed TBIs have the potential to increase the reach and efficacy of SUD treatment (**Table 3**).

Advances in biosensor technology have contributed to the emergence of novel interventional approaches. To date, the most work has been conducted with transdermal alcohol sensors such as the commercially available Secure Continuous Remote Alcohol Monitoring device (SCRAM; Alcohol Monitoring Systems, Inc, Littleton, CO). SCRAM takes measurements every 30 minutes and is able to wirelessly convey transdermal readings to a remote server. Although frequently used in the criminal justice system, SCRAM, especially in conjunction with contingency management interventions, has resulted in promising drinking outcomes among outpatients engaged in alcohol treatment.[62–64] Other transdermal sensors include the WrisTAS (Giner, Inc, Newton, MA). The WrisTAS, unlike the SCRAM, is worn on the wrist and takes measurements every minute and has shown high sensitivity and specificity.[65]

Table 2 Online support forums	
Program	**Web Site**
Sober Recovery	www.soberrecovery.com/forums/
12 Step Recovery Forums	www.12stepforums.net
Women for Sobriety	womenforsobriety.org
Rational Recovery	rational.org
SMART Recovery	https://www.smartrecovery.org/community/forums/6-Tools-and-Discussions

Abbreviation: SMART, Self-Management and Recovery Training.

Table 3 Emerging technologies			
Secure Continuous Remote Alcohol Monitoring Device (Alcohol Monitoring Systems, Inc)	Sensor	(1) Alcohol	www.scramsystems.com/
WrisTAS (Giner, Inc)	Sensor	(1) Alcohol	www.ginerinc.com/wrist-transdermal-alcohol-sensor
Wisepill device (Wisepill Technologies)	Pillbox plus smartphone app	(1) Medication adherence	www.wisepill.com
Soberlink device (Soberlink, Inc)	Portable breathalyzer	(1) Alcohol	www.soberlink.com/

Other emerging technologies have focused on the ability to obtain real-time feedback, thereby increasing the potential to intervene more promptly. Examples of this include technological approaches for monitoring medication adherence. The Wisepill device (Wisepill Technologies, Cape Town, South Africa), the size of a pack of cards, stores pills, tracks when the device has been opened, and wirelessly sends information to an external server (eg, to a researcher or clinician). In addition, the Wisepill device can also be paired with text message reminders to help facilitate patient adherence. The Wisepill device and messages have been used successfully to increase adherence to antiretroviral therapy in patients with HIV and has been used to monitor naltrexone adherence in methamphetamine users and binge drinkers.[66,67] Because of concerns about whether patients actually ingest a medication when opening such monitoring devices, researchers have explored the use of inert radiofrequency emitters attached to the medication to create an ingestible digital pill that communicates with a cloud-based server while in the stomach.[68,69] Another real-time monitoring approach involves the use of a Soberlink device (Soberlink, Inc, CA), equipped with facial recognition software to verify identity, that allows patients to provide breath sample data on breath alcohol levels, which are wirelessly sent to treating providers.[70] The clinician is then able to promptly respond to positive results and provide the patient who continues to drink with appropriate intervention. Alternatively, others have explored pairing breathalyzer results with a smartphone app to provide feedback and encourage skill building.[71]

Although the technologies described earlier involve obtaining objective information on alcohol and drug use from patients, there are several emerging technologies that can be used to predict potentially risky behaviors before they happen. For example, Boyer and colleagues[72] (2012) argued that, in concert, technologies including artificial intelligence, continuous physiologic monitoring, wireless connectivity, and smartphone computation would be able to detect when an individual is experiencing craving for alcohol or drug use and could receive a just-in-time intervention to prevent substance use. Acute changes in negative affect and craving (known risk factors for relapse) are associated with concomitant changes in physiologic arousal; namely, heart rate and electrodermal activity (EDA).[73–76] Both research-grade devices and commercially available smartwatches that communicate wirelessly with smartphones are equipped with medical-grade biosensors that provide continuous monitoring of heart rate, temperature, and EDA. Physiologic data that include EDA and temperature, measured by a portable biosensor wristwatch (Q sensor; Affectiva, Waltham, MA), have been shown to be associated with cocaine and opiate use in both laboratory and ambulatory environments.[77,78] Work is currently underway to identify drug use cravings and, through machine learning approaches, develop algorithms for predicting drug use so that personalized relapse prevention interventions can be delivered during the time of greatest need.[72]

Machine learning approaches have also been proposed to aid in the prediction of whether an individual is intoxicated. For example, Arnold and colleagues[79] argue that data collected from the smartphone accelerometer and gyroscope (called Alcogait) coupled with information on how much an individual has consumed alcohol could, through machine learning, reliably predict blood alcohol levels. In doing so, when this information can be used to deliver feedback to an individual about their ability to drive, for example, alcohol-related risk behaviors may be decreased or avoided.

These emerging technologies can be integrated into individuals' everyday lives, with passive collection of data that can be computationally processed for available feedback to the at-risk individual, without much additional effort from the individual. As these technologies enter the next stage of experimental investigation and efficacy testing, clinicians will have a greater understanding of their impact on reducing the overall public health risk associated with SUDs.

IMPORTANT CONSIDERATIONS RELATED TO TECHNOLOGY-BASED INTERVENTIONS FOR SUBSTANCE USE DISORDERS
Technology-Based Interventions for Dual-Diagnosis Populations

Comorbid SUD and psychiatric disorder is common. Although efforts have been made to address psychiatric comorbidity in patients with SUD, few treatments exist that effectively address multiple comorbidities. Because individuals with comorbid disorders experience more treatment access barriers, including social deficits and stigma,[80] the use of TBIs in dual-diagnosis populations may be a particularly effective strategy.

In a recent systematic review of TBIs for substance use and comorbid disorders, Sugarman and colleagues[81] (2017) identified only 9 studies, with the largest number being for depression comorbidity. The TBI with the most empirical testing has been the SHADE, a 9-session MI plus CBT computer-delivered intervention that has shown reduction in alcohol and cannabis use as well as decreases in depressive symptoms.[82] An abbreviated version of SHADE has been developed for young adults with alcohol and depressive comorbidity, called DEAL.[83] Short-term decreases in drinking and depression were found but not sustained, and adherence to the intervention was challenging. There is an ongoing study of DEAL that adds a social networking component for depressed, binge drinking young adults.[84] There are also several studies examining TBIs for individuals with comorbid trauma experiences and SUDs, with or without a diagnosis of posttraumatic stress disorder. In a recent review of these studies, Gilmore and colleagues[85] (2016) found that TBIs are feasible for this population and are likely to be efficacious in reducing either trauma symptoms or substance use.

As reported by Sugarman and colleagues[81] (2017), there are several special considerations when developing and testing TBIs for a dual-diagnosis population. First, the more effective interventions tend to be longer and more intensive. Adherence to the intervention is therefore a challenge and the investigators suggested that financial incentives, gamification of TBIs, and some clinical involvement may be necessary to increase engagement with the intervention. Also, because there is always a concern for clinical deterioration and suicidal ideation, there is a need to consider strategies for incorporating clinical monitoring in the delivery of TBIs in dual-diagnosis patients.

Factors Influencing the Fidelity of Technology-Based Interventions

If well-designed, TBIs can minimize the burden on delivery systems and reduce net spending for SUDs while expanding the use of underused addiction pharmacotherapies and psychosocial interventions. Translating evidence-based TBIs into mainstream health care settings will rely on a reorganization of clinical practices that consider patient-level factors to sustained engagement with emerging platforms (eg, socioeconomic and clinical barriers to care), privacy and regulatory concerns, on-boarding delivery systems and providers that have limited experience with TBIs, and reimbursement mechanisms.[24,86]

Patient-level barriers to treatment entry for SUDs (eg, race/ethnicity, socioeconomic status, less education, impaired cognition, severe mental illness)[8,80] mirror the barriers to access to mobile phones, computers, and Internet.[19,87,88] However, offering free mobile phones or in-clinic access to computers ensures open access to evidence-based interventions and improved clinical outcomes (eg, cognitive functioning, abstinence, and treatment retention).[12,23,49,89,90] Additional strategies for dissemination of evidence-based TBIs include subsidizing Internet or mobile phone plans, offering instructions on intervention use, and tailoring intervention content and design features to user preferences.

The spread of unvalidated, commercially driven smartphone applications, social media pages, and Web-based interventions has dampened the dissemination of effective TBIs. Developers often claim medical expertise and offer unsubstantiated claims of intervention efficacy, and may sell user data to third parties for commercial use.[91] The monetization of digital data and risks for compromised patient health information require clinicians to caution patients regarding commercially driven TBIs. The US Food and Drug Administration (FDA) has increased oversight of emerging TBIs, including mobile medical applications but may have difficulties in regulating product claims unrelated to specific medical conditions (eg, promotes reduced stress, concentration, behavior control).[92] Nonetheless, clinicians should help patients navigate the marketplace by confirming device approval via the FDA (eg, https://www.accessdata.fda.gov/scripts/cdrh/cfdocs/cfRL/rl.cfm) and existing literature.

Privacy and Regulatory Considerations to Technology-Based Intervention Integration

Adoption of effective TBIs in mainstream and addiction treatment settings remains slow because concerns over social, legal, and ethical implications remain unanswered. Potential issues for patients and providers include:

1. Open access to indefinitely stored content in mobile phones, emails, IVR platforms, online forums, or mobile sensors requires protocols for deletion
2. Inability for physicians or patients to confirm the authenticity of authorship of content transmitted between one another
3. Interception of content exchanged between providers and patients
4. Lack of familiarity with the Health Insurance Portability and Accountability Act (HIPAA)[93]

Risk management of compromising patient health information includes the removal of any patient's identifiers or stigmatizing content (eg, HIV, addict, methadone), restricting patient contact to only 1 provider or software, password protecting all mobile phones and devices, obtaining security certifications from mobile phone service providers, using encryption technologies for transmitted content, and regularly deleting transmitted content.[24,93]

Clarifying Intervention Design and Clinical Impact

Interventions that are overly complex, contain redundant or ineffective components, and seem homogenous can lead to a reduction in treatment efficacy with every type of intervention. To preempt such problems, software that incorporates graded approaches, such as adjusting the frequency of TM prompts based on the patient's clinical condition and level of responsiveness with the intervention, sustains engagement during the different stages of recovery.[12,49] In addition, intervention development based on mixed-methods research and usability testing (eg, intervention mapping approach, multiphase optimization strategy testing) improves the reach, long-term engagement, and effectiveness of newly introduced platforms.[12,94,95] Meta-analysis and recent reviews have also found that integrating patient-tailored design features and effective psychosocial interventions enhances engagement with the TBI, is associated with greater effect sizes, and optimizes behavior change and clinical outcomes.[12,13,18,96] In addition, linking TBIs with immediate access to health care providers or supportive peers is preferable to interventions that lack any human contact because of the demotivating nature of some automated interactions.[12,18,21]

Although TBIs may be tailored to the patient's clinical needs, studies are needed to assess the appropriate level of exposure or dose of TBIs versus clinician-delivered psychosocial interventions, the effectiveness of computer-based versus mobile phone–based interventions, and smartphone-based compared with TM-based platforms. In addition, the clinical effectiveness of adding TBI-delivered psychosocial interventions to existing addiction pharmacotherapies (eg, buprenorphine, naltrexone) in traditional primary care settings remains limited.

SUMMARY

In the last 2 decades, advances in TBIs addressing SUDs, most often in addiction treatment settings, have made possible effective point of service data gathering, adherence management, reinforcement of evidence-based psychosocial interventions, improved patient-physician communication, retention in office-based treatment, and increased abstinence with minimal disruption to health care personnel and clinical workflow. For TBIs to reach their full potential to reduce the burden of SUDs, strategies are needed to facilitate their dissemination and implementation in primary care: addressing clinician adoption of TBIs, financial reimbursement, adaptability of hardware in primary care, integration and interoperability, and user engagement.[97]

ACKNOWLEDGMENTS

The authors wish to thank Sarah Lord, Geisel School of Medicine at Dartmouth College, and Christopher W. Shanahan, Boston Medical Center/Boston University, for providing a critical review of this article.

REFERENCES

1. Florence CS, Zhou C, Luo F, et al. The economic burden of prescription opioid overdose, abuse, and dependence in the United States, 2013. Med Care 2016; 54(10):901–6.

2. Bauer UE, Briss PA, Goodman RA, et al. Prevention of chronic disease in the 21st century: elimination of the leading preventable causes of premature death and disability in the USA. Lancet 2014;384(9937):45–52.

3. Sacks JJ, Gonzales KR, Bouchery EE, et al. 2010 national and state costs of excessive alcohol consumption. Am J Prev Med 2015;49(5):e73–9.

4. Nosyk B, Anglin MD, Brissette S, et al. A call for evidence-based medical treatment of opioid dependence in the United States and Canada. Health Aff 2013; 32(8):1462–9.

5. Anton RF, O'Malley SS, Ciraulo DA, et al. Combined pharmacotherapies and behavioral interventions for alcohol dependence: the COMBINE study: a randomized controlled trial. Jama 2006;295(17):2003–17.

6. Bhatraju EP, Grossman E, Tofighi B, et al. Public sector low threshold office-based buprenorphine treatment: outcomes at year 7. Addict Sci Clin Pract 2017;12(1):7.

7. Saitz R, Horton NJ, Larson MJ, et al. Primary medical care and reductions in addiction severity: a prospective cohort study. Addiction 2005;100(1):70–8.

8. Hansen HB, Siegel CE, Case BG, et al. Variation in use of buprenorphine and methadone treatment by racial, ethnic, and income characteristics of residential social areas in New York City. J Behav Health Serv Res 2013;40(3):367–77.

9. Teruya C, Schwartz RP, Mitchell SG, et al. Patient perspectives on buprenorphine/naloxone: a qualitative study of retention during the Starting Treatment with Agonist Replacement Therapies (START) study. J Psychoactive Drugs 2014; 46(5):412–26.

10. Kermack A, Flannery M, Tofighi B, et al. Buprenorphine prescribing practice trends and attitudes among New York providers. J Subst Abuse Treat 2017;74: 1–6.

11. Duncan LG, Mendoza S, Hansen H. Buprenorphine maintenance for opioid dependence in public sector healthcare: benefits and barriers. J Addict Med Ther Sci 2015;1(2):31.

12. Tofighi B, Nicholson JM, McNeely J, et al. Mobile phone messaging for illicit drug and alcohol dependence: a systematic review of the literature. Drug Alcohol Rev 2017;36(4):477–91.

13. Bickel WK, Christensen DR, Marsch LA. A review of computer-based interventions used in the assessment, treatment, and research of drug addiction. Subst Use Misuse 2011;46(1):4–9.

14. Copeland J, Martin G. Web-based interventions for substance use disorders: a qualitative review. J Subst Abuse Treat 2004;26(2):109–16.

15. Free C, Phillips G, Galli L, et al. The effectiveness of mobile-health technology-based health behaviour change or disease management interventions for health care consumers: a systematic review. PLoS Med 2013;10(1):e1001362.

16. Muessig KE, Nekkanti M, Bauermeister J, et al. A systematic review of recent smartphone, Internet and Web 2.0 interventions to address the HIV continuum of care. Curr HIV/AIDS Rep 2015;12(1):173–90.

17. Buller DB, Borland R, Bettinghaus EP, et al. Randomized trial of a smartphone mobile application compared to text messaging to support smoking cessation. Telemed J E Health 2014;20(3):206–14.

18. Litvin EB, Abrantes AM, Brown RA. Computer and mobile technology-based interventions for substance use disorders: an organizing framework. Addict Behav 2013;38(3):1747–56.

19. Cole-Lewis H, Kershaw T. Text messaging as a tool for behavior change in disease prevention and management. Epidemiol Rev 2010;32(1):56–69.

20. Hall MJ, Tidwell WC. Internet recovery for substance abuse and alcoholism: an exploratory study of service users. J Substance Abuse Treat 2003;24(2):161–7.

21. Tofighi B, Grossman E, Buirkle E, et al. Mobile phone use patterns and preferences in safety net office-based buprenorphine patients. J Addict Med 2015; 9(3):217.

22. Reid MC, Fiellin DA, O'Connor PG. Hazardous and harmful alcohol consumption in primary care. Arch Intern Med 1999;159(15):1681–9.

23. Gustafson DH, McTavish FM, Chih M-Y, et al. A smartphone application to support recovery from alcoholism: a randomized clinical trial. JAMA Psychiatry 2014;71(5):566–72.

24. Tofighi B, Grossman E, Sherman S, et al. Mobile phone messaging during unobserved "home" induction to buprenorphine. J Addict Med 2016;10(5):309–13.

25. Rooke S, Thorsteinsson E, Karpin A, et al. Computer-delivered interventions for alcohol and tobacco use: a meta-analysis. Addiction 2010;105(8):1381–90.

26. Moore BA, Fazzino T, Garnet B, et al. Computer-based interventions for drug use disorders: a systematic review. J substance abuse Treat 2011;40(3):215–23.

27. Riper H, Blankers M, Hadiwijaya H, et al. Effectiveness of guided and unguided low-intensity internet interventions for adult alcohol misuse: a meta-analysis. PLoS One 2014;9(6):e99912.

28. Riper H, Spek V, Boon B, et al. Effectiveness of E-self-help interventions for curbing adult problem drinking: a meta-analysis. J Med Internet Res 2011; 13(2):e42.

29. White A, Kavanagh D, Stallman H, et al. Online alcohol interventions: a systematic review. J Med Internet Res 2010;12(5):e62.

30. Kay-Lambkin FJ, Baker AL, Lewin TJ, et al. Computer-based psychological treatment for comorbid depression and problematic alcohol and/or cannabis use: a randomized controlled trial of clinical efficacy. Addiction 2009;104(3):378–88.

31. Bickel WK, Marsch LA, Buchhalter AR, et al. Computerized behavior therapy for opioid-dependent outpatients: a randomized controlled trial. Exp Clin Psychopharmacol 2008;16(2):132.

32. Roozen HG, Boulogne JJ, van Tulder MW, et al. A systematic review of the effectiveness of the community reinforcement approach in alcohol, cocaine and opioid addiction. Drug and alcohol dependence 2004;74(1):1–13.

33. Stitzer ML, Bigelow GE, Liebson I. Reinforcement of drug abstinence: a behavioral approach to drug abuse treatment. Behavioral analysis and treatment of substance abuse 1979;25(68).

34. Carroll KM, Ball SA, Martino S, et al. Computer-assisted delivery of cognitive-behavioral therapy for addiction: a randomized trial of CBT4CBT. Am J Psychiatry 2008;165(7):881–8.

35. Olmstead TA, Ostrow CD, Carroll KM. Cost-effectiveness of computer-assisted training in cognitive-behavioral therapy as an adjunct to standard care for addiction. Drug and alcohol dependence 2010;110(3):200–7.

36. Marsch LA, Guarino H, Acosta M, et al. Web-based behavioral treatment for substance use disorders as a partial replacement of standard methadone maintenance treatment. J Substance Abuse Treat 2014;46(1):43–51.

37. Postel MG, de Haan HA, ter Huurne ED, et al. Effectiveness of a web-based intervention for problem drinkers and reasons for dropout: randomized controlled trial. J Med Internet Res 2010;12(4):e68.

38. Postel MG, ter Huurne ED, de Haan HA, et al. A 9-month follow-up of a 3-month web-based alcohol treatment program using intensive asynchronous therapeutic support. Am J Drug Alcohol Abuse 2015;41(4):309–16.

39. Campbell AN, Nunes EV, Matthews AG, et al. Internet-delivered treatment for substance abuse: a multisite randomized controlled trial. Am J Psychiatry 2014;171(6):683–90.

40. Whittaker R, McRobbie H, Bullen C, et al. Mobile phone-based interventions for smoking cessation. Cochrane Database Syst Rev 2016;(4):CD006611.

41. Guerriero C, Cairns J, Roberts I, et al. The cost-effectiveness of smoking cessation support delivered by mobile phone text messaging: Txt2stop. Eur J Health Econ 2013;14(5):789–97.

42. Rainie L. Internet, broadband, and cell phone statistics. Pew Internet & American Life Project 2010;5:3–8.

43. Stoner SA, Arenella PB, Hendershot CS. Randomized controlled trial of a mobile phone intervention for improving adherence to naltrexone for alcohol use disorders. PLoS One 2015;10(4):e0124613.

44. Tofighi B, Grazioli F, Bereket S, et al. Text message reminders for improving patient appointment adherence in an office-based buprenorphine program: a feasibility study. Am J Addict 2017;26(6):581–6.

45. Keoleian V, Polcin D, Galloway GP. Text messaging for addiction: a review. J psychoactive Drugs 2015;47(2):158–76.

46. Gonzales R, Ang A, Murphy DA, et al. Substance use recovery outcomes among a cohort of youth participating in a mobile-based texting aftercare pilot program. J substance abuse Treat 2014;47(1):20–6.

47. Lucht MJ, Hoffman L, Haug S, et al. A surveillance tool using mobile phone short message service to reduce alcohol consumption among alcohol-dependent patients. Alcohol Clin Exp Res 2014;38(6):1728–36.

48. Agyapong VI, McLoughlin DM, Farren CK. Six-months outcomes of a randomised trial of supportive text messaging for depression and comorbid alcohol use disorder. J Affect Disord 2013;151(1):100–4.

49. Reback CJ, Fletcher JB, Shoptaw S, et al. Exposure to theory-driven text messages is associated with HIV risk reduction among methamphetamine-using men who have sex with men. AIDS Behav 2015;19(2):130–41.

50. Abu-Hasaballah K, James A, Aseltine RH. Lessons and pitfalls of interactive voice response in medical research. Contemp Clin Trials 2007;28(5):593–602.

51. Piette JD. Interactive voice response systems in the diagnosis and management of chronic disease. Am J Manag Care 2000;6(7):817–27.

52. Regan S, Reyen M, Lockhart AC, et al. An interactive voice response system to continue a hospital-based smoking cessation intervention after discharge. Nicotine Tob Res 2011;13(4):255–60.

53. Toll BA, Cooney NL, McKee SA, et al. Correspondence between Interactive Voice Response (IVR) and Timeline Followback (TLFB) reports of drinking behavior. Addict behaviors 2006;31(4):726–31.

54. Mundt JC, Moore HK, Bean P. An interactive voice response program to reduce drinking relapse: a feasibility study. J substance abuse Treat 2006;30(1):21–9.

55. Andersson C, Öjehagen A, Olsson MO, et al. Interactive voice response with feedback intervention in outpatient treatment of substance use problems in adolescents and young adults: a randomized controlled trial. Int J Behav Med 2017; 24(5):789–97.

56. Dulin PL, Gonzalez VM, King DK, et al. Development of a smartphone-based, self-administered intervention system for alcohol use disorders. Alcohol Treat Q 2013;31(3):321–36.

57. Patrick H, Williams GC. Self-determination theory: its application to health behavior and complementarity with motivational interviewing. Int J Behav Nutr Phys Act 2012;9:18.
58. Larimer ME, Palmer RS, Marlatt GA. Relapse prevention. An overview of Marlatt's cognitive-behavioral model. Alcohol Res Health 1999;23(2):151–60.
59. Barak A, Klein B, Proudfoot JG. Defining internet-supported therapeutic interventions. Ann Behav Med 2009;38(1):4–17.
60. Monico LB, Gryczynski J, Mitchell SG, et al. Buprenorphine treatment and 12-step meeting attendance: conflicts, compatibilities, and patient outcomes. J substance abuse Treat 2015;57:89–95.
61. NIDA. Using social media to better understand, prevent, and treat substance use. In: NIDA, editor. Bethesda (MD): National Institute on Drug Abuse; 2014. Available at: https://www.drugabuse.gov/news-events/news-releases/2014/10/using-social-media-to-better-understand-prevent-treat-substance-use. Accessed October 1, 2017.
62. Alessi SM, Barnett NP, Petry NM. Experiences with SCRAMx alcohol monitoring technology in 100 alcohol treatment outpatients. Drug and Alcohol Dependence 2017;178:417–24.
63. Barnett NP, Celio MA, Tidey JW, et al. A preliminary randomized controlled trial of contingency management for alcohol use reduction using a transdermal alcohol sensor. Addiction 2017;112:1025–35.
64. Dougherty DM, Hill-Kapturczak N, Liang Y, et al. Use of continuous transdermal alcohol monitoring during a contingency management procedure to reduce excessive alcohol use. Drug Alcohol Depend 2014;142:301–6.
65. Greenfield TK, Bond J, Kerr WC. Biomonitoring for improving alcohol consumption surveys: the new gold standard? Alcohol Res 2014;36:39–45.
66. Orrell C, Cohen K, Mauff K, et al. A randomized controlled trial of real-time electronic adherence monitoring with text message dosing reminders in people starting first-line antiretroviral therapy. J Acquir Immune Defic Syndr 2015;70:495–502.
67. Santos G, Coffin P, Santos D, et al. Feasibility, acceptability and tolerability of targeted naltrexone for non-dependent methamphetamine-using and binge drinking men who have sex with men. JAIDS J Acquired Immune Deficiency Syndromes 2016;72:21–30.
68. Carreiro S, Chai PR, Carey J, et al. Integrating personalized technology in toxicology: sensors, smart glass, and social media applications in toxicology research. J Med Toxicol 2017;13:166–72.
69. Chai PR, Rosen RK, Boyer EW, et al. Ingestible biosensors for real-time medical adherence monitoring: MyTMed. Proc Annu Hawaii Int Conf Syst Sci 2016;2016:3416–23.
70. Gordon A, Jaffe A, McLellan AT, et al. How should remote clinical monitoring be used to treat alcohol use disorders? J Addict Med 2017;11:145–53.
71. You CW, Chen YC, Chen CH, et al. Smartphone-based support system (SoberDiary) coupled with a Bluetooth breathalyser for treatment-seeking alcohol-dependent patients. Addict Behaviors 2017;65:174–8.
72. Boyer EW, Fletcher R, Fay RJ, et al. Preliminary efforts directed toward the detection of craving of illicit substances: the iHeal project. J Med Toxicol 2012;8:5–9.
73. Ebner-Priemer UW, Kuo J, Schlotz W, et al. Distress and affective dysregulation in patients with borderline personality disorder: a psychophysiological ambulatory monitoring study. J Nerv Ment Dis 2008;196(4):314–20.

74. Feldman G, Dunn E, Stemke C, et al. Mindfulness and rumination as predictors of persistence with a distress tolerance task. Pers Individ Dif 2014;56:154–8.

75. Herrero N, Gadea M, Rodriguez-Alarcon G, et al. What happens when we get angry? Hormonal, cardiovascular and asymmetrical brain responses. Horm Behav 2010;57(3):276–83.

76. Kobele R, Koschke M, Schulz S, et al. The influence of negative mood on heart rate complexity measures and baroreflex sensitivity in healthy subjects. Indian J Psychiatry 2010;52(1):42–7.

77. Carreiro S, Fang H, Zhang J, et al. iMStrong: deployment of a biosensor system to detect cocaine use. J Med Syst 2015;39:1–14.

78. Carreiro S, Wittbold K, Indic P, et al. Wearable biosensors to detect physiologic change during opioid use. J Med Toxicol 2016;12:255–62.

79. Arnold Z, LaRose D, Agu E. Smartphone inference of alcohol consumption levels from gait. Proceedings - 2015 IEEE International Conference on Healthcare Informatics, ICHI 2015 2015. Verona, Italy, September 15 – 17, 2014. p. 417–26.

80. Priester MA, Browne T, Iachini A, et al. Treatment access barriers and disparities among individuals with co-occurring mental health and substance use disorders: an integrative literature review. J Substance Abuse Treat 2016;61:47–59.

81. Sugarman DE, Campbell ANC, Iles BR, et al. Technology-based interventions for substance use and comorbid disorders. Harv Rev Psychiatry 2017;25:123–34.

82. Kay-Lambkin FJ, Simpson AL, Bowman J, et al. Dissemination of a computer-based psychological treatment in a drug and alcohol clinical service: an observational study. Addict Sci Clin Pract 2014;9(1):15.

83. Deady M, Mills KL, Teesson M, et al. An online intervention for co-occurring depression and problematic alcohol use in young people: primary outcomes from a randomized controlled trial. J Med Internet Res 2016;18:1–12.

84. Kay-Lambkin F, Baker A, Geddes J, et al. The iTreAD project: a study protocol for a randomised controlled clinical trial of online treatment and social networking for binge drinking and depression in young people. BMC Public Health 2015; 15(1):1025.

85. Gilmore AK, Wilson SM, Skopp NA, et al. A systematic review of technology-based interventions for co-occurring substance use and trauma symptoms. J Telemed Telecare 2017;23(8):701–9.

86. Buntin MB, Burke MF, Hoaglin MC, et al. The benefits of health information technology: a review of the recent literature shows predominantly positive results. Health Aff 2011;30(3):464–71.

87. Eyrich-Garg KM. Mobile phone technology: a new paradigm for the prevention, treatment, and research of the non-sheltered "street" homeless? J Urban Health 2010;87(3):365–80.

88. Tofighi B, Campbell A, Pavlicova M, et al. Recent internet use and associations with clinical outcomes among patients entering addiction treatment involved in a web-delivered psychosocial intervention study. J Urban Health 2016;93(5): 871–83.

89. Acosta MC, Marsch LA, Xie H, et al. A web-based behavior therapy program influences the association between cognitive functioning and retention and abstinence in clients receiving methadone maintenance treatment. J Dual Diagn 2012;8(4):283–93.

90. Bates ME, Buckman JF, Nguyen TT. A role for cognitive rehabilitation in increasing the effectiveness of treatment for alcohol use disorders. Neuropsychol Rev 2013; 23(1):27–47.

91. Lupton D, Jutel A. 'It's like having a physician in your pocket!' A critical analysis of self-diagnosis smartphone apps. Social Sci Med 2015;133:128–35.

92. Administration USFD. Mobile medical applications. 2017. Available at: https://www.fda.gov/MedicalDevices/DigitalHealth/MobileMedicalApplications/default.htm. Accessed September 8, 2017.

93. Karasz HN, Eiden A, Bogan S. Text messaging to communicate with public health audiences: how the HIPAA Security Rule affects practice. Am J Public Health 2013;103(4):617–22.

94. Bartholomew LK, Parcel GS, Kok G. Intervention mapping: a process for developing theory and evidence-based health education programs. Health Educ Behav 1998;25(5):545–63.

95. Collins LM, Murphy SA, Strecher V. The Multiphase Optimization Strategy (MOST) and the Sequential Multiple Assignment Randomized Trial (SMART): new methods for more potent eHealth interventions. Am J Prev Med 2007;32(5):S112–8.

96. Webb TL, Joseph J, Yardley L, et al. Using the internet to promote health behavior change: a systematic review and meta-analysis of the impact of theoretical basis, use of behavior change techniques, and mode of delivery on efficacy. J Med Internet Res 2010;12(1):e4.

97. Bates DW, Bitton A. The future of health information technology in the patient-centered medical home. Health Aff 2010;29(4):614–21.

Sleep Management Among Patients with Substance Use Disorders

Subhajit Chakravorty, MD[a],*, Ryan G. Vandrey, PhD[b],
Sean He, BS[c,d], Michael D. Stein, MD[e]

KEYWORDS

- Sleep initiation and maintenance disorders • Substance-related disorders
- Alcoholism • Cocaine-related disorders • Marijuana abuse
- Opioid-related disorders

KEY POINTS

- Insomnia is linked with substance use and withdrawal.
- Cognitive behavioral therapy for insomnia has shown promise as an intervention for insomnia in individuals with alcohol and possibly other drug use disorders.
- Sleep-disordered breathing should be considered in the differential diagnosis of sleep maintenance insomnia, especially for patients misusing opioids and alcohol.
- Abstinence from substance use should be recommended for those with short-term insomnia.
- A referral to a sleep medicine clinic should be considered for insomnia disorder or other intrinsic sleep disorders, especially during abstinence.

Disclosure Statement: Dr S. Chakravorty has received research support from AstraZeneca and Teva Pharmaceuticals. Dr R.G. Vandrey is a paid consultant or serves on the advisory board of Zynerba Pharmaceuticals, Insys Therapeutics Inc, Battelle Memorial Institute, and several small US businesses engaged in state medicinal cannabis programs. The study was supported by VA grant IK2CX000855 (S. Chakravorty), U01 DA031784 (R.G. Vandrey), R01 DA034261, R01 NR015977 R34 DA032800 R21 DA031369 (M.D. Stein). The content of this publication does not represent the views of the Department of Veterans Affairs or any other institution.
[a] Department of Psychiatry, Perelman School of Medicine, Corporal Michael J. Crescenz VA Medical Center, MIRECC, 2nd Floor, Postal Code 116, 3900 Woodland Avenue, Philadelphia, PA 19104, USA; [b] Behavioral Pharmacology Research Unit, Johns Hopkins University School of Medicine, 5510 Nathan Shock Drive, Baltimore, MD 21224, USA; [c] Post-baccalaureate studies program, College of Liberal Arts and Professional Studies, University of Pennsylvania, 3440 Market Street Suite 100, Philadelphia, PA 19104, USA; [d] Department of R & D, Corporal Michael J. Crescenz VA Medical Center, 3900 Woodland Avenue, Philadelphia, PA 19104, USA; [e] Department of Health Law, Policy and Management, Boston University School of Public Health, 715 Albany Street, Boston, MA 02118, USA
* Corresponding author.
E-mail address: Subhajit.Chakravorty@uphs.upenn.edu

INTRODUCTION: SLEEP AND ITS ASSOCIATION WITH SUBSTANCE USE DISORDERS

A disturbance of sleep continuity has effects on next-day functioning and behavior. One such behavior is the use of psychoactive substances. Disturbed sleep is also a frequent complaint among persons using alcohol and illicit drugs. Further, sleep dysfunction in the context of substance misuse may contribute to increased severity of substance use disorder (SUD), impaired quality of life, comorbid psychiatric complaints, suicidal behavior, and psychosocial problems.[1,2] This narrative review focuses on the identification and treatment of sleep disorders in persons with comorbid SUDs.

ASSESSMENT AND DIAGNOSIS OF SUBSTANCE USE AND SLEEP DISORDERS
Substance Use and Substance Use Disorder

Various aspects of substance use are relevant to sleep. Drugs can have an acute impact on sleep by either increasing or decreasing arousal. Pharmacologically specific sleep-related withdrawal symptoms may occur on cessation or reduction of heavy, sustained periods of substance use.[3] Problematic patterns of substance use also may lead to distress, which may in turn impact sleep via nonpharmacological mechanisms. Commonly used substances in the context of sleep-related problems include alcohol, cocaine, cannabis (marijuana), opioids, and sedative-hypnotic-anxiolytic medications.

APPROACH TO THE ASSESSMENT OF PATIENTS WITH SLEEP DISORDERS

Patient complaints related to sleep most often consist of difficulty falling asleep, difficulty staying asleep, or impaired daytime functioning. Symptoms of impaired daytime functioning may include mood disturbance, fatigue, problems with concentration, or daytime sleepiness. The common sleep-related disorders evaluated in the context of substance use include the following:

1. Insomnia
2. Circadian rhythm disorder–delayed sleep phase type (CRSD-DSP)
3. Sleep-related breathing disorder (SRBD)

Fig. 1 explains a strategy for screening patients in a clinical setting, especially in the context of a primary care setting when substance use is suspected or confirmed.

Insomnia

Insomnia is a disorder characterized by complaints of poor sleep continuity (ie, difficulty falling asleep and/or staying asleep), early morning awakening, and impairment of daytime functioning.[4] Insomnia may be assessed using a structured rating instrument, such as the Insomnia Severity Index or a sleep diary. The sleep diary should be prospectively completed for a week or more and yields multiple indices, see **Table 1**. Acute insomnia denotes a recent onset of insomnia, less than 3 months in duration and commonly precipitated by a psychosocial stressor, that may be treated with reassurance, close monitoring, or with medications. Acute insomnia also is common in the acute withdrawal phase from substances. However, most of the hypnotic medications approved by the Food and Drug Administration (FDA), such as temazepam or zolpidem, may be contraindicated in patients with SUD. For those with chronic insomnia ($\geq$3 months in duration), behavioral interventions, such as cognitive behavioral therapy for insomnia (CBT-I), are the recommended first-line intervention. Insomnia comorbid with active substance use is optimally treated in a substance misuse program or primary care setting staffed by clinicians with experience in

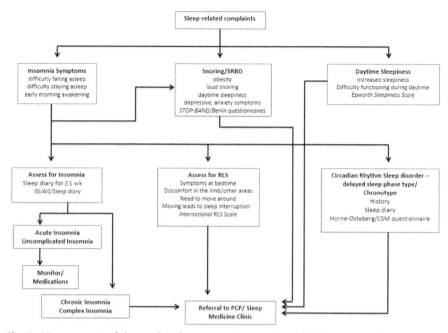

Fig. 1. Management of sleep-related symptoms in a patient with SUD. AIS, Athens insomnia scale; CSM questionnaire, composite scale of morningness questionnaire; ISI, Insomnia Severity Index scale; PCP, primary care provider; STOP-BANG questionnaire, a screening questionnaire for OSA.

substance-related problems. In contrast, chronic insomnia in patients with remitted SUD are best treated by referral to a sleep medicine clinic (see **Fig. 1**).

Circadian Rhythm Sleep Disorder–Delayed Sleep Phase Type

CRSDs are generated as a consequence of a mismatch between the individual's internal (biological) rhythm and the required environmental schedule. CRSD-DSP is a particular subtype of CRSD that is characterized by going to bed later in the night and awakening later in the morning. This later sleep-wake timing may interfere with daily activities, and patients may present with complaints of insomnia, sleepiness, and impaired daytime functioning. CRSDs may be easily assessed in a clinic setting using sleep diaries, actigraphy, or with the help of rating scales that evaluate the patient's propensity for sleep at a particular time during the 24-hour period. Prior research has linked alcohol use with the blunting of circadian rhythms in healthy adults,[5] and, alcohol use disorder (AUD) with insomnia and a nocturnal delay in the rise of melatonin level (a marker of circadian activity).[6,7]

Sleep-Related Breathing Disorder

SRBDs are characterized by disruption of sleep by respiratory events. An individual may be screened for SRBD either using an in-laboratory clinical polysomnogram or home sleep monitoring using a portable sleep monitor. Obstructive sleep apnea (OSA) is condition characterized by loud snoring, breath interruptions, and polysomnographic evidence of obstructive apneas and/or obstructive hypopneas, see **Table 1**. Central sleep apnea (CSA) syndrome may present similarly, but mostly consists of events with complete cessation of airflow along with cessation of thoracic and

Table 1
Commonly used terminologies in sleep medicine

Acronym	Term	Description
SE	Sleep efficiency (%)	The proportion of time spent sleeping through the night
NREM	NREM sleep	The initial stages of sleep (N1 + N2 + SWS); approximately 80% of sleep
N1	Stage 1 sleep	Characterized by low eye movements, waves with low amplitude, and, mostly 4–7-Hz frequency
N2	Stage 2 sleep	The sleep stage that demonstrates sleep spindles and K complexes
N3/SWS	Slow-wave sleep (stages 3 + 4)	The presence of high amplitude and low frequency (0.5–2.0 Hz), $\geq$20% of the epoch
REM	Rapid eye movement sleep	Sleep with sawtooth waveforms, rapid eye movements, and low muscle tone
SOL	Sleep-onset latency (min)	Time from "lights out" until the onset of sleep in the reading pane
REM-L	REM-onset latency (min)	Interval of time from onset of sleep to the appearance of the first epoch of REM sleep
S1	Stage 1 (%)	The fraction of sleep that is spent in N1 (total Stage 1 sleep/TST × 100); usually approximately 4%–5%
S2	Stage 2 (%)	The fraction of sleep that is spent in N2 (total Stage 2 sleep/TST × 100); usually approximately 45%–55%
SWS	Slow-wave sleep (%)	The percentage of sleep that is spent in SWS (total SWS sleep/TST × 100); usually approximately 16%–21%
REM	REM (%)	The percentage of sleep that is spent in REM (total REM sleep/TST × 100); usually approximately 20%–25%
Apnea	(polysomnography or home sleep test)	A complete cessation of airflow for $\geq$10 s
Hypopnea	(polysomnography or home sleep test)	A partial cessation of airflow for $\geq$10 s, and either a $\geq$4% drop in SpO_2, or, an arousal (as seen on electroencephalogram)
AHI	Apnea Hypopnea Index (events/h)	Total number of apneas and hypopneas per hour of sleep; that is, total number of apneas and hypopneas/TST
Advance	Phase advance	Shift of the sleep cycle to an earlier time during a circadian period (24 h)
Delay	Phase delay	Shift of the sleep cycle to a later time during a circadian period (24 h)
SRBD	Sleep-related breathing disorder	Abnormalities of respiration during sleep; include OSA, CSA, and obesity hypoventilation and hypoventilation syndromes
OSA	Obstructive sleep apnea	A syndrome with symptoms (loud snoring and breathing interruptions)/cardio-metabolic syndrome + AHI $\geq$5 events/h of sleep
CSA	Central sleep apnea	A syndrome with symptoms (sleepiness, insomnia, snoring, and witnessed apneas)/atrial fibrillation/CHF + $\geq$5 central events/h of sleep
CPAP	Continuous positive airway pressure	A machine delivering air at a continuous pressure to prevent collapse of the air passage during sleep

(continued on next page)

Table 1 (continued)		
Acronym	**Term**	**Description**
BiPAP	Bi-level positive airway pressure	A machine delivering air at 2 pressures: a higher pressure during inspiration and a lower pressure during expiration
ASV	Adaptive servo-ventilation	A specialized form of positive airway pressure support in which the delivered pressure changes when respiratory events are detected
CBT-I	Cognitive behavioral therapy for insomnia	A manualized behavioral treatment for insomnia, consisting of sleep restriction, stimulus control, and cognitive therapy, for ≤8 wk

Abbreviation: CHF, congestive heart failure; NREM, non–rapid eye movement; TST, total sleep time.
   Data from American Academy of Sleep Medicine (AASM). The AASM manual for the scoring of sleep and associated events. 2007; and American Academy of Sleep Medicine (AASM). 2012. Available at: http://www.sleepnet.com/definition.html. Accessed October 28, 2017.

abdominal wall movements for ≥10 seconds. **Fig. 1** elaborates on ways to screen for SRBD in an outpatient setting. The management of SRBD requires referral to a sleep medicine service.

Limb Movement Disorders in Sleep

This category of sleep disorders includes restless leg syndrome (RLS) and periodic limb movement disorder. A patient with RLS presents with "an urge to move the legs usually accompanied by or thought to be caused by uncomfortable and unpleasant sensation in the legs," which in turn leads to difficulty falling asleep at bedtime.[4] Patients in whom these disorders are suspected also should be referred to a sleep center.

It should be noted that an individual might have multiple comorbid sleep and/or SUDs. Complex case presentations may require cotreatment in substance use and sleep medicine clinics.

ALCOHOL AND SLEEP DISORDERS
Alcohol and Insomnia

Acute alcohol use has sedating effects, particularly on the descending limb of the blood-alcohol concentration curve, and is sometimes used for its sleep-promoting effects. However, alcohol may disrupt sleep by interfering with homeostatic and circadian balance, disrupting local sleep mechanisms, and distorting the electrophysiology of sleep.[1]

Risky alcohol use and AUD have been associated with subjective insomnia as well as objective sleep continuity disturbance. In those with AUD, the prevalence of insomnia ranges from 36% to 91% as compared with the 10% prevalence in the general population, and is prevalent in all stages of AUD.[1] The prevalence of insomnia decreases once alcohol-dependent individuals transition from active drinking to abstinence, with persisting insomnia possibly being a risk factor for relapse.[1] However, in heavy drinkers with AUD, sleep dysfunction may persist up to 2 years into recovery in a subset of individuals and is a risk factor for relapse.[8] Those who screen positive for AUD should be educated about the association of insomnia with AUD.

Behavioral and pharmacologic interventions for insomnia in AUD have been studied. Behavioral interventions have consistently demonstrated efficacy in treating insomnia among individuals with AUD.[1] CBT-I is the recommended first-line treatment for insomnia.[9] Prior studies have demonstrated conflicting results with gabapentin and trazodone.[1] Other drugs that have demonstrated an improvement in insomnia among alcohol-dependent patients have included acamprosate, agomelatine, and quetiapine.[1]

If insomnia persists despite continued abstinence, patients should be referred to a sleep medicine clinic. If a behavioral sleep medicine specialist is unavailable in the sleep clinic, bibliotherapy, online sleep treatment programs, or evidence-based psychopharmacologic interventions should be considered, such as gabapentin or ramelteon.

Most of the currently approved hypnotic medications, such as zolpidem or eszopiclone, are contraindicated in those with current AUD due to the potential risk of dependence and drug-drug interactions secondary to polypharmacy in this population. Therefore, gabapentin may be an alternative for those who continue to drink, although risks and benefits should be carefully reviewed.

Alcohol and Sleep-Related Breathing Disorder

Alcohol relaxes the musculature of the upper airway and impairs protective arousal response during sleep. These effects may lead to an aggravation of snoring, fragmentation of sleep, and worsening of preexisting SRBD. Treatment-seeking persons with AUD have a higher intensity of sleep-disordered breathing during alcohol withdrawal and a high prevalence of SRBD.[1] Continuous positive airway pressure (CPAP) is the first-line treatment modality, although alternatives to CPAP are also available depending on severity.

OPIOIDS AND SLEEP DISORDERS

Opioid prescriptions for chronic pain analgesia, along with opioid morbidity, have increased dramatically over the past 2 decades. Hassamal and colleagues[10] demonstrated that prescription opioid receipt and increasing opioid dose were associated with greater self-reported sleep disturbance among individuals with chronic pain, suggesting opioids worsen sleep beyond the disruptive sleep effects of pain. Insomnia and SRBD are the primary sleep disorders reported in those using opioids. Because pain and respiratory control are mediated by the endogenous opioid system, opioid-induced impairment in breathing must be a central concern of clinical evaluation in sleep-impaired persons.

Opioids and Insomnia

Most persons receiving opioids for chronic pain have insomnia, and approximately three-quarters of persons receiving methadone maintenance treatment (MMT) or buprenorphine for opioid use disorder (OUD) have sleep complaints. Acute dosing of opioids for the treatment of pain appears to improve aspects of sleep quality.[11] But as use continues, there appears to be a significant association between prescription opioid dose and self-reported sleep dysfunction. The most frequent complaints include increased sleep latency and increased time awake after sleep onset.[12]

Among individuals with OUD, sleep gradually improves during the first 90 days after initiating treatment with buprenorphine/naltrexone.[13] Factors contributing to persisting sleep complaints in opioid users are pain, depression,[14] benzodiazepine (BZD) use, and cigarette smoking. It should be noted that use of medications in the BZD class is common in this population and is associated with longer sleep time estimates by patients than is demonstrated during sleep studies. Still, many opioid users will use

BZDs to facilitate sleep,[15] increasing their risk for overdose, as both substances suppress respiration.[16,17]

CBT-I treatment has been shown to improve sleep-related outcomes,[18–20] including patients who had previously been prescribed medications for sleep[21] and among patients whose impaired sleep was secondary to pain.[22] Trazodone has failed to show efficacy in one study,[23] and no data exist on other medications like doxepin or suvorexant.

Opioids and Sleep-Related Breathing Disorder

Opioid-induced impairment of breathing includes central depression of the respiratory rate, amplitude and reflex responses, reduced brain arousal, and upper airway dysfunction.[24] SRBDs occur in most chronic opioid users.[25] OSA was observed in 39% of 140 patients with chronic pain taking opioids,[26] whereas the prevalence of OSA in the general population is estimated at 9% in women and 24% in men.[27] Risk factors for SRBD in patients with OUD include smoking, female gender, and increased body weight.[10] OSA in this population is likely due to opioid-induced reductions in airway muscle activation.[28] CSA may arise from depression of hypoxic and hypercapnic ventilatory drives, which are already reduced during sleep.[24] This effect has been reported to occur in 0% to 60% of MMT patients,[10] although it is rarely observed in the general population. CSA has been associated with methadone dose and concomitant BZD use, and with higher methadone blood concentration.[10] Cases in which CSA reverses after discontinuation of opioid treatment have been reported.[10] Although very little information exists on SRBD associated with buprenorphine/naloxone, 1 study demonstrated incidence rates of 63% for mild, 16% for moderate, and 17% for severe OSA.[29]

Treatment recommendations for opioid-induced SRBD are limited by a lack of research on the topic. As a first step, the option of discontinuing opioids should be considered in the context of risks and benefits with this decision. When long-term treatment with opioid therapy is continued, and SRBD is identified, treatment options include CPAP, adaptive servo-ventilation, and bi-level spontaneous timed therapy.[24] An alternative option is switching to an injectable formulation of depot-Naltrexone, a mu-opioid receptor antagonist.

CANNABIS AND SLEEP DISORDERS

Acute cannabis or tetrahydrocannabinol (THC) administration is associated with reduced latency to sleep onset, a decrease in rapid eye movement sleep and an increase in Stage 3 sleep.[30] The hypnotic properties of cannabis are often reported as a reason for use of cannabis, and may drive sustained use patterns among individuals with underlying sleep dysfunction.[2] However, there is evidence of tolerance developing to the hypnotic effects of cannabis use, likely due to neurobiological changes in the endocannabinoid system.[30]

Daily cannabis users self-report greater sleep disturbance compared with nonusers and less-frequent users, and treatment-seeking cannabis users have high rates of disordered sleep.[31,32] However, it remains unclear whether increased sleep problems among daily and treatment-seeking cannabis users reflects a direct impact of heavy cannabis use or that the sleep dysfunction in this population is due to an underlying psychiatric or sleep pathology that predated, and possibly contributed to the development of cannabis use disorder (CUD). Notably, one of the defining features of CUD is a cannabis withdrawal syndrome, in which sleep difficulty and an increase in vivid/strange dreams are hallmark features.[33] Sleep difficulty typically lasts 2 to 3 weeks before returning to baseline levels, but the increase in vivid/strange dreams appears to persist indefinitely, suggesting that cannabis suppresses the recall or vividness of dreams rather than this being a true withdrawal effect.[33]

Sleep difficulty during cannabis abstinence is a commonly reported barrier to cessation, with individuals reporting relapse to cannabis use, increased alcohol use, or use of sedative/hypnotic drugs to mitigate abstinence-induced sleep problems.[33] Treatment-seeking cannabis users often exhibit clinically significant sleep dysfunction, and poor sleep at the beginning of treatment predicts relapse early in a quit attempt.[32,34] Pilot studies suggest that behavioral and pharmacologic interventions that can improve sleep during treatment for CUD may improve cannabis use outcomes.[35,36]

The medicinal use of cannabis in the treatment of pain, multiple sclerosis, or post-traumatic stress disorder (PTSD) can result in improved sleep. In some cases, the sleep improvement may contribute to better clinical outcomes and an improved quality of life. However, long-term use of cannabis or THC primarily as a hypnotic agent is not recommended due to the development of tolerance to its hypnotic properties, risk of long-term sleep disturbance, and subsequent withdrawal symptoms on abrupt cessation, which can exacerbate symptoms of certain illnesses (eg, PTSD).

COCAINE AND ITS ASSOCIATED SLEEP DISORDERS

Acute cocaine use increases arousal, and binge use often occurs when the individual does not sleep. Persons with cocaine use disorder (CoUD) seldom seek help for insomnia; however, recent studies that included objective measures indicate sleep dysfunction is common during cocaine withdrawal.[33]

In a controlled trial of CoUD, modafinil (an FDA-approved medication for sleepiness in adequately treated OSA, narcolepsy, and shift work sleep disorder) was superior to placebo in improving the total sleep time, Stage 3 sleep, and abstinence from cocaine.[33] Other medications investigated for sleep continuity disturbance in individuals with CoUD have included lorazepam, tiagabine, and mirtazapine. In a comparative efficacy trial of lorazepam and tiagabine, both drugs decreased sleep latency, but tiagabine increased slow-wave sleep in recently abstinent persons with CoUD.[37] Mirtazapine, compared with placebo, transiently improved sleep-onset latency in depressed subjects with CoUD after 4 weeks of treatment, but did not reduce cocaine consumption.[38]

SEDATIVE-HYPNOTIC-ANXIOLYTIC DRUGS AND SLEEP DISORDERS

Sedative-hypnotic-anxiolytic medications include BZD medications and newer non-BZD Z-drugs. Long-term use of BZDs may lead to dependence and characteristic withdrawal symptoms on discontinuation that include autonomic hyperactivity, insomnia, anxiety, and agitation. Similarly, reports also exist for unhealthy use of non-BZD Z-drugs, although the rate of misuse of these medications is lower than for BZDs.

BZD use has been associated with other SUDs, including alcohol and opioid use, conditions that are also independently linked with insomnia symptoms.[39–41] Abrupt cessation of these medications has been associated with sleep complaints, such as decreased total sleep time and a poor sleep quality. Among the sedative-hypnotic medications, the intensity of withdrawal-induced insomnia is higher in those using BZD-class drugs as compared with the newer Z-drugs. In fact, withdrawal insomnia may be mild or nonexistent after cessation of use of these Z-drugs. Sleep disturbances following abstinence from hypnotic medications typically improve over time during recovery, suggesting it is a true withdrawal effect.[42]

There is scant literature on the treatment of sleep problems in patients with sedative-hypnotic use disorder. Pregabalin has shown promise in decreasing insomnia and the use of BZDs and to bolster abstinence.[43,44] In addition to medications, behavioral interventions, such as relaxation therapy and CBT-I, have demonstrated promise in treating the insomnia.[45]

SUMMARY AND FUTURE DIRECTIONS

Sleep and SUDs are commonly comorbid conditions. Use of psychoactive substances often leads to the development of complaints of disturbed sleep, insomnia disorder, or circadian rhythm sleep disorders. Abrupt cessation of substances of unhealthy use commonly results in sleep disruption, which may be treated with behavioral or pharmacologic interventions as a means of improving cessation attempt outcomes. Other sleep disorders, such as SRBD should be considered in the differential diagnosis for insomnia, especially in those with opioid use or AUD. When chronic insomnia or another intrinsic sleep disorder is suspected, a referral to the local sleep center is recommended. Chronic insomnia may be optimally treated with CBT-I. Acute insomnia or insomnia in the context of active substance use may be best treated in an addiction medicine or a primary care setting in which the preliminary focus should be to target abstinence.

ACKNOWLEDGMENTS

The editors thank Deirdre A. Conroy, University of Michigan, and Bhanu Prakash Kolla, Mayo Clinic, Rochester, MN, for providing a critical review of this article.

REFERENCES

1. Chakravorty S, Chaudhary NS, Brower KJ. Alcohol dependence and its relationship with insomnia and other sleep disorders. Alcohol Clin Exp Res 2016;40(11): 2271–82.
2. Vandrey R, Babson KA, Herrmann ES, et al. Interactions between disordered sleep, post-traumatic stress disorder, and substance use disorders. Int Rev Psychiatry 2014;26(2):237–47.
3. DSM-5. Diagnostic and statistical manual of mental disorders, 5th edition. Arlington (VA): American Psychiatric Publishing; 2013.
4. International classification of sleep disorders - 3rd edition. Darien (IL): American Academy of Sleep Medicine; 2014.
5. Danel T, Libersa C, Touitou Y. The effect of alcohol consumption on the circadian control of human core body temperature is time dependent. Am J Physiol Regul Integr Comp Physiol 2001;281(1):R52–5.
6. Kuhlwein E, Hauger RL, Irwin MR. Abnormal nocturnal melatonin secretion and disordered sleep in abstinent alcoholics. Biol Psychiatry 2003;54(12):1437–43.
7. Conroy DA, Hairston IS, Arnedt JT, et al. Dim light melatonin onset in alcohol-dependent men and women compared with healthy controls. Chronobiol Int 2012;29(1):35–42.
8. Brower KJ. Insomnia, alcoholism and relapse. Sleep Med Rev 2003;7(6):523–39.
9. Schutte-Rodin S, Broch L, Buysse D, et al. Clinical guideline for the evaluation and management of chronic insomnia in adults. J Clin Sleep Med 2008;4(5):487–504.
10. Hassamal S, Miotto K, Wang T, et al. A narrative review: the effects of opioids on sleep disordered breathing in chronic pain patients and methadone maintained patients. Am J Addict 2016;25(6):452–65.

11. Dimsdale JE, Norman D, DeJardin D, et al. The effect of opioids on sleep architecture. J Clin Sleep Med 2007;3(1):33–6.
12. Peles E, Schreiber S, Adelson M. Variables associated with perceived sleep disorders in methadone maintenance treatment (MMT) patients. Drug Alcohol Depend 2006;82(2):103–10.
13. Zheng WH, Wakim RJ, Geary RC, et al. Self-reported sleep improvement in buprenorphine MAT (Medication Assisted Treatment) population. Austin J Drug Abuse Addict 2016;3(1) [pii: 1009].
14. Tsuno N, Besset A, Ritchie K. Sleep and depression. J Clin Psychiatry 2005; 66(10):1254–69.
15. Stein MD, Kanabar M, Anderson BJ, et al. Reasons for benzodiazepine use among persons seeking opioid detoxification. J Subst Abuse Treat 2016;68: 57–61.
16. Li L, Sangthong R, Chongsuvivatwong V, et al. Lifetime multiple substance use pattern among heroin users before entering methadone maintenance treatment clinic in Yunnan, China. Drug Alcohol Rev 2010;29(4):420–5.
17. Stein MD, Herman DS, Bishop S, et al. Sleep disturbances among methadone maintained patients. J Subst Abuse Treat 2004;26(3):175–80.
18. Backhaus J, Hohagen F, Voderholzer U, et al. Long-term effectiveness of a short-term cognitive-behavioral group treatment for primary insomnia. Eur Arch Psychiatry Clin Neurosci 2001;251(1):35–41.
19. Montgomery P, Dennis J. Cognitive behavioural interventions for sleep problems in adults aged 60+. Cochrane Database Syst Rev 2003;(1):CD003161.
20. Trauer JM, Qian MY, Doyle JS, et al. Cognitive behavioral therapy for chronic insomnia: a systematic review and meta-analysis. Ann Intern Med 2015;163(3): 191–204.
21. Dolan DC, Taylor DJ, Bramoweth AD, et al. Cognitive-behavioral therapy of insomnia: a clinical case series study of patients with co-morbid disorders and using hypnotic medications. Behav Res Ther 2010;48(4):321–7.
22. Currie SR, Wilson KG, Pontefract AJ, et al. Cognitive-behavioral treatment of insomnia secondary to chronic pain. J Consult Clin Psychol 2000;68(3):407–16.
23. Stein MD, Kurth ME, Sharkey KM, et al. Trazodone for sleep disturbance during methadone maintenance: a double-blind, placebo-controlled trial. Drug Alcohol Depend 2012;120(1–3):65–73.
24. Van Ryswyk E, Antic NA. Opioids and sleep-disordered breathing. Chest 2016; 150(4):934–44.
25. Correa D, Farney RJ, Chung F, et al. Chronic opioid use and central sleep apnea: a review of the prevalence, mechanisms, and perioperative considerations. Anesth Analg 2015;120(6):1273–85.
26. Webster LR, Choi Y, Desai H, et al. Sleep-disordered breathing and chronic opioid therapy. Pain Med 2008;9(4):425–32.
27. Young T, Palta M, Dempsey J, et al. The occurrence of sleep-disordered breathing among middle-aged adults. N Engl J Med 1993;328(17):1230–5.
28. Hajiha M, DuBord MA, Liu H, et al. Opioid receptor mechanisms at the hypoglossal motor pool and effects on tongue muscle activity in vivo. J Physiol 2009;587(Pt 11):2677–92.
29. Farney RJ, McDonald AM, Boyle KM, et al. Sleep disordered breathing in patients receiving therapy with buprenorphine/naloxone. Eur Respir J 2013;42(2): 394–403.
30. Schierenbeck T, Riemann D, Berger M, et al. Effect of illicit recreational drugs upon sleep: cocaine, ecstasy and marijuana. Sleep Med Rev 2008;12(5):381–9.

31. Conroy DA, Kurth ME, Strong DR, et al. Marijuana use patterns and sleep among community-based young adults. J Addict Dis 2016;35(2):135–43.
32. Pacek LR, Herrmann ES, Smith MT, et al. Sleep continuity, architecture and quality among treatment-seeking cannabis users: an in-home, unattended polysomnographic study. Exp Clin Psychopharmacol 2017;25(4):295–302.
33. Angarita GA, Emadi N, Hodges S, et al. Sleep abnormalities associated with alcohol, cannabis, cocaine, and opiate use: a comprehensive review. Addict Sci Clin Pract 2016;11(1):9.
34. Babson KA, Boden MT, Bonn-Miller MO. The impact of perceived sleep quality and sleep efficiency/duration on cannabis use during a self-guided quit attempt. Addict Behav 2013;38(11):2707–13.
35. Babson KA, Ramo DE, Baldini L, et al. Mobile app-delivered cognitive behavioral therapy for insomnia: feasibility and initial efficacy among veterans with cannabis use disorders. JMIR Res Protoc 2015;4(3):e87.
36. Mason BJ, Crean R, Goodell V, et al. A proof-of-concept randomized controlled study of gabapentin: effects on cannabis use, withdrawal and executive function deficits in cannabis-dependent adults. Neuropsychopharmacology 2012;37(7): 1689–98.
37. Morgan PT, Malison RT. Pilot study of lorazepam and tiagabine effects on sleep, motor learning, and impulsivity in cocaine abstinence. Am J Drug Alcohol Abuse 2008;34(6):692–702.
38. Afshar M, Knapp CM, Sarid-Segal O, et al. The efficacy of mirtazapine in the treatment of cocaine dependence with comorbid depression. Am J Drug Alcohol Abuse 2012;38(2):181–6.
39. Kroll DS, Nieva HR, Barsky AJ, et al. Benzodiazepines are prescribed more frequently to patients already at risk for benzodiazepine-related adverse events in primary care. J Gen Intern Med 2016;31(9):1027–34.
40. Hackman DT, Greene MS, Fernandes TJ, et al. Prescription drug monitoring program inquiry in psychiatric assessment: detection of high rates of opioid prescribing to a dual diagnosis population. J Clin Psychiatry 2014;75(7):750–6.
41. Manthey L, Lohbeck M, Giltay EJ, et al. Correlates of benzodiazepine dependence in the Netherlands Study of Depression and Anxiety. Addiction 2012; 107(12):2173–82.
42. Lichstein KL. Behavioral intervention for special insomnia populations: hypnotic-dependent insomnia and comorbid insomnia. Sleep Med 2006;7(Suppl 1): S27–31.
43. Oulis P, Konstantakopoulos G. Efficacy and safety of pregabalin in the treatment of alcohol and benzodiazepine dependence. Expert Opin Investig Drugs 2012; 21(7):1019–29.
44. Cho YW, Song ML. Effects of pregabalin in patients with hypnotic-dependent insomnia. J Clin Sleep Med 2014;10(5):545–50.
45. Beaulieu-Bonneau S, Ivers H, Guay B, et al. Long-term maintenance of therapeutic gains associated with cognitive-behavioral therapy for insomnia delivered alone or combined with zolpidem. Sleep 2017;40(3).

Pain and Addiction
An Integrative Therapeutic Approach

Ajay Manhapra, MD[a,b,c,*], William C. Becker, MD[d,e,f]

KEYWORDS

- Substance use disorder • Addiction • Opioid use disorder • Pain • Chronic pain
- Multimorbidity • Treatment • Management

KEY POINTS

- Treating "pain and addiction" as 2 separate problems is often unsuccessful, because this clinical condition is often more than the sum of its parts.
- Patients with pain and addiction often have multiple psychological, psychiatric, and medical comorbidities with associated polypharmacy, all interacting with each other in complex ways (multimorbidity).
- Multimorbidity appears to be the key driver of "chronification" of pain (evolution of acute pain to severely disabling chronic pain) and associated adverse outcomes, rather than the persistence of injuries.
- The authors suggest an integrative approach that involves reexplaining the pain based on multimorbidity as the driver, followed by concurrent coordinated management of addiction/dependence, comorbidities, and chronic pain, and polypharmacy reduction.

INTRODUCTION

The current opioid crisis, partly fueled by the excess availability of prescription opioids for pain management, has highlighted the enormous challenge of managing disabling chronic pain intertwined with physiologic dependence to medications

Funding: A. Manhapra was supported by the Research in Addiction Medicine Scholars Research in Addiction Medicine Scholars (RAMS) Program, Grant number R25DA033211 from the National Institute on Drug Abuse, and VA/OAA Interprofessional Advanced Fellowship in Addiction Treatment. The funding organizations had no role in the design and conduct of the study; collection, management, analysis, and interpretation of the data; preparation, review, or approval of the article; and decision to submit the article for publication.

[a] Veteran Affairs New England Mental Illness Research, Education and Clinical Center (MIR-ECC), West Haven, CT, USA; [b] Advanced PACT Pain Clinic, VA Hampton Medical Center, 100 Emancipation Drive, PRIME 5, Hampton, VA 23667, USA; [c] Department of Psychiatry, Yale School of Medicine, New Haven, CT, USA; [d] Opioid Reassessment Clinic, VA Connecticut Healthcare System, 950 Campbell Avenue, Mailstop 151B, West Haven, CT 06516, USA; [e] Pain Research, Informatics, Multimorbidities and Education (PRIME) Center, West Haven, CT, USA; [f] Department of Medicine, Yale School of Medicine, New Haven, CT, USA
* Corresponding author. 100 Emancipation Drive, PRIME 5, Hampton, VA 23667.
E-mail address: ajay.manhapra@yale.edu

Med Clin N Am 102 (2018) 745–763
https://doi.org/10.1016/j.mcna.2018.02.013
medical.theclinics.com

(here forward termed "medication dependence") and substance use disorders (SUDs) and other medical and psychiatric disorders.[1,2] It is also now clear that long-term opioid therapy (LTOT), especially at high doses, is neither as safe nor as effective for treating chronic pain as once considered.[3] Many patients continue to have disabling pain despite high-dose LTOT and yet may be unable to discontinue opioids without major challenges.[4] Also, the prevalence of prior SUDs and psychiatric and medical comorbidities is high among these patients.[5,6] Given this complex context, there is an urgent need for better paradigms for the clinical conceptualization of disabling chronic pain among patients with dependence and addiction to opioids and other substances.[1]

Clinicians evaluating patients with the dual problem of pain and addiction often face the question, "Is this pain or is this addiction?" However, constricted focus on chronic pain and SUD as separate treatment entities often misses the complexity of the whole individual who suffers from the 2 maladies. These patients may also have high psychiatric and medical illness burden and may also use multiple substances or medications to manage their symptoms. These coexisting multiple problems interact with each other and pain and addiction in complex ways (multimorbidity), making clinical management challenging. In a nutshell, the problem of "pain and addiction" is more than the sum of its parts and thus necessitates an integrated, multidimensional therapeutic approach.

In this article, the authors first describe the complex interconnections of pain with dependence, opioid use disorder (OUD), and other SUDs. They then seek to draw attention to the critical role of multimorbidity (multiple illnesses existing together and interacting with each other in complex ways).[7] In light of the complexity of the current opioid epidemic, the authors propose an integrative multidimensional pharmacobehavioral model to manage these complex, commonly cooccurring conditions.

PAIN AND ADDICTION, A COMPLEX PROBLEM
Prevalence of Pain, Opioid Use Disorder, and Other Substance Use Disorders

Pain and SUD, including OUD, have a complicated reciprocal relationship with a myriad of interconnections (**Fig. 1**). Although a large proportion of patients with SUD have chronic pain compared with those without SUD, a smaller, nonetheless

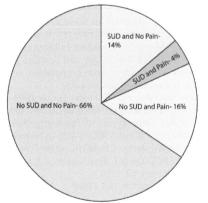

Fig. 1. Key information regarding pain and SUD including OUD. AUD/DUD, Alcohol use disorder and drug use disorder; NESARC, National Epidemiologic Survey on Alcohol and Related Conditions; PI, pain interference. (*Data from* Refs.[2,9,12–24,116])

significant proportion of patients with chronic pain tends to report SUD.[8] In the National Comorbidity Survey Replication (NCS-R), 35% of those with lifetime SUD reported chronic spinal pain, whereas only 4.8% of those with chronic spinal pain had SUD in the past year.[2] Although 38% of those with prescription OUD (pOUD) reported pain to the level that it interferes with life (pain interference) in a US national sample, only 18.9% of those without pOUD reported pain interference. Among those reporting pain interference, approximately 20% reported any SUD and 0.6% reported pOUD.[9] The prevalence of chronic pain and pain interference is even higher among those engaging in treatment of SUD,[10–18] with rates as high as 75% among patients with OUD treated with methadone or buprenorphine.[11,14,16,19–27]

Opioid Use Disorder, Pain, and Prescription Opioid Use

An estimated 12.5% of the 91.8 million US adults who used prescription opioids in 2015 misused them, with substantially higher misuse rates among those with pOUD and other SUDs.[28] Although those without pOUD reported pain as the most common reason for misuse (63%), more than half of those with pOUD and other SUDs reported other reasons, such as relaxing and getting high. Prescription opioid misuse among patients entering treatment for SUD appears to be largely for withdrawal prevention and getting high,[29,30] with slightly higher misuse for pain relief among those using heroin.[30,31]

The demographics of heroin use have changed over time. Those who started heroin use in the 1960s were mostly racially heterogeneous young people who initiated with heroin, whereas those who used heroin use in subsequent decades tended to be mostly older Caucasian men who started with prescription opioids.[32,33] More recently, this trend seems to be reversing because of decreased availability and increased cost of prescription opioids and increased availability of the often cheaper option of heroin. Between 2005 and 2013, opioid initiation with prescription opioids among treatment-seeking heroin users decreased from 84% to 52%, whereas opioid initiation with heroin increased from 8.7% to 33%.[34,35] Because the use of prescription opioids alone is waning among those with OUD, their concurrent use with heroin is steadily increasing.[34]

Pain and Substance Use Disorders: Which Starts First?

Although it is often assumed that chronic pain precedes onset of SUDs, it appears that SUD typically precedes the onset of chronic pain among those with both. However, the less common pathway, pain before SUD, is by no means rare. Among those with pain and SUD in the NCS-R, SUD preceded pain in 58.2%, and pain preceded SUD in 35.4%.[36] A similar temporal pattern of OUD more often preceding chronic pain is also seen among those using prescription opioids, in both clinical trial data and epidemiologic studies.[9–11]

Pain, a Driver of Opioid Use Disorder in Individuals

Pain drives increased craving for opioids[37] and use of multiple substances for pain relief among individuals engaged in SUD treatment.[38,39] Although a higher intensity of pain has only shown limited association with OUD outcomes,[25,26,30] higher variability in pain fluctuations (pain volatility) is associated with higher relapse rates and poor outcomes after detoxification.[14,40,41] A high level of persistent pain is often observed after opioid use cessation among patients with OUD and predicts a high level of craving and substance use.[13,14,42] Also, those with a history of SUD show lower improvement with pain treatments.[43]

These data suggest that although persistent pain and its volatility could be a symptom reflective of the severity of ongoing opioid use and OUD, it could also be a symptom of protracted abstinence syndrome after opioid cessation or dose reduction.[4,44] This dual role of pain in different treatment phases of OUD can often be perplexing to patients and providers.[4] Other SUDs also show a similar relationship to pain as seen with OUD.[38,45–48]

Opioid Use Disorder in Long-Term Opioid Therapy for Pain

The data regarding OUD among patients on LTOT are somewhat confusing because of the nonuniform methodologies in studies. The prevalence of current OUD (Diagnostic and Statistical Manual of Mental Disorders, 5th Edition [DSM-5]) among those on LTOT was 8% to 12% in a recent systematic review.[49] An earlier review with stricter inclusion criteria reported that the median incidence of opioid dependence (DSM-IV) was only 0.5% (range 0%–24%) and the median prevalence was 4.5% (range 0%–32%).[50] Both studies reported substantial methodological heterogeneity among individual studies as a serious limitation. The influential 2016 Centers for Disease Control and Prevention Guideline for Prescribing Opioids for Chronic Pain[3] reported that the rates of opioid abuse or dependence diagnoses (DSM-IV) were 0.7% with a low daily dose of opioids and 6.1% with a higher daily dose versus 0.004% among those without LTOT.

LONG-TERM OPIOID THERAPY, OPIOID USE DISORDER DIAGNOSIS, AND COMPLEX PERSISTENT OPIOID DEPENDENCE

OUD diagnosis among patients on LTOT for pain can be clinically challenging for 2 main reasons:

1. Many of the DSM-5 criteria for OUD can also be attributed to pain
2. The procurement of opioids is within a therapeutic context

One study on LTOT reported 31% prevalence of DSM-IV opioid dependence when pain-related symptoms were included in the criteria-based diagnosis and 2% when they were excluded.[51] Ballantyne and colleagues[52,53] have suggested that despite lacking a DSM-5 diagnosis of OUD, many patients with pain on LTOT have complex persistent dependence (CPD), which is qualitatively more severe than simple physical dependence. One of the clinical hallmarks of this condition is that the patients are unwilling or unable to taper LTOT despite medical or functional deterioration, and classic OUD-like behaviors often emerge with opioid dose reduction or cessation.[4,52,53] About 20% of patients on LTOT in a primary care practice who tend to have high pain interference, addictive behaviors, high daily opioid doses, and significant psychiatric comorbidity[6] can be characterized as having significant CPD, the gray area between the uncomplicated physical dependence and full opioid addiction (**Fig. 2**).[4,52,53] The management principles in the gray area of CPD is currently being clarified.[4]

CHRONIC PAIN AND SUBSTANCE USE DISORDERS: THE MULTIMORBIDITY UNDERNEATH
Multimorbidity in Chronic Pain and Substance Use Disorders

As pointed out before, patients with pain and addiction are often suffering many other maladies, too. For example, in an analysis of NCS-R, 87.1% of the people with chronic spinal pain reported that at least one other comorbid condition, including other chronic pain conditions (68.6%), chronic physical conditions (55.3%), and mental disorders (35.0%). In a study of patients with OUD, pain, physical illness, psychiatric disorders, and polysubstance use were frequent even among younger patients, but the severity

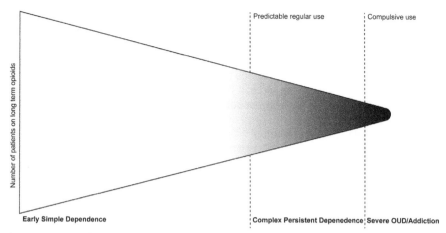

Predictable regular use   Compulsive use

Number of patients on long term opioids

Early Simple Dependence   Complex Persistent Depenedence   Severe OUD/Addiction

Fig. 2. A pictorial representation of the continuum of opioid dependence among LTOT patients.

of these grew with age, with 75% of those older than 45 years of age having significant pain and psychiatric problems.[54] Similar high levels of comorbidities and polypharmacy/polysubstance use have been reported by many other studies related to SUD, including OUD,[8,45,55–61] and among patients on LTOT for chronic pain.[62–65] A higher level of comorbidity and polypharmacy has been linked with higher frequency of pain, too.[66] In summary, the presence of significant chronic pain with SUD in an individual often reveals a complex, multifaceted clinical scenario involving multiple other illnesses: a multimorbid disease state underneath.

Consequences of Multimorbidity in Chronic Pain and Substance Use Disorder (Including Opioid Use Disorder)

The multimorbidity seen in association with chronic pain and substance use has significant consequences. Two separate analyses from NCS-R suggested that the excess risk of suicidal ideations, plans, and attempts among those with chronic pain is substantially mediated by comorbidities, including SUDs, mental illness, and medical illness.[67,68] Recently, Oliva and colleagues[5] reported that SUDs, mental health disorders, medical comorbidity, and nonopioid psycho-polypharmacy are more predictive of the increased risk of overdose, suicide, and suicide-related event associated with opioids than the higher opioid dose level.

Although heroin overdose deaths are often conceptualized as the consumption of a quantity or purity of opioid in excess of the person's tolerance, most overdose deaths occur among experienced users with low levels of heroin detected at autopsy,[69] but in combination with multiple substances and medications.[69–71] The recent fentanyl-related overdose deaths also largely seem to be among experienced users with polysubstance use and polypharmacy.[72–74]

Autopsy examination of heroin deaths has revealed a growing pattern of systemic disease burden, especially among older individuals.[69,75] Chronic medical illness–related morbidity and mortality are substantially higher among individuals with long-term heroin use compared with the general population, and more than half of the years of potential life lost before 65 years of age among them is due to chronic diseases,[76] with only about a third of the deaths due to overdose and accidents.[77,78]

The impact of chronic medical diseases also seems to compound with increasing age. Overdose declines as a cause of death, and chronic diseases become the more common cause for death among those with OUD those older than 45 years of age. Indeed, the median age of death among persons with OUD is steadily increasing over time.[75,76,78–80] Suicide also increases with age, but at a lower rate.[78,79]

Patients on LTOT for chronic pain also seem to experience substantially higher all-cause mortalities and chronic disease mortality than those who are not on opioids, with only a small portion of the excess mortality (about 20%) due to direct opioid-related causes.[81–83] LTOT is also associated with poor overall physical health on long-term follow-up.[84,85]

On a larger scale, Case and Deaton[86,87] have reported that midlife mortality is selectively increasing among white non-Hispanics in the United States because of a significant contribution from drug and alcohol poisoning, suicide, liver disease, and a slowing of the historic decline in cardiovascular mortality. They also reported a parallel increase in disabling chronic pain and the self-reported decline in mental and physical health in this subpopulation.

In summary, there is ample evidence that multimorbidity involving chronic pain, SUD, psychiatric illness, and medical comorbidities is associated with declining overall health and increasing mortality due to suicide, overdose, and systemic causes.

Multimorbidity and Evolution from Acute to Chronic to Disabling Chronic Pain (Chronification of Pain)

Acute pain is defined by a peripheral injurious or inflammatory focus initiating the neural processing of nociceptive stimuli by the central nervous system resulting in the perception of pain with assigned severity and salience; **Box 1** provides a definition of pain and chronic pain. Although many patients and practitioners view and manage chronic pain as persistent or recurrent acute pain, modern neurobiological research suggests this is a flawed approach. Chronic pain is by definition a pain that persists beyond tissue repair following an injury and has no known adaptive utility with regards to preservation of life and prevention of injury (see **Box 1** for definition).

Chronification of Pain

The progression from acute pain to disabling chronic pain, the "chronification" of pain, is a complex process. Only a small proportion of the patients progress from an acute injury to established chronic pain with normal function and even fewer to disabling chronic pain (**Fig. 3**). Neurobiologically, pain chronification involves neuroplasticity (central nervous system learning and adapting) in pain-processing central nervous pathways and downward pain-inhibition pathways. Such neuroplasticity causes changes in several domains related to pain, including perception, cognition, attention, emotion, learning, memory, and motivation. The pain processing also shows an overall shift from pain pathways to emotional pathways.[88–90] These neurobiological changes drive the chronic pain experience through various mechanisms. The threshold for nociception at the site of pain is often reduced, and the severity and the extent of pain sensation are amplified as it ascends the pain pathways. The endogenous pain

---

Box 1
Definition of pain and chronic pain

Pain: An unpleasant sensory and emotional experience associated with actual or potential tissue damage, or described in terms of such damage.

Chronic pain: A pain without apparent biological value that has persisted beyond the normal tissue healing time (usually taken to be 3 months).

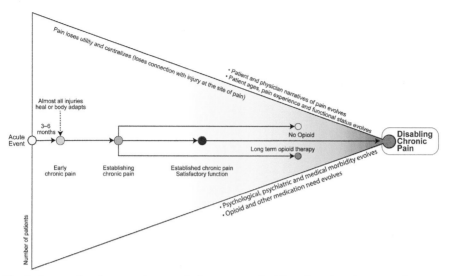

Fig. 3. Progression from persistent pain in many to disabling chronic pain among few.

inhibition through the downward pathways is also altered. At the cognitive level, there are maladaptive modifications of the assigned salience of pain, associated negative affect, and behavioral response.

Multimorbidity and Pain Chronification

A multitude of factors influence pain chronification,[91] and for clinical utility, this complex array of factors can be categorized into 3 main groups (**Fig. 4, Box 2**):

1. Psychosocial factors
2. Comorbidities with psychological impact (psychiatric and medical)
3. Dependencies (SUD, SUD recovery, and medication dependence)

Decades of research have established that several demographic, social, and psychological factors (see **Box 2**) can drive chronification of pain, and many of them are amenable to psychological treatment.[91,92] Although the severity of initial pain and associated disability play a role in chronification, it is confined to the early part of chronification.[91,93]

Extensive available literature supports the notion that preexisting psychiatric comorbidities (see **Box 2**) are key drivers of pain chronification, and pain, in turn, worsens psychiatric status.[8,91,92,94–96] It is less appreciated that medical comorbidities (see **Box 2**) also greatly influence pain chronification, especially among older individuals.[91,94,97–101] Recently, there is also growing recognition of the increased burden of chronic pain and opioid use following recovery from life-threatening medical illness,[102] traumatic brain injury and concussions,[103,104] and cancer.[105] As the population, including those with SUD, ages, multimorbidity and chronic pain prevalence are simultaneously increasing.[99–101] In addition, several infectious and noninfectious sequelae like hepatitis C, HIV, liver disease, pancreatitis, and infectious arthritis can all lead to chronic pain. Multiple painful conditions due to different initiating abnormalities are also common among those with chronic pain.[2,100]

As detailed in prior sections, regular use of substances that can cause dependence is a key driver in the development of disabling chronic pain. Often, those substances

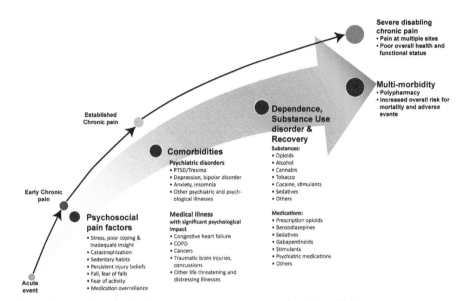

Fig. 4. Progression to disabling chronic pain: the role of multimorbidity.

are medications for pain and accompanying symptoms like insomnia, lack of focus, anxiety and mood disorders, and other medical comorbidities, often leading to a dizzying array of polypharmacy. This, in turn, can adversely affect pain and disability.[5,30,54,64–66,106,107]

Thus, disabling chronic pain, especially among those with SUD, often evolves and presents as multimorbidity involving varying combinations of several chronic pain conditions, psychiatric and medical comorbidities, polysubstance and medication dependencies, and a complex set of pain-related maladaptive psychopathologies influenced by all the comorbidities (see **Fig. 4**). Such patients with consequential severe disabilities and excess risk of suicide, overdose, and all-cause mortality are becoming increasingly common in physician practices, posing a great challenge to providers and health systems. Isolated focus on a single issue or limited set of issues like pain and SUD without coordinated treatment of multiple comorbidities is unlikely to lead to sustained benefit. Recently, there is growing recognition of the need for multidimensional approaches to successfully manage patients with such complex clinical conditions.[108–110]

MULTIDIMENSIONAL PHARMACOBEHAVIORAL MODEL FOR COMPLEX CHRONIC PAIN MANAGEMENT

The authors propose a multidimensional, pharmacobehavioral model for medical management of complex chronic pain with a whole person focus, rooted in the biopsychosocial framework (**Fig. 5**). This model divides the overall management of the patient into categories or steps:

1. Patient education and activation: Reexplaining pain based on modern conceptualization of the chronification of pain and shifting the locus of control to the patient
2. Dependence treatment
3. Comorbidity treatment
4. Polypharmacy reduction
5. Chronic pain treatment

Patients with disabling chronic pain and SUD/medication dependence often present in a state of personal crisis, and the initial goal of management is often achieving clinical stability. Crisis stabilization is followed by a slow transition from disease-focused, provider-based management to a whole person–focused paradigm with

---

Box 2
Various factors involved in chronification of pain

Demographic factors

Age

Gender

Education level

Smoking

Overweight

Disability

Receiving Workers' compensation

Higher work dissatisfaction

Higher physical work demand

Psychological pain factors

Maladaptive coping

Fear avoidance (of work, movements, activities)

Falls, fear of falls

Catastrophization (excessive negative thoughts about future in relation to pain)

Low self-efficacy

Pain hypervigilance

Overreliance on pain medications

Initial pain severity (confined to early part of chronification)

Comorbidities with psychological impact

Psychiatric
  Trauma, posttraumatic stress disorder (PTSD)
  Depression, anxiety
  Bipolar disorder
  Other severe mental illnesses
  Personality disorder

Medical
  Poor overall health
  Congestive heart failure, chronic obstructive pulmonary disease, cancer diagnosis, critical illness recovery
  Traumatic brain injury and concussions

Dependencies to various agents

Active substance use & recovery from SUD
  Tobacco, alcohol, opioid, cocaine, stimulants, cannabis, barbiturates, benzodiazepines, and other drugs

Medications
  Opioids, benzodiazepines, stimulants, anti-depressants, anti-psychotics, anticonvulsants, barbiturates, other psychoactive medications
  Nonsteroidal anti-inflammatory agents

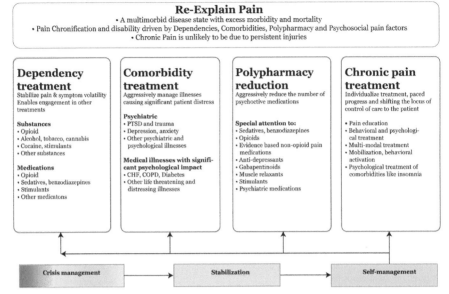

Fig. 5. Multidimensional pharmacobehavioral model for management of disabling pain among those with substance dependence. CHF, congestive heart failure; COPD, chronic obstructive pulmonary disease.

self-management of pain and comorbidities. This model could be implemented using an adequately trained single medical provider or an interdisciplinary team, both within primary care settings when feasible. A detailed discussion of each element of this complex process is beyond the scope of this review, but the authors broadly discuss each of the management categories. Although as a learning heuristic, these are described as discrete components; the management in each of these categories usually progresses simultaneously, and often one treatment intervention can impact multiple components, both positively and negatively.

Reexplaining Pain

The first and arguably most important step in treatment is developing a shared clinical conceptualization of the complex reasons for the disabling pain, or developing a more nuanced diagnosis beyond the common explanation of persistent injury, tissue damage, or disease. Such a shared conceptualization requires an initial detailed longitudinal diagnostic formulation of chronic pain as a condition caused by the persistence of perceived need to protect body tissue, driven by central nervous system neuroplasticity, under the influence of pain factors, comorbidities, dependencies, and polypharmacy (chronification of pain).

Over time, patients may acquire injury/disease-focused beliefs and cognitive narratives related to pain-driving maladaptive behaviors that sustain painful disability and suffering.[111,112] Such maladaptive beliefs and narratives are no doubt also sustained by health care systems that promote passive treatments (medications, procedures) over active self-management. Patients (and the multiple providers caring for them) are often unaware of the complex connection between pain and SUDs, and about the further contribution of multimorbidity to the chronification of pain. For example, a patient with disabling chronic back pain, failed spinal surgeries, and OUD may see the continued pain-related opioid use as a consequence of the inability to "fix" the back and may seek out additional procedures. This patient might be uninformed that persistent spine injury/disease is an unlikely explanation for disabling chronic pain, and that the comorbid SUD, PTSD, and insomnia are much more important drivers of pain chronification. This example patient may also be unaware that the polypharmacy developing from the fragmented treatment of multiple problems will also affect pain and health deleteriously. Education of patients, families, and other providers based on a nuanced longitudinal narrative enables them to integrate this new understanding into their wider pain- and function-related beliefs, attitudes, behaviors, treatment, and lifestyle choices.[113] This psychological/cognitive approach commonly known as "explaining pain" (therapeutic neuroscience or pain neuroscience education) has been shown to be an effective mode of pain treatment.[113]

Dependence Treatment

The most logical next step after the "reexplaining pain" is the treatment of significant SUD and medication dependence, which often restricts the ability of patients to engage in treatments for pain and comorbidities.

It is often difficult to control pain and other symptoms without effective treatment of SUD and medication dependencies that often drive the intensity and volatility of these symptoms. In the case of OUD or opioid medication dependence, buprenorphine treatment that can effectively manage both dependence and pain offers a viable pharmacologic treatment path.[114] Methadone is another treatment option, but can cause increasing levels of dependence with long-term use that could worsen pain and associated symptoms.[115] A more detailed description of the influence of dependence on pain and its management is beyond the scope of this review and can be found elsewhere.[4]

The influence of alcohol, tobacco, cannabis, and cocaine use in pain chronification is not often recognized; they require equal attention as other substances. Many patients often use these substances to get relief from pain. Nonopioid SUD and medication dependence are much more difficult to manage as pharmacologic treatment, like anticonvulsants, naltrexone, and antidepressants, may have limited impact on pain associated with dependence. The authors often have to judiciously use prescription opioids and/or interventional procedures to control overwhelming pain to facilitate SUD/dependence treatment engagement.

Many patients with pain often have multiple SUDs and medication dependencies, making the management even more challenging. In these situations, a nuanced individualized approach based on the longitudinal diagnostic formulation is often the way forward. The authors recommend an integrative simultaneous treatment of multiple SUDs and medication dependencies with a harm reduction approach, engaging patients at the level they are willing to engage. In addition, the authors strongly believe treaters should not deny treatment of one SUD to patients because they have another active SUD or medication dependence. It is critical not to abandon patients if their behaviors become difficult under the influence of polysubstance use. Such patients tend to be at higher risk of adverse outcomes, including overdose, suicide, and death.

Comorbidity Treatment

As noted above, psychiatric comorbidities, medical comorbidities, and pain are commonly seen as separate treatment entities with little recognition of the complex reciprocal interconnections between them. This is especially the case with medical comorbidities that often generate a sustained sense of mortality dread and anxiety (eg, congestive heart failure, coronary artery disease, chronic obstructive pulmonary disease, and cancer). Simultaneous, effective management of these comorbidities often leads to better control of pain, and effective dependence treatment often allows patients to engage in better management of comorbidities.

Polypharmacy Reduction

Patients and providers are often unaware that polypharmacy from the nonintegrated treatment of individual symptoms associated with chronic pain, SUDs, and comorbidities often worsens chronic pain and disability. Polypharmacy reduction is often an important component of chronic pain treatment. Patients are often reluctant to leave the perceived safety of taking a pill to control overwhelming symptoms. Managing patient expectation around the need for polypharmacy reduction can be extremely challenging, but is crucial to maintaining a therapeutic alliance. Patient education, psychotherapies focused on treatment of coping, insomnia, anxiety, and depression, and effective treatment of medication dependencies and SUD all can reduce medication need.

Pain Treatment

It is essential to recognize that traditional biomedically oriented treatment with a focus on pharmacotherapy and passive interventions should be abandoned as the primary treatment of chronic pain, especially among those with comorbid SUD/medication dependence. "Reexplaining pain" followed by the effective management of SUD/ medication dependence, comorbidities, and polypharmacy, combined with simple behavioral activation (eg, walking 30 minutes 2 times a day at a comfortable speed), are effective for many patients. This basic approach *may* obviate evidence-based professional psychological treatments like cognitive behavioral therapy (CBT), acceptance and commitment therapy (ACT), and mindfulness,[92] which are often difficult to access currently. Also, many elements of psychological treatment of pain like motivational interviewing, goal setting, cognitive reframing, basic mindfulness, and behavioral activation are deployable in primary care clinics; models to build capacity and expand reach are under development. CBT, ACT, and mindfulness-based psychological treatment are more successful when combined with "Reexplaining pain" beyond what is offered traditionally within the respective treatment protocols.[113] Other comorbidities can create their own psychological challenges (eg, emotional volatility in SUDs, constant dread of mortality in cancer or CHF) can complicate overall treatment and may require further health psychology treatment.

Pain medications and procedural interventions to control overwhelming pain can enable engagement in the multidimensional treatment. Structured opioid therapy with close attention to patient safety can often be helpful in allaying overwhelming distress associated with pain. Structured opioid therapy, in turn, enables engagement in further treatment of multimorbidity, thus improving functionality and reducing overall risk. Although seemingly contrary to the current climate of frenzied opioid restriction, this is consistent with the whole-person approach to the treatment of SUD and chronic pain. It is also vital to recognize that surgical procedures are less likely to show sustained effectiveness in patients who have uncontrolled comorbidities, and postsurgical pain can develop into yet another chronic pain. Hence, it is important to engage in multidimensional treatment if surgical treatment of chronic pain is considered.

SUMMARY

Chronic pain combined with SUD and medication dependence often presents as a disabling multimorbid disease state with polypharmacy or polysubstance use associated with excess risk of adverse outcomes, including death. It is becoming increasingly clear that simple strategies like opioid tapering and nonpharmacologic treatment of pain are insufficient by themselves. Health systems and clinical teams must develop resources to manage this vulnerable population. Categorization of patient problems and treatment options in a multidimensional pharmacobehavioral model can help both patients and physicians to engage in more effective treatment. Acquisition of knowledge and skills spanning multiple fields of pain, addiction, psychiatry, and complex medical multimorbidity required to manage these complex conditions can be challenging, but eminently possible with effective provider education and training. Clinical and research foci in this area must shift from management of individual conditions to development of effective methods to manage multimorbidities in association with dependence.

ACKNOWLEDGMENTS

The editors wish to thank Stefan G. Kertesz, Birmingham Veterans Affairs Medical Center and University of Alabama at Birmingham, for providing a critical review of this article.

REFERENCES

1. Volkow ND, Collins FS. The role of science in addressing the opioid crisis. N Engl J Med 2017;377(4):391–4.
2. Von Korff M, Crane P, Lane M, et al. Chronic spinal pain and physical-mental comorbidity in the United States: results from the national comorbidity survey replication. Pain 2005;113(3):331–9.
3. Dowell D, Haegerich TM, Chou R. CDC guideline for prescribing opioids for chronic pain—United States, 2016. MMWR Recomm Rep 2016;65(1):1–49.
4. Manhapra A, Arias AJ, Ballantyne JC. The conundrum of opioid tapering in long-term opioid therapy for chronic pain: a commentary. Subst Abuse 2017;1–10.
5. Oliva EM, Bowe T, Tavakoli S, et al. Development and applications of the Veterans Health Administration's Stratification Tool for Opioid Risk Mitigation (STORM) to improve opioid safety and prevent overdose and suicide. Psychol Serv 2017;14(1):34–49.
6. Banta-Green CJ, Merrill JO, Doyle SR, et al. Opioid use behaviors, mental health and pain–development of a typology of chronic pain patients. Drug Alcohol Depend 2009;104(1–2):34–42.
7. Viana MC, Lim CCW, Pereira FG, et al. Previous mental disorders and subsequent onset of chronic back or neck pain: findings from 19 countries. J Pain 2017;19(1):99–110.
8. Howe CQ, Sullivan MD. The missing 'P' in pain management: how the current opioid epidemic highlights the need for psychiatric services in chronic pain care. Gen Hosp Psychiatry 2014;36(1):99–104.
9. Blanco C, Wall MM, Okuda M, et al. Pain as a predictor of opioid use disorder in a nationally representative sample. Am J Psychiatry 2016;173(12):1189–95.
10. Weiss RD, Potter JS, Griffin ML, et al. Reasons for opioid use among patients with dependence on prescription opioids: the role of chronic pain. J Subst Abuse Treat 2014;47(2):140–5.
11. Weiss RD, Rao V. The prescription opioid addiction treatment study: what have we learned. Drug Alcohol Depend 2017;173(Suppl 1):S48–54.

12. Dhingra L, Perlman DC, Masson C, et al. Longitudinal analysis of pain and illicit drug use behaviors in outpatients on methadone maintenance. Drug Alcohol Depend 2015;149:285–9.

13. Larson MJ, Paasche-Orlow M, Cheng DM, et al. Persistent pain is associated with substance use after detoxification: a prospective cohort analysis. Addiction 2007;102(5):752–60.

14. Potter JS, Chakrabarti A, Domier CP, et al. Pain and continued opioid use in individuals receiving buprenorphine-naloxone for opioid detoxification: secondary analyses from the Clinical Trials Network. J Subst Abuse Treat 2010;38(Suppl 1): S80–6.

15. Potter JS, Prather K, Weiss RD. Physical pain and associated clinical characteristics in treatment-seeking patients in four substance use disorder treatment modalities. Am J Addict 2008;17(2):121–5.

16. Rosenblum A, Joseph H, Fong C, et al. Prevalence and characteristics of chronic pain among chemically dependent patients in methadone maintenance and residential treatment facilities. JAMA 2003;289(18):2370–8.

17. Sheu R, Lussier D, Rosenblum A, et al. Prevalence and characteristics of chronic pain in patients admitted to an outpatient drug and alcohol treatment program. Pain Med 2008;9(7):911–7.

18. Caldeiro RM, Malte CA, Calsyn DA, et al. The association of persistent pain with out-patient addiction treatment outcomes and service utilization. Addiction 2008;103(12):1996–2005.

19. Barry DT, Beitel M, Joshi D, et al. Pain and substance-related pain-reduction behaviors among opioid dependent individuals seeking methadone maintenance treatment. Am J Addict 2009;18(2):117–21.

20. Barry D, Beitel M, Cutter C, et al. Allopathic, complementary, and alternative medical treatment utilization for pain among methadone-maintained patients. Am J Addict 2009;18(5):379–85.

21. Jamison RN, Kauffman J, Katz NP. Characteristics of methadone maintenance patients with chronic pain. J Pain Symptom Manage 2000;19(1):53–62.

22. Nordmann S, Vilotitch A, Lions C, et al. Pain in methadone patients: time to address undertreatment and suicide risk (ANRS-Methaville trial). PLoS One 2017;12(5):e0176288.

23. Peles E, Schreiber S, Gordon J, et al. Significantly higher methadone dose for methadone maintenance treatment (MMT) patients with chronic pain. Pain 2005;113(3):340–6.

24. Dhingra L, Masson C, Perlman DC, et al. Epidemiology of pain among outpatients in methadone maintenance treatment programs. Drug Alcohol Depend 2013;128(1–2):161–5.

25. Chakrabarti A, Woody GE, Griffin ML, et al. Predictors of buprenorphine-naloxone dosing in a 12-week treatment trial for opioid-dependent youth: secondary analyses from a NIDA Clinical Trials Network study. Drug Alcohol Depend 2010;107(2–3):253–6.

26. Fox AD, Sohler NL, Starrels JL, et al. Pain is not associated with worse office-based buprenorphine treatment outcomes. Subst Abuse 2012;33(4):361–5.

27. Griffin ML, McDermott KA, McHugh RK, et al. Longitudinal association between pain severity and subsequent opioid use in prescription opioid dependent patients with chronic pain. Drug Alcohol Depend 2016;163:216–21.

28. Han B, Compton WM, Blanco C, et al. Prescription opioid use, misuse, and use disorders in U.S. Adults: 2015 national survey on drug use and health. Ann Intern Med 2017;167(5):293–301.

29. Bohnert AS, Eisenberg A, Whiteside L, et al. Prescription opioid use among addictions treatment patients: nonmedical use for pain relief vs. other forms of nonmedical use. Addict Behav 2013;38(3):1776–81.

30. Trafton JA, Oliva EM, Horst DA, et al. Treatment needs associated with pain in substance use disorder patients: implications for concurrent treatment. Drug Alcohol Depend 2004;73(1):23–31.

31. Dahlman D, Kral AH, Wenger L, et al. Physical pain is common and associated with nonmedical prescription opioid use among people who inject drugs. Subst Abuse Treat Prev Pol 2017;12(1):29.

32. Cicero TJ, Ellis MS, Surratt HL, et al. The changing face of heroin use in the United States: a retrospective analysis of the past 50 years. JAMA Psychiatry 2014;71(7):821–6.

33. Martins SS, Sarvet A, Santaella-Tenorio J, et al. Changes in US lifetime heroin use and heroin use disorder: prevalence from the 2001-2002 to 2012-2013 National Epidemiologic Survey on alcohol and related conditions. JAMA Psychiatry 2017;74(5):445–55.

34. Cicero TJ, Ellis MS, Harney J. Shifting patterns of prescription opioid and heroin abuse in the United States. N Engl J Med 2015;373(18):1789–90.

35. Cicero TJ, Ellis MS, Kasper ZA. Increased use of heroin as an initiating opioid of abuse. Addict behaviors 2017;74:63–6.

36. Ilgen MA, Perron B, Czyz EK, et al. The timing of onset of pain and substance use disorders. Am J Addict 2010;19(5):409–15.

37. Tsui JI, Lira MC, Cheng DM, et al. Chronic pain, craving, and illicit opioid use among patients receiving opioid agonist therapy. Drug Alcohol Depend 2016; 166:26–31.

38. Alford DP, German JS, Samet JH, et al. Primary care patients with drug use report chronic pain and self-medicate with alcohol and other drugs. J Gen Intern Med 2016;31(5):486–91.

39. Brennan PL, Schutte KK, Moos RH. Pain and use of alcohol to manage pain: prevalence and 3-year outcomes among older problem and non-problem drinkers. Addiction 2005;100(6):777–86.

40. Worley MJ, Heinzerling KG, Shoptaw S, et al. Pain volatility and prescription opioid addiction treatment outcomes in patients with chronic pain. Exp Clin Psychopharmacol 2015;23(6):428–35.

41. Worley MJ, Heinzerling KG, Shoptaw S, et al. Volatility and change in chronic pain severity predict outcomes of treatment for prescription opioid addiction. Addiction 2017;112(7):1202–9.

42. Ren ZY, Shi J, Epstein DH, et al. Abnormal pain response in pain-sensitive opiate addicts after prolonged abstinence predicts increased drug craving. Psychopharmacology 2009;204(3):423–9.

43. Morasco BJ, Corson K, Turk DC, et al. Association between substance use disorder status and pain-related function following 12 months of treatment in primary care patients with musculoskeletal pain. J Pain 2011;12(3):352–9.

44. Heilig M, Egli M, Crabbe JC, et al. Acute withdrawal, protracted abstinence and negative affect in alcoholism: are they linked? Addict Biol 2010;15(2):169–84.

45. Zale EL, Maisto SA, Ditre JW. Interrelations between pain and alcohol: an integrative review. Clin Psychol Rev 2015;37:57–71.

46. Jakubczyk A, Ilgen MA, Kopera M, et al. Reductions in physical pain predict lower risk of relapse following alcohol treatment. Drug Alcohol Depend 2016; 158:167–71.

47. Riley JL 3rd, King C. Self-report of alcohol use for pain in a multi-ethnic community sample. J Pain 2009;10(9):944–52.
48. Rohilla J, Desai G, Chan P. Prevalence of chronic pain in patients with alcohol dependence syndrome in tertiary care center in India. Asian J Psychiatr 2016; 17(2):199–208.
49. Vowles KE, McEntee ML, Julnes PS, et al. Rates of opioid misuse, abuse, and addiction in chronic pain: a systematic review and data synthesis. Pain 2015; 156(4):569–76.
50. Minozzi S, Amato L, Davoli M. Development of dependence following treatment with opioid analgesics for pain relief: a systematic review. Addiction 2013; 108(4):688–98.
51. Elander J, Lusher J, Bevan D, et al. Pain management and symptoms of substance dependence among patients with sickle cell disease. Social Sci Med 2003;57(9):1683–96.
52. Ballantyne JC, Stannard C. New addiction criteria: diagnostic challenges persist in treating pain with opioids. Pain 2013;1:1–7.
53. Ballantyne JC, Sullivan MD, Kolodny A. Opioid dependence vs addiction: a distinction without a difference? Arch Intern Med 2012;172(17):1342–3.
54. Cicero TJ, Surratt HL, Kurtz S, et al. Patterns of prescription opioid abuse and comorbidity in an aging treatment population. J Subst Abuse Treat 2012; 42(1):87–94.
55. Saunders K, Merikangas K, Low NC, et al. Impact of comorbidity on headache-related disability. Neurology 2008;70(7):538–47.
56. Polatin PB, Kinney RK, Gatchel RJ, et al. Psychiatric illness and chronic low-back pain. The mind and the spine–which goes first? Spine (Phila Pa 1976) 1993;18(1):66–71.
57. Grant BF, Saha TD, Ruan WJ, et al. Epidemiology of DSM-5 drug use disorder: results from the National Epidemiologic Survey on alcohol and related conditions-III. JAMA Psychiatry 2016;73(1):39–47.
58. Fayaz A, Ayis S, Panesar SS, et al. Assessing the relationship between chronic pain and cardiovascular disease: a systematic review and meta-analysis. Scand J Pain 2016;13:76–90.
59. Heimer R, Zhan W, Grau LE. Prevalence and experience of chronic pain in suburban drug injectors. Drug Alcohol Depend 2015;151:92–100.
60. Mellbye A, Karlstad O, Skurtveit S, et al. Co-morbidity in persistent opioid users with chronic non-malignant pain in Norway. Eur J Pain 2014;18(8):1083–93.
61. Hser YI, Gelberg L, Hoffman V, et al. Health conditions among aging narcotics addicts: medical examination results. J Behav Med 2004;27(6):607–22.
62. Cicero TJ, Wong G, Tian Y, et al. Co-morbidity and utilization of medical services by pain patients receiving opioid medications: data from an insurance claims database. Pain 2009;144(1–2):20–7.
63. Morasco BJ, Duckart JP, Carr TP, et al. Clinical characteristics of veterans prescribed high doses of opioid medications for chronic non-cancer pain. Pain 2010;151(3):625–32.
64. Hudson TJ, Edlund MJ, Steffick DE, et al. Epidemiology of regular prescribed opioid use: results from a national, population-based survey. J Pain Symptom Manage 2008;36(3):280–8.
65. Parsells Kelly J, Cook SF, Kaufman DW, et al. Prevalence and characteristics of opioid use in the US adult population. Pain 2008;138(3):507–13.

66. Robinson KT, Bergeron CD, Mingo CA, et al. Factors associated with pain frequency among adults with chronic conditions. J Pain Symptom Manage 2017; 54(5):619–27.

67. Braden JB, Sullivan MD. Suicidal thoughts and behavior among adults with self-reported pain conditions in the national comorbidity survey replication. J Pain 2008;9(12):1106–15.

68. Ilgen MA, Zivin K, McCammon RJ, et al. Pain and suicidal thoughts, plans and attempts in the United States. Gen Hosp Psychiatry 2008;30(6):521–7.

69. Darke S, Ross J, Zador D, et al. Heroin-related deaths in New South Wales, Australia, 1992-1996. Drug Alcohol Depend 2000;60(2):141–50.

70. Coffin PO, Galea S, Ahern J, et al. Opiates, cocaine and alcohol combinations in accidental drug overdose deaths in New York City, 1990-98. Addiction 2003; 98(6):739–47.

71. Lyndon A, Audrey S, Wells C, et al. Risk to heroin users of polydrug use of pregabalin or gabapentin. Addiction 2017;112(9):1580–9.

72. Slavova S, Costich JF, Bunn TL, et al. Heroin and fentanyl overdoses in Kentucky: epidemiology and surveillance. Int J Drug Policy 2017;46:120–9.

73. Tomassoni AJ, Hawk KF, Jubanyik K, et al. Multiple fentanyl overdoses - New Haven, Connecticut, June 23, 2016. MMWR Morb Mortal Wkly Rep 2017; 66(4):107–11.

74. Marshall BDL, Krieger MS, Yedinak JL, et al. Epidemiology of fentanyl-involved drug overdose deaths: a geospatial retrospective study in Rhode Island, USA. Int J Drug Policy 2017;46:130–5.

75. Webb L, Oyefeso A, Schifano F, et al. Cause and manner of death in drug-related fatality: an analysis of drug-related deaths recorded by coroners in England and Wales in 2000. Drug Alcohol Depend 2003;72(1):67–74.

76. Hser YI, Evans E, Grella C, et al. Long-term course of opioid addiction. Harv Rev Psychiatry 2015;23(2):76–89.

77. Smyth B, Hoffman V, Fan J, et al. Years of potential life lost among heroin addicts 33 years after treatment. Prev Med 2007;44(4):369–74.

78. Degenhardt L, Larney S, Randall D, et al. Causes of death in a cohort treated for opioid dependence between 1985 and 2005. Addiction 2014;109(1):90–9.

79. Larney S, Bohnert AS, Ganoczy D, et al. Mortality among older adults with opioid use disorders in the Veteran's Health Administration, 2000-2011. Drug Alcohol Depend 2015;147:32–7.

80. Beynon C, McVeigh J, Hurst A, et al. Older and sicker: changing mortality of drug users in treatment in the North West of England. Int J Drug Policy 2010; 21(5):429–31.

81. Solomon DH, Rassen JA, Glynn RJ, et al. The comparative safety of analgesics in older adults with arthritis. Arch Intern Med 2010;170(22):1968–76.

82. Solomon DH, Rassen JA, Glynn RJ, et al. The comparative safety of opioids for nonmalignant pain in older adults. Arch Intern Med 2010;170(22):1979–86.

83. Gomes T, Juurlink DN, Dhalla IA, et al. Trends in opioid use and dosing among socio-economically disadvantaged patients. Open Med 2011;5(1):e13–22.

84. Eriksen J, Sjogren P, Bruera E, et al. Critical issues on opioids in chronic non-cancer pain: an epidemiological study. Pain 2006;125(1–2):172–9.

85. Ekholm O, Kurita GP, Hojsted J, et al. Chronic pain, opioid prescriptions, and mortality in Denmark: a population-based cohort study. Pain 2014;155(12): 2486–90.

86. Case A, Deaton A. Rising morbidity and mortality in midlife among white non-Hispanic Americans in the 21st century. Proc Natl Acad Sci U S A 2015; 112(49):15078–83.

87. Case A, Deaton A. Mortality and morbidity in the 21st century. Brookings Pap Econ Act 2017;397–476.

88. Apkarian AV, Baliki MN, Geha PY. Towards a theory of chronic pain. Prog Neurobiol 2009;87(2):81–97.

89. Simons LE, Elman I, Borsook D. Psychological processing in chronic pain: a neural systems approach. Neurosci Biobehav Rev 2014;39:61–78.

90. Pelletier R, Higgins J, Bourbonnais D. Is neuroplasticity in the central nervous system the missing link to our understanding of chronic musculoskeletal disorders? BMC Musculoskelet Disord 2015;16:25.

91. Chou R, Shekelle P. Will this patient develop persistent disabling low back pain? JAMA 2010;303(13):1295–302.

92. Edwards RR, Dworkin RH, Sullivan MD, et al. The role of psychosocial processes in the development and maintenance of chronic pain. J Pain 2016; 17(9 Suppl):T70–92.

93. Castillo RC, Wegener ST, Heins SE, et al. Longitudinal relationships between anxiety, depression, and pain: results from a two-year cohort study of lower extremity trauma patients. Pain 2013;154(12):2860–6.

94. Kroenke K, Outcalt S, Krebs E, et al. Association between anxiety, health-related quality of life and functional impairment in primary care patients with chronic pain. Gen Hosp Psychiatry 2013;35(4):359–65.

95. Tegethoff M, Belardi A, Stalujanis E, et al. Comorbidity of mental disorders and chronic pain: chronology of onset in adolescents of a national representative cohort. J Pain 2015;16(10):1054–64.

96. Gebhardt S, Heinzel-Gutenbrunner M, Konig U. Pain relief in depressive disorders: a meta-analysis of the effects of antidepressants. J Clin Psychopharmacol 2016;36(6):658–68.

97. Mundal I, Grawe RW, Bjorngaard JH, et al. Prevalence and long-term predictors of persistent chronic widespread pain in the general population in an 11-year prospective study: the HUNT study. BMC Musculoskelet Disord 2014;15:213.

98. van Hecke O, Torrance N, Smith BH. Chronic pain epidemiology and its clinical relevance. Br J Anaesth 2013;111(1):13–8.

99. Butchart A, Kerr EA, Heisler M, et al. Experience and management of chronic pain among patients with other complex chronic conditions. Clin J Pain 2009; 25(4):293–8.

100. Patel KV, Guralnik JM, Dansie EJ, et al. Prevalence and impact of pain among older adults in the United States: findings from the 2011 National Health and Aging Trends Study. Pain 2013;154(12):2649–57.

101. Sharpe L, McDonald S, Correia H, et al. Pain severity predicts depressive symptoms over and above individual illnesses and multimorbidity in older adults. BMC Psychiatry 2017;17(1):166.

102. Battle CE, Lovett S, Hutchings H. Chronic pain in survivors of critical illness: a retrospective analysis of incidence and risk factors. Crit Care 2013;17(3):R101.

103. Khoury S, Benavides R. Pain with traumatic brain injury and psychological disorders. Prog Neuropsychopharmacology Biol Psychiatry 2017. [Epub ahead of print].

104. Seal KH, Bertenthal D, Barnes DE, et al. Association of traumatic brain injury with chronic pain in Iraq and Afghanistan veterans: effect of comorbid mental health conditions. Arch Phys Med Rehabil 2017;98(8):1636–45.

105. Sutradhar R, Lokku A, Barbera L. Cancer survivorship and opioid prescribing rates: a population-based matched cohort study among individuals with and without a history of cancer. Cancer 2017;123(21):4286–93.
106. Hsu ES. Medication overuse in chronic pain. Curr Pain Headache Rep 2017; 21(1):2.
107. Menzies V, Thacker LR 2nd, Mayer SD, et al. Polypharmacy, opioid use, and fibromyalgia: a secondary analysis of clinical trial data. Biol Res Nurs 2016; 19(1):97–105.
108. Liu NH, Daumit GL, Dua T, et al. Excess mortality in persons with severe mental disorders: a multilevel intervention framework and priorities for clinical practice, policy and research agendas. World Psychiatry 2017;16(1):30–40.
109. Gallagher RM. Rational integration of pharmacologic, behavioral, and rehabilitation strategies in the treatment of chronic pain. Am J Phys Med Rehabil 2005; 84(3):S64–76.
110. Castillo RC, Archer KR, Newcomb AB, et al. Pain and psychological distress following orthopedic trauma: a call for collaborative models of care. Tech Orthop 2016;31(4):228–34.
111. Garland EL, Froeliger B, Zeidan F, et al. The downward spiral of chronic pain, prescription opioid misuse, and addiction: cognitive, affective, and neuropsychopharmacologic pathways. Neurosci biobehavioral Rev 2013;37(10 Pt 2): 2597–607.
112. Langer EJ. Matters of mind: mindfulness/mindlessness in perspective. Conscious Cogn 1992;1(3):289–305.
113. Moseley GL, Butler DS. Fifteen years of explaining pain: the past, present, and future. J Pain 2015;16(9):807–13.
114. Daitch D, Daitch J, Novinson D, et al. Conversion from high-dose full-opioid agonists to sublingual buprenorphine reduces pain scores and improves quality of life for chronic pain patients. Pain Med 2014;15(12):2087–94.
115. Rhodin A, Gronbladh L, Nilsson LH, et al. Methadone treatment of chronic nonmalignant pain and opioid dependence–a long-term follow-up. Eur J Pain 2006; 10(3):271–8.
116. Rosenblum A, Parrino M, Schnoll SH, et al. Prescription opioid abuse among enrollees into methadone maintenance treatment. Drug Alcohol Depend 2007; 90(1):64–71.

Weighing the Risks and Benefits of Electronic Cigarette Use in High-Risk Populations

Deepa R. Camenga, MD, MHS[a],*, Hilary A. Tindle, MD, MPH[b]

KEYWORDS

- E-cigarette • Tobacco • Smoking cessation
- Electronic nicotine delivery systems (ENDS)

KEY POINTS

- The evidence surrounding the efficacy of electronic (e)-cigarettes for smoking cessation is inconclusive.
- Early evidence suggests that e-cigarette use among adults with cardiovascular or pulmonary disease may have less risk than continued cigarette smoking; however, it also most likely has more adverse health outcome risk than tobacco abstinence. Long-term health effects of e-cigarettes are unknown.
- Among adults with serious mental illness, initial findings support the possibility that e-cigarettes may help some smokers with smoking reduction.
- Primary care providers should continue to screen all adults and adolescents for tobacco use, including e-cigarette use, and offer evidence-based smoking cessation therapies including medications approved by the US Food and Drug Administration to all cigarette smokers.

INTRODUCTION

Electronic cigarettes (e-cigarettes) are battery-operated devices typically designed to deliver nicotine and other additives via aerosol.[1] Since the introduction of e-cigarettes into the US market more than a decade ago, rates of current (ie, past month) and ever e-cigarette use among US adults have increased, especially among cigarette smokers.[2] A recent analysis of the nationally representative sample of US adults in the Population Assessment of Tobacco and Health Study found that 5.5% of US

Disclosure Statement: The authors report no disclosures.
[a] Yale School of Medicine, 464 Congress Avenue Suite 260, New Haven, CT 06519, USA;
[b] Vanderbilt University Medical Center, 2525 West End, Suite 370, Nashville, TN 37203, USA
* Corresponding author.
E-mail address: deepa.camenga@yale.edu

adults reported current e-cigarette use and many (44%) of persons who currently use e-cigarette reported regular use some or most days of the week.[2] Among adults and youth who use more than 1 tobacco product, dual use of cigarettes and e-cigarettes is the most common pattern.[2] Thus, e-cigarette use rates are higher among cigarette smokers than nonsmokers, with 12.7% of daily cigarette smokers reporting concomitant e-cigarette use in 2015.[3]

Recent studies have found that more than half of cigarette smokers in primary care and about 20% of hospitalized smokers have ever used e-cigarettes, with the most popular reasons for use being cigarette smoking reduction or cessation and perceptions of reduced harm.[4–6] As awareness of e-cigarettes continues to increase among US adults and youth,[2] clinical discussions about e-cigarettes are also becoming more common.[7] Among 1500 primary care and specialty physicians surveyed, most reported regularly fielding patient questions about e-cigarettes.[7] Given the abundant scientific evidence demonstrating the numerous short-term and long-term health consequences of cigarette smoking and other tobacco use,[8,9] provider-patient discussions about the safety and efficacy of e-cigarettes for smoking cessation or reduction are likely to increase.

Public Health England and the Royal College of Physicians have published expert opinions that e-cigarettes are likely to be about 95% safer than conventional cigarettes.[10] This estimate has been widely contested in the literature and was based on the speculation that e-cigarettes have 5% of the risk of cigarettes because the levels of carcinogens in e-cigarette vapor are 5% of that in cigarette smoke.[11] In contrast, US professional organizations have been more cautious in affirming the safety of e-cigarettes because there is little direct evidence to assess their long-term health impact.[12] Additionally, given emerging evidence that e-cigarette experimentation is associated with cigarette smoking initiation among youth, and concerns that e-cigarettes may promote dual use or renormalize smoking, there is an ongoing debate about whether these products will indeed improve the health of the population.[13–15] These concerns are particularly salient for the more than 16 million Americans at risk for or with an existing smoking-attributable illness, including those with cardiovascular disease (CVD) and pulmonary disease.[9] Other high risk populations include adults with serious mental illness (SMI) and adolescents because they may have unique vulnerabilities to the potential risks and benefits of e-cigarettes.

Thus, in an effort to inform clinical counseling around e-cigarette use in primary care, this article reviews the evidence about e-cigarette safety and efficacy for smoking cessation. Given the burden of tobacco-related morbidity among smokers with cardiac disease, pulmonary disease, or SMI, this article also reviews the current evidence assessing the potential health impact of e-cigarette use in these populations, as well as among adolescents who are uniquely vulnerable to developing nicotine dependence. In addition, current recommendations for managing e-cigarette use in primary care are reviewed.

WHAT ARE ELECTRONIC CIGARETTES OR ELECTRONIC NICOTINE DELIVERY SYSTEMS?

E-cigarettes have been recognized by the US Food and Drug Administration (FDA) as a type of electronic nicotine delivery system (ENDS) that is a tobacco product.[16] There are more than 400 different brands of e-cigarettes available for purchase via retail stores and online, and several different types of products, including disposable, cartridge, and tank-style e-cigarettes; and personal vaporizers (**Fig. 1**).[17] Of note, tobacco companies produce several popular brands of e-cigarettes.[18]

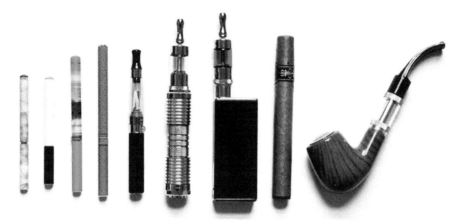

Fig. 1. There are several different types of e-cigarettes available, including disposable, cartridge and tank style, and personal vaporizers. (*From* US Department of Health and Human Services. US Food and Drug Administration (FDA). Tobacco products: vaporizers, e-cigarettes, and other Electronic Nicotine Delivery Systems (ENDS). Available at: https://www.fda.gov/TobaccoProducts/Labeling/ProductsIngredientsComponents/ucm456610.htm. Accessed February 15, 2018.)

In general, an ENDS consists of a power source (ie, rechargeable lithium ion battery), heating element, and reservoir for e-liquid solution. The solution contains nicotine, propylene glycol and/or vegetable glycerin, flavorants, and other additives. Persons who use ENDSs can use prefilled cartridges of e-liquid or can pour the e-liquid directly into the device's chamber. When a person puffs on an e-cigarette, the e-liquid is heated and vaporized into a mist that is inhaled.[19] The act of inhaling is often called vaping rather than smoking because e-cigarettes do not burn tobacco and, therefore, do not produce smoke.

Patients may refer to e-cigarettes by a variety of names, including vape pens, e-pens, e-hookah, vape sticks, and mods.[20] ENDSs can resemble traditional cigarettes (cig-a-like models); however, newer products (also called advanced generation products) are especially popular among adult smokers and come in a variety of shapes, colors, and sizes.[21,22] Advanced generation products have been shown to deliver nicotine more efficiently than cig-a-like models,[23] and experienced adult who use them report that the ability to customize flavors and nicotine concentrations in advanced generation e-cigarettes helps promote traditional cigarette reduction or abstinence.[24,25]

SAFETY CONCERNS WITH ELECTRONIC NICOTINE DELIVERY SYSTEMS AND ELECTRONIC CIGARETTE LIQUIDS

Although the public may perceive that e-cigarettes contain only water vapor, the main ingredients in the e-cigarette (e)-liquid (e-juice) are nicotine, propylene glycol, vegetable glycerin, flavorants, and various additives.[1] E-liquid nicotine concentrations can vary from 0 to 24 or more mg per milliliter of e-liquid. The nicotine in many e-liquids has been shown to have vasoactive effects, although some studies suggest that the tobacco smoke compounds, rather than the nicotine, primarily contribute to increased cardiovascular risk.[9] Cardiovascular toxicants present in tobacco smoke, such as formaldehyde, acetaldehyde, acetone, acrolein, and butanol, have been found in e-cigarettes, although typically at lower concentrations than those found in combustible cigarettes.[26,27]

There are several safety concerns that have arisen in relation to e-liquids. First, studies have shown that the e-liquid nicotine content can be mislabeled, raising the concern that patients may unknowingly expose themselves to higher levels of nicotine than intended.[28,29] However, it is possible that mislabeling will become less of a problem as the FDA enacts regulations to standardize e-cigarette product labeling.[16] Second, although the e-liquids are intended to be consumed via inhalation, there are case reports of both e-liquid ingestion and transdermal poisonings. In fact, between 2012 and 2015 poison control centers reported a near 15-fold increase in the monthly number of exposures associated with e-cigarettes among children younger than 6 years (from 16 to 223 exposures).[30] Given that a 5-mL vial of an 18 mg per milliliter solution may contain up to 90 mg of nicotine, exposure to a vial of nicotine-containing e-liquid could result in intoxication or death.[16]

The potential for e-cigarette battery explosions has also risen as a safety concern.[31] Persons who use e-cigarette can inadvertently overheat the lithium ion battery, which results in explosion and fire due to the inherent flammability of the e-liquid.[32] Recent case series have reported burns and traumatic injuries of the oral or maxillofacial region (from explosions during e-cigarette use) and the extremities (from spontaneous explosions while the devices were stored in pockets).[33–38] Specific injuries to the oral cavity include intraoral burns, luxation injuries, and chipped and fractured teeth.[34] In addition, sight-threatening ocular injuries from ENDS explosions have been reported, including a penetrating corneoscleral laceration with iris prolapse, hyphema, and bilateral thermal and/or chemical corneal burns.[39,40] There is also a case report of ocular chemical injury due to inadvertent administration of the e-liquid (which was mistaken for antibiotic drops) to the eye.[41] To prevent the potential for explosion, some manufactured e-cigarettes have built-in timers to prevent battery overheating; however, these safety features are not regulated or standardized, and are not present in the modified devices.

ELECTRONIC CIGARETTES AND SMOKING CESSATION

In 2015, 68% of current smokers reported that they wanted to stop smoking completely; however, only 7% of adults reported success with smoking cessation in the past year.[42] Given well-documented obstacles to smoking cessation, many smokers are interested in trying e-cigarettes during efforts to quit or reduce smoking.[4–6] Hence, the role of e-cigarettes in smoking cessation is currently among the leading issues relevant to clinical and public health, and tobacco regulatory practice and policy.

Less than one-third of smokers use evidence-based medications during cigarette quit attempts.[43] Although not FDA-approved as a pharmacotherapy or device for smoking cessation, proponents of e-cigarettes argue that they help promote smoking cessation by providing a more attractive, and potentially effective, alternative to the 7 FDA-approved smoking cessation medications.[44,45] Both adolescents and adult smokers report that e-cigarettes are appealing because they are customizable, are available in a variety of flavors, can be used in traditionally smoke-free venues, and have fewer toxins than cigarettes.[46–50] Furthermore, unlike most FDA-approved smoking cessation therapies, persons who use e-cigarettes can mimic smoking behaviors (eg, via hand-to-mouth behaviors), which can provide a coping mechanism for conditioned smoking cues such as smoking when eating or consuming alcohol.[51]

To date, 2 randomized controlled clinical trials have examined the effectiveness of e-cigarettes for smoking cessation in adults. Bullen and colleagues[52] randomized 689 adult cigarette smokers in New Zealand who smoked more than 10 cigarettes per day to nicotine-containing (10–16 mg/mL) e-cigarettes, placebo (containing no nicotine) e-cigarettes, or nicotine patches (21 mg/24 h). At 6 months, the biochemically verified continuous abstinence rate was 7.3% in the e-cigarette group, 5.8% in the patch group, and 4.1% in the placebo e-cigarette group; however, the study was not statistically powered to detect a difference between the abstinence rates. Caponnetto and colleagues[19] randomized 300 smokers in Italy who were not intending to quit to placebo e-cigarettes, 7.2 mg nicotine-containing e-cigarettes, or e-cigarettes tapered from 7.2 to 5.4 mg nicotine. Twelve-month quit rates were statistically nonsignificant (13% for 7.2 mg nicotine e-cigarette, 9% for the e-cigarette tapered from 7.2 to 5.4 mg, and 4% for nonnicotine e-cigarettes).

A recent meta-analysis of 8 observational cohorts comparing e-cigarette use with no e-cigarette use failed to show a difference between the odds of cigarette abstinence between the 2 groups (odds ratio 0.74, $P = .051$, I^2 statistic $= 56\%$).[53] Of note, a variety of types and brands of e-cigarettes were provided or used by participants in both the randomized controlled trials and the observational studies, reducing the ability to determine if certain types of e-cigarette devices may be more helpful than others. Furthermore, the cohort studies are also limited because they generally did not report on other important predictors of successful smoking cessation, such as motivation to quit. By following a cohort of smokers, they may have underestimated the impact of e-cigarettes because they did not include smokers who had already successfully quit. Overall, given the small numbers of published clinical trials and the inherent limitations of observational studies, it is currently not possible for clinicians to determine whether e-cigarettes promote cessation from tobacco products among the general population of adult smokers.

SPECIAL POPULATIONS
Patients with Cardiovascular Disease

About 29% of the smoking-attributable deaths in the United States between 2005 and 2009 were due to CVD.[9] Among patients with established CVD, continued cigarette smoking is associated with poorer treatment outcomes; however, smoking cessation is a powerful secondary prevention technique and reduces mortality rates.[9,54] Data from the 2014 and 2015 National Interview Survey found that 21.9% of adult smokers ages 45 to 64 years with self-reported CVD and 14% of those with hypertension reported current e-cigarette use.[3] Adult smokers with CVD have a 1.54 increased likelihood of current e-cigarette use compared with smokers without any self-reported comorbidity.[3] These data indicate that it is especially important to understand how e-cigarette use affects overall cardiovascular health.

Currently, well-designed trials examining the efficacy of e-cigarettes for smoking cessation in adult smokers with CVD are lacking. Due to the vasoactive effects of nicotine and the presence of cardiovascular toxicants in e-liquids, there is ongoing concern in the field that long-term exposure to e-cigarette vapor may induce cardiac injury.[12,55] These toxicants can increase CVD risk by affecting blood pressure (BP) regulation, and promoting coagulation and atherosclerotic inflammation.[56–58] However, a recent longitudinal study showed that some persons who use e-cigarette have significantly lower levels of these carcinogens and toxins in their urine than cigarette smokers.[59]

Studies have yet to directly compare cardiovascular risk between cigarette smokers and persons who use e-cigarettes but early evidence suggests there is potential that e-cigarette use is associated with a range of cardiovascular effects. A recent study of 23 healthy adult volunteers who regularly use e-cigarette found that heart rate variability was shifted toward sympathetic predominance, a pattern associated with increased cardiovascular risk.[60] On the other hand, other small studies have reported positive effects on hypertension. For example, a medical record review of 43 patients with hypertension found that regular e-cigarette use reported on at least 2 occasions over a year was associated with a significant reduction in systolic and diastolic BP.[61] Another study of 52 adults with elevated systolic BP at baseline found that smoking reduction or abstinence via switching to e-cigarettes resulted in lower systolic BP at 1-year follow-up.[62] Furthermore, although the health effects of long-term exposure to nicotine among patients with CVD raises concern, studies have shown that patients with known CVD can tolerate short-term nicotine replacement therapy, raising the possibility that temporary e-cigarette use would be safe in this population.[63,64] These studies and others have led some experts to suggest that, although e-cigarette use may pose some heightened cardiovascular risk, especially among adults with existing CVD, the risk is likely to be less than that of cigarettes and, therefore, may result in reduced harm at the individual and population levels.[56]

Patients with Pulmonary Disease

E-cigarette use is also highly prevalent among adults with pulmonary disease such as asthma and chronic obstructive pulmonary disease (COPD), necessitating an understanding of the potential health effects in this group.[3] In 2015, about 12.5% of cigarette smokers with asthma and 15.8% of those with COPD reported past-month use of e-cigarettes.[3,65] Multiple studies demonstrate the relationship between cigarette smoking and worsened asthma symptoms, increased acute care utilization, missed days of school or work, and increased need for medications, which begs the question of whether e-cigarettes could result in harm reduction in this population if these individuals were able to completely stop using combustible tobacco.[66–68] Tobacco smoking is the leading cause of COPD globally. Cigarette smoking increases the risk of COPD exacerbations and lung function declines over time.[69,70]

There is emerging evidence that certain e-liquid flavorants have toxic pulmonary effects.[71] Cinnamon-flavored (ie, cinnamaldehyde) e-liquids and aerosols have been shown to be cytotoxic at low concentrations in human lung cells.[72] Recent studies have demonstrated that several flavorings induce expression of inflammatory cytokines in lung cell cultures.[73] One case report documented respiratory bronchiolitis interstitial lung disease, confirmed by open lung biopsy, in a person who uses e-cigarette who also smoked cigarettes.[74] Diacetyl is present in many e-cigarette liquids (found in caramel, butterscotch, watermelon, piña colada, and strawberry) and has been shown to be a cause of bronchiolitis obliterans (popcorn lung) in the occupational setting.[72,75]

There are few studies that tested the effect of e-cigarettes on human pulmonary function. Among healthy volunteers, several studies have shown short-term increases in airway hyperreactivity and airway resistance after using nicotine-containing e-cigarettes.[76,77] Studies have also shown that smokers with COPD who completely switched to e-cigarettes had a reduction in symptoms and an improved quality of life.[78] A small group of asthmatic smokers (18) who switched to e-cigarettes were followed prospectively and found to have improvements in spirometry and Asthma Control Questionnaire scores up to 2 years later.[79,80] Overall, the evidence regarding pulmonary outcomes is scant and future research is needed to understand the long-term impact of e-cigarettes on pulmonary health.

Patients with Serious Mental Illness

Primary care providers have an important role in improving health and care coordination of patients with SMI. Although smoking rates have declined significantly in the general population, they remain disproportionately high in individuals with mental health conditions.[81] Adults with SMI are those who have a current or past-year behavioral, mental, or emotional disorder that seriously impairs participation in major life activities.[82] Schizophrenia, schizoaffective disorder, bipolar disorder, or major depressive disorder, as well as other disorders, have the potential to produce impairment to a degree that a person would have SMI.[82] People with SMI generally have poorer physical health and life expectancy, which is partially attributed to the high prevalence of tobacco use in this population.[83] Smokers with SMI have greater difficulty quitting tobacco than those without SMI, which has been attributed to variety of factors, including higher levels of nicotine dependence, comorbid substance use, and psychosocial stress.[84]

The prevalence of e-cigarette use among adults with SMI varies, and studies have reported prevalence rates of current e-cigarette use from 11% to greater than 30%.[14,85,86] Prevalence rates are higher among adults with multiple mental health diagnoses compared with those with a single diagnosis.[87] A 2015 examination of a large representative sample of US adults found that 1 in 5 adults with SMI reported current e-cigarette use, and adults with mental health conditions were almost 2 times more likely to report past-month use of e-cigarettes than those without mental health conditions.[87]

Initial findings support the possibility that e-cigarettes may help with smoking reduction, whereas it is unknown how e-cigarette use will affect smoking cessation.[14] Thus, there is growing concern that e-cigarette use in this population may encourage dual e-cigarette and cigarette use. A 2015 study of a national representative sample of more than 6000 adult smokers found that adults with SMI were more likely than those without SMI to substitute some cigarettes with e-cigarettes during a quit attempt; however, they were also more likely to have completely switched to e-cigarettes during a smoking quit attempt.[87] However, a secondary analysis of the Bullen and colleagues[52] trial, which randomized 657 smokers to 16 mg nicotine e-cigarettes, 21 mg nicotine patches, or 0 mg nicotine e-cigarettes, with minimal behavioral support, found no differences in cessation rates (patches 14%, 16 mg e-cigarettes 5%, 0 mg e-cigarettes 0%, $P = .245$) among the subsample of 86 smokers with mental illness.[88]

More specific to SMI, a feasibility study of 14 smokers with schizophrenia not intending to quit found that 50% of the sample reported smoking 50% fewer cigarettes per day after 52 weeks, 14% had quit smoking, and schizophrenia symptoms did not increase with smoking.[19] Another pilot study provided e-cigarettes to 19 daily smokers with SMI for 4 weeks and found that self-reported use of combustible tobacco declined from 192 to 67 cigarettes per week ($P = .005$), confirmed by a reduction in breath carbon monoxide.[89] This initial evidence suggests that e-cigarette use is associated with reductions in cigarette smoking; however, future studies are needed in larger populations to validate these findings.

Considerations in Adolescents

When weighing the potential benefits of e-cigarette use in adult smokers, public health advocates and clinicians must also consider the potential risks if widespread use in adults facilitates youth exposure to nicotine through e-cigarettes and other tobacco products. Adolescents have heighted neurodevelopmental vulnerability to the development of nicotine addiction. A recognition of this enhanced vulnerability has led the United States to develop and implement multifaceted and comprehensive tobacco control efforts aimed at reducing youth access to tobacco.[90] As a result, rates of cigarette smoking among US adolescents have fallen in the last decade. In 2016, only 8.6% of high school students reported past-month cigarette smoking, whereas 19.6%

reported this in 2006.[90-92] However, during this same period, rates of e-cigarette use have increased from less than 2% in 2011 to 11.3% of high school and 4.3% of middle school students reported current e-cigarette use in 2016.[91] Thus, whereas cigarettes are the most popular tobacco product used by US adults, e-cigarettes have surpassed cigarettes as the most common tobacco product used by youth.[20,91]

A recent meta-analysis of 9 longitudinal studies of 17,389 adolescents and young adults ages 14 to 30 years found that pooled probabilities of cigarette smoking initiation were 30.4% for baseline persons who ever used e-cigarette and 7.9% for baseline persons who never used e-cigarette.[13] The analysis reported that the baseline of ever using e-cigarettes (vs never using e-cigarettes) increased the odds of cigarette smoking initiation, with a pooled odds ratio of 3.62 (95% CI 2.42–5.41) when adjusting for known demographic, psychosocial, and behavioral risk factors for cigarette smoking. This raised the concern that e-cigarette use in youth may increase the burden of tobacco-related morbidity and mortality in future generations.[13] Several observational studies have found no association between e-cigarette use and smoking cessation in adolescents[93,94]; however, longitudinal studies in this area are lacking. Taken together, these findings led to the 2016 US Surgeon General's report, *E-cigarette Use Among Youth and Young Adults*, which recommended that "The use of products containing nicotine in any form among youth, including in e-cigarettes, is unsafe."[20]

ELECTRONIC CIGARETTES IN THE CONTEXT OF TOBACCO PRODUCT REGULATION AND PROPOSED POLICY CHANGES FOR TOBACCO CONTROL

In 2016, the FDA exercised its authority, as outlined in the 2009 Family Smoking Prevention and Tobacco Control Act, to regulate e-cigarettes as tobacco products with a goal of improving population health.[16,95] Building on this goal, the FDA has affirmed its commitment to encourage tobacco product innovations that offer smokers safer alternatives to cigarettes.[96] Additionally, the FDA has proposed a strategy that could reduce the nicotine content in cigarettes to levels that are low enough to be minimally addictive or even nonaddictive.[95] This strategy is aimed at encouraging millions of adult smokers to cease their use of combustible tobacco products but could also prompt the continued use or even initiation of less harmful, noncombustible nicotine delivery systems, such as e-cigarettes. For some populations, such as those with CVD, pulmonary disease, or SMI, this strategy offers both opportunities and challenges. Although harm reduction is expected with the complete cessation of combustible tobacco, chronic exposure to nicotine in e-cigarettes may not be totally benign due to the pharmacologic effects of nicotine on the cardiovascular system or the inflammatory effects of e-liquids on the lung. Furthermore, there could be unintended consequences for adolescents and young adults, especially if this policy encourages young people to erroneously view e-cigarettes as harmless instead of less harmful than combustible tobacco. Overall, the proposed US policy change will be considered successful if it achieves a similar outcome to that seen in the United Kingdom, where widespread use of e-cigarettes has been credited with reducing prevalence of cigarette smoking.[97]

SYNTHESIS OF THE EVIDENCE TO INFORM CLINICAL MANAGEMENT OF ELECTRONIC CIGARETTE USE IN PRIMARY CARE

Several professional organizations have put forth clinical policy statements that include e-cigarettes (**Box 1**). Of note, the US Preventative Services Task Force states the evidence is insufficient to determine the efficacy of e-cigarettes for smoking cessation, and the American Academy of Pediatrics recommends against e-cigarette use for smoking cessation.[98,99] However, the American Heart Association does point

> **Box 1**
> **Resources for current recommendations from US professional organizations**
>
> US Preventive Services Task Force (2015)[98]
>   https://www.uspreventiveservicestaskforce.org/
>
> American Heart Association (2015)[12]
>   http://www.heart.org/HEARTORG/
>
> The Forum of International Respiratory Society Position Statement (2014)[101]
>   https://www.firsnet.org/
>
> American Academy of Pediatrics (2015)[99]
>   https://www.aap.org/en-us/Pages/Default.aspx
>
> American Society of Clinical Oncology (2015)[102]
>   https://www.asco.org/

out that it is reasonable to support patients who use e-cigarettes for smoking cessation in settings in which the patient has repeatedly failed or is intolerant of guideline-based treatment or refuses conventional, FDA-approved smoking cessation medications.[12] In these cases, the clinician should advise patients about the potential risks of e-cigarette exposure and the lack of evidence to support their efficacy for smoking cessation.

COUNSELING ADULTS WHO USE ELECTRONIC CIGARETTES

When discussing e-cigarettes, primary care providers should educate patients about potential risks and benefits of e-cigarettes and specific concerns relevant to adults with heightened vulnerability tobacco-induced illnesses. In general, primary care providers should listen openly to patients' views on e-cigarettes and convey that there is not enough medical evidence to recommend e-cigarettes as a safe or efficacious product for smoking cessation. Based on the data presented in this article, medical professionals may tailor advice based on the patient's comorbid conditions. For example, patients with CVD should be counseled about the potential adverse effects of nicotine on cardiovascular health, whereas patients with pulmonary disease should be aware there is some inconclusive evidence of symptom improvement, as well as increased pulmonary inflammation, with e-cigarettes. Patients with SMI should learn that the current evidence supports the possibility that e-cigarettes may help with smoking reduction, whereas it is unknown how e-cigarette use will affect smoking cessation.[14] Nonetheless, all patients should be counseled on the potentially superior health impact of tobacco abstinence compared with prolonged e-cigarette use.

Primary care providers should continue to screen all adults for tobacco use, including e-cigarette use, and offer evidence-based smoking cessation therapies, including FDA-approved medications, to all cigarette smokers.[100] Additionally, e-cigarette use in smokers should be viewed as a step toward cessation, and trigger a deeper discussion between the physician and patient about goals for smoking cessation and the use of evidence-based medications. Overall, there is a great ongoing need to understand the potential impact of e-cigarettes on both individual smoking cessation and population health.

FUTURE CONSIDERATIONS AND SUMMARY

Tobacco exposure continues to be the leading cause of preventable morbidity and mortality in the United States. As a result, clinicians, policy makers, and public health professionals continue to strive to reduce cigarette and tobacco smoking rates. E-cigarettes are used by smokers in efforts to quit smoking; however, to date, the evidence regarding their efficacy for smoking cessation is inconclusive and does not meet the standard for evidence-based practice recommendations.

ACKNOWLEDGMENTS

The editors wish to thank Sara Kalkhoran, Massachusetts General Hospital and Harvard Medical School, for providing a critical review of this article.

REFERENCES

1. Grana R, Benowitz N, Glantz SA. E-cigarettes: a scientific review. Circulation 2014;129(19):1972–86.
2. Kasza KA, Ambrose BK, Conway KP, et al. Tobacco-product use by adults and youths in the United States in 2013 and 2014. N Engl J Med 2017;376(4): 342–53.
3. Kruse GR, Kalkhoran S, Rigotti NA. Use of electronic cigarettes among U.S. Adults with medical comorbidities. Am J Prev Med 2017;52(6):798–804.
4. De Genna NM, Ylioja T, Schulze AE, et al. Electronic cigarette use among counseled tobacco users hospitalized in 2015. J Addict Med 2017;11(6):449–53.
5. Kalkhoran S, Alvarado N, Vijayaraghavan M, et al. Patterns of and reasons for electronic cigarette use in primary care patients. J Gen Intern Med 2017; 32(10):1122–9.
6. Coleman BN, Rostron B, Johnson SE, et al. Electronic cigarette use among US adults in the Population Assessment of Tobacco and Health (PATH) Study, 2013–2014. Tob Control 2017;26(e2):e117–26.
7. Nickels AS, Warner DO, Jenkins SM, et al. Beliefs, practices, and self-efficacy of us physicians regarding smoking cessation and electronic cigarettes: a national survey. Nicotine Tob Res 2017;19(2):197–207.
8. U.S Department of Health and Human Services. How tobacco smoke causes disease: the biology and behavioral basis for smoking-attributable disease: a report of the Surgeon General. Atlanta (GA): U.S Department of Health and Human Services, Centers for Disease Control and Prevention, National Center for Chronic Disease Prevention and Health Promotion, Office on Smoking and Health; 2010.
9. US Department of Health and Human Services. The health consequences of smoking–50 years of progress: a report of the surgeon general. Atlanta (GA): US Department of Health and Human Services, Centers for Disease Control and Prevention, National Center for Chronic Disease Prevention and Health Promotion, Office on Smoking and Health; 2014.
10. McNeill A, Brose L, Calder R, et al. E-cigarettes: an evidence update. Public Health Engl 2015;3:76–80.
11. Hajek P. Underpinning evidence for the estimate that e-cigarette use is around 95% safer than smoking: authors' note. 2015. Available at: https://www.gov.uk/government/uploads/system/uploads/attachment_data/file/456704/McNeill-Hajek_report_authors_note_on_evidence_for_95_estimate.pdf. Accessed October 1, 2017.
12. Bhatnagar A, Whitsel LP, Ribisl KM, et al. Electronic cigarettes. A policy statement from the American Heart Association 2014;129(1):28–41.
13. Soneji S, Barrington-Trimis JL, Wills TA, et al. Association between initial use of e-cigarettes and subsequent cigarette smoking among adolescents and young

adults: a systematic review and meta-analysis. JAMA Pediatr 2017;171(8): 788–97.

14. Hefner K, Valentine G, Sofuoglu M. Electronic cigarettes and mental illness: Reviewing the evidence for help and harm among those with psychiatric and substance use disorders. Am J Addict 2017;26(4):306–15.

15. Choi K, Grana R, Bernat D. Electronic nicotine delivery systems and acceptability of adult cigarette smoking among Florida youth: renormalization of smoking? J Adolesc Health 2017;60(5):592–8.

16. Food and Drug Administration, Health and Human Services. Deeming Tobacco Products To Be Subject to the Federal Food, Drug, and Cosmetic Act, as Amended by the Family Smoking Prevention and Tobacco Control Act; Restrictions on the Sale and Distribution of Tobacco Products and Required Warning Statements for Tobacco Products. Final rule. Fed Regist 2016;81(90): 28973–9106.

17. Grana RA, Ling PM. "Smoking revolution": a content analysis of electronic cigarette retail websites. Am J Prev Med 2014;46(4):395–403.

18. Richtel M. A bolder effort by big tobacco on e-cigarettes. New York Times, June 17, 2014. p. A1.

19. Caponnetto P, Campagna D, Cibella F, et al. EffiCiency and safety of an eLectronic cigAreTte (ECLAT) as tobacco cigarettes substitute: a prospective 12-month randomized control design study. PLoS One 2013;8(6):e66317.

20. US Department of Health and Human Services. E-cigarette use among youth and young adults: a report of the surgeon general. Atlanta (GA): US Department of Health and Human Services, Centers for Disease Control and Prevention, National Center for Chronic Disease Prevention and Health Promotion, Office on Smoking and Health; 2016.

21. Chen C, Zhuang YL, Zhu SH. E-cigarette design preference and smoking cessation: a U.S. population study. Am J Prev Med 2016;51(3):356–63.

22. Yingst JM, Veldheer S, Hrabovsky S, et al. Factors associated with electronic cigarette users' device preferences and transition from first generation to advanced generation devices. Nicotine Tob Res 2015;17(10):1242–6.

23. Lechner WV, Meier E, Wiener JL, et al. The comparative efficacy of first- versus second-generation electronic cigarettes in reducing symptoms of nicotine withdrawal. Addiction 2015;110(5):862–7.

24. Etter JF. Characteristics of users and usage of different types of electronic cigarettes: findings from an online survey. Addiction 2016;111(4):724–33.

25. Farsalinos KE, Romagna G, Tsiapras D, et al. Impact of flavour variability on electronic cigarette use experience: an internet survey. Int J Environ Res Public Health 2013;10(12):7272–82.

26. Goniewicz ML, Knysak J, Gawron M, et al. Levels of selected carcinogens and toxicants in vapour from electronic cigarettes. Tob Control 2014;23(2):133–9.

27. Goniewicz ML, Gawron M, Smith DM, et al. Exposure to nicotine and selected toxicants in cigarette smokers who switched to electronic cigarettes: a longitudinal within-subjects observational study. Nicotine Tob Res 2017;19(2):160–7.

28. Buettner-Schmidt K, Miller DR, Balasubramanian N. Electronic cigarette refill liquids: child-resistant packaging, nicotine content, and sales to minors. J Pediatr Nurs 2016;31(4):373–9.

29. Goniewicz ML, Kuma T, Gawron M, et al. Nicotine levels in electronic cigarettes. Nicotine Tobac Res 2013;15(1):158–66.

30. Kamboj A, Spiller HA, Casavant MJ, et al. Pediatric exposure to e-cigarettes, nicotine, and tobacco products in the United States. Pediatrics 2016;137(6) [pii:e20160041].

31. Ramirez JI, Ridgway CA, Lee JG, et al. The unrecognized epidemic of electronic cigarette burns. J Burn Care Res 2017;38(4):220–4.

32. Treitl D, Solomon R, Davare DL, et al. Full and partial thickness burns from spontaneous combustion of e-cigarette lithium-ion batteries with review of literature. J Emerg Med 2017;53(1):121–5.

33. Archambeau BA, Young S, Lee C, et al. E-cigarette blast injury: complex facial fractures and pneumocephalus. West J Emerg Med 2016;17(6):805–7.

34. Harrison R, Hicklin D Jr. Electronic cigarette explosions involving the oral cavity. J Am Dent Assoc 2016;147(11):891–6.

35. Hassan S, Anwar MU, Muthayya P, et al. Burn injuries from exploding electronic cigarette batteries: an emerging public health hazard. J Plast Reconstr Aesthet Surg 2016;69(12):1716–8.

36. Meernik C, Williams FN, Cairns BA, et al. Burns from e-cigarettes and other electronic nicotine delivery systems. BMJ 2016;354:i5024.

37. Goverman J, Schulz JT. Thigh burns from exploding E-cigarette. Burns 2016; 42(7):1618.

38. Colaianni CA, Tapias LF, Cauley R, et al. Injuries caused by explosion of electronic cigarette devices. Eplasty 2016;16:ic9.

39. Paley GL, Echalier E, Eck TW, et al. Corneoscleral laceration and ocular burns caused by electronic cigarette explosions. Cornea 2016;35(7):1015–8.

40. Khairudin MN, Mohd Zahidin AZ, Bastion ML. Front to back ocular injury from a vaping-related explosion. BMJ Case Rep 2016;2016 [pii:bcr2016214964].

41. Jamison A, Lockington D. Ocular chemical injury secondary to electronic cigarette liquid misuse. JAMA Ophthalmol 2016;134(12):1443.

42. Quitting smoking among adults–United States, 2001-2010. MMWR Morb Mortal Wkly Rep 2011;60(44):1513–9.

43. Babb S, Malarcher A, Schauer G, et al. Quitting smoking among adults - United States, 2000-2015. MMWR Morb Mortal Wkly Rep 2017;65(52):1457–64.

44. Correa JB, Ariel I, Menzie NS, et al. Documenting the emergence of electronic nicotine delivery systems as a disruptive technology in nicotine and tobacco science. Addict Behav 2017;65:179–84.

45. Pechacek TF, Nayak P, Gregory KR, et al. The potential that electronic nicotine delivery systems can be a disruptive technology: results from a national survey. Nicotine Tob Res 2016;18(10):1989–97.

46. Patrick ME, Miech RA, Carlier C, et al. Self-reported reasons for vaping among 8th, 10th, and 12th graders in the US: Nationally-representative results. Drug Alcohol Depend 2016;165:275–8.

47. Bold KW, Kong G, Cavallo DA, et al. Reasons for trying E-cigarettes and risk of continued use. Pediatrics 2016;138(3) [pii:e20160895].

48. Patel D, Davis KC, Cox S, et al. Reasons for current E-cigarette use among U.S. adults. Prev Med 2016;93:14–20.

49. Berg CJ. Preferred flavors and reasons for e-cigarette use and discontinued use among never, current, and former smokers. Int J Public Health 2016;61(2): 225–36.

50. Kong G, Morean ME, Cavallo DA, et al. Reasons for electronic cigarette experimentation and discontinuation among adolescents and young adults [published online ahead of print Dec 6 2014]. Nicotine Tob Res 2015;17(7):847–54.

51. Caponnetto P, Russo C, Bruno CM, et al. Electronic cigarette: a possible substitute for cigarette dependence. Monaldi Arch Chest Dis 2013;79(1):12–9.
52. Bullen C, Howe C, Laugesen M, et al. Electronic cigarettes for smoking cessation: a randomised controlled trial. Lancet 2013;382(9905):1629–37.
53. El Dib R, Suzumura EA, Akl EA, et al. Electronic nicotine delivery systems and/or electronic non-nicotine delivery systems for tobacco smoking cessation or reduction: a systematic review and meta-analysis. BMJ Open 2017;7(2): e012680.
54. Rigotti NA, Clair C. Managing tobacco use: the neglected cardiovascular disease risk factor. Eur Heart J 2013;34(42):3259–67.
55. Bhatnagar A. Are electronic cigarette users at increased risk for cardiovascular disease? JAMA Cardiol 2017;2(3):237–8.
56. Benowitz NL, Fraiman JB. Cardiovascular effects of electronic cigarettes. Nat Rev Cardiol 2017;14(8):447–56.
57. Rigotti NA, Clair C. Managing tobacco use: the neglected cardiovascular disease risk factor. Eur Heart J 2013;34(42):3259–67.
58. Morris PB, Ference BA, Jahangir E, et al. Cardiovascular effects of exposure to cigarette smoke and electronic cigarettes. J Am Coll Cardiol 2015;66(12): 1378–91.
59. Shahab L, Goniewicz ML, Blount BC, et al. Nicotine, carcinogen, and toxin exposure in long-term e-cigarette and nicotine replacement therapy users: a cross-sectional study. Ann Intern Med 2017;166(6):390–400.
60. Moheimani RS, Bhetraratana M, Yin F, et al. Increased cardiac sympathetic activity and oxidative stress in habitual electronic cigarette users: Implications for cardiovascular risk. JAMA Cardiol 2017;2(3):278–84.
61. Polosa R, Morjaria JB, Caponnetto P, et al. Blood Pressure Control in Smokers with Arterial Hypertension Who Switched to Electronic Cigarettes. International Journal of Environmental Research and Public Health 2016;13(11):1123.
62. Farsalinos K, Cibella F, Caponnetto P, et al. Effect of continuous smoking reduction and abstinence on blood pressure and heart rate in smokers switching to electronic cigarettes. Intern Emerg Med 2016;11(1):85–94.
63. Meine TJ, Patel MR, Washam JB, et al. Safety and effectiveness of transdermal nicotine patch in smokers admitted with acute coronary syndromes. Am J Cardiol 2005;95(8):976–8.
64. Mills EJ, Thorlund K, Eapen S, et al. Cardiovascular events associated with smoking cessation pharmacotherapies a network meta-analysis. Circulation 2014;129(1):28–41.
65. Centers for Disease Control. National current asthma prevalence (2015). 2017. Available at: https://www.cdc.gov/asthma/most_recent_data.htm. Accessed April 6, 2017.
66. Thomson NC, Chaudhuri R, Heaney LG, et al. Clinical outcomes and inflammatory biomarkers in current smokers and exsmokers with severe asthma. J Allergy Clin Immunol 2013;131(4):1008–16.
67. Thomson NC, Chaudhuri R. Asthma in smokers: challenges and opportunities. Curr Opin Pulm Med 2009;15(1):39–45.
68. Chaudhuri R, McSharry C, McCoard A, et al. Role of symptoms and lung function in determining asthma control in smokers with asthma. Allergy 2008;63(1): 132–5.
69. Rabe KF, Watz H. Chronic obstructive pulmonary disease. Lancet 2017; 389(10082):1931–40.

70. Jimenez-Ruiz CA, Andreas S, Lewis KE, et al. Statement on smoking cessation in COPD and other pulmonary diseases and in smokers with comorbidities who find it difficult to quit. Eur Respir J 2015;46(1):61–79.

71. Shields PG, Berman M, Brasky TM, et al. A review of pulmonary toxicity of electronic cigarettes in the context of smoking: a focus on inflammation. Cancer Epidemiol Biomarkers Prev 2017;26(8):1175–91.

72. Behar RZ, Wang Y, Talbot P. Comparing the cytotoxicity of electronic cigarette fluids, aerosols and solvents. Tob Control 2017. [Epub ahead of print].

73. Chun LF, Moazed F, Calfee CS, et al. Pulmonary toxicity of E-cigarettes. Am J Physiol Lung Cell Mol Physiol 2017;313(2):L193–206.

74. Flower M, Nandakumar L, Singh M, et al. Respiratory bronchiolitis-associated interstitial lung disease secondary to electronic nicotine delivery system use confirmed with open lung biopsy. Respirol Case Rep 2017;5(3):e00230.

75. Allen JG, Flanigan SS, LeBlanc M, et al. Flavoring chemicals in E-cigarettes: diacetyl, 2,3-pentanedione, and acetoin in a sample of 51 products, including fruit-, candy-, and cocktail-flavored E-cigarettes. Environ Health Perspect 2016;124(6):733–9.

76. Palamidas A, Gennimata SA, Kaltsakas G, et al. Acute effect of an e-cigarette with and without nicotine on lung function. Tob Ind Dis 2014;12(1):A34.

77. Vardavas CI, Anagnostopoulos N, Kougias M, et al. Short-term pulmonary effects of using an electronic cigarette: impact on respiratory flow resistance, impedance, and exhaled nitric oxide. Chest 2012;141(6):1400–6.

78. Polosa R, Morjaria JB, Caponnetto P, et al. Evidence for harm reduction in COPD smokers who switch to electronic cigarettes. Respir Res 2016;17(1):166.

79. Campagna D, Cibella F, Caponnetto P, et al. Changes in breathomics from a 1-year randomized smoking cessation trial of electronic cigarettes. Eur J Clin Invest 2016;46(8):698–706.

80. Cibella F, Campagna D, Caponnetto P, et al. Lung function and respiratory symptoms in a randomized smoking cessation trial of electronic cigarettes. Clin Sci 2016;130(21):1929.

81. Cook BL, Wayne GF, Kafali EN, et al. Trends in smoking among adults with mental illness and association between mental health treatment and smoking cessation. JAMA 2014;311(2):172–82.

82. SAMSHA's registry of evidence based practices and programs. Behind the term: serious mental illness. 2016. Available at: http://www.nrepp.samhsa.gov/Docs/Literatures/Behind_the_Term_Serious%20%20Mental%20Illness.pdf. Accessed August 2, 2017.

83. Sharma R, Gartner CE, Castle DJ, et al. Should we encourage smokers with severe mental illness to switch to electronic cigarettes? Aust N Z J Psychiatry 2017;51(7):663–4.

84. Sharma R. The challenge of reducing smoking in people with serious mental illness. Lancet Respir Med 2016;4(10):835–44.

85. Chen LS, Baker T, Brownson RC, et al. Smoking cessation and electronic cigarettes in community mental health centers: patient and provider perspectives. Community Ment Health J 2017;53(6):695–702.

86. Prochaska JJ, Grana RA. E-cigarette use among smokers with serious mental illness. PLoS One 2014;9(11):e113013.

87. Spears CA, Jones DM, Weaver SR, et al. Use of electronic nicotine delivery systems among adults with mental health conditions, 2015. Int J Environ Res Public Health 2016;14(1) [pii:E10].

88. O'Brien B, Knight-West O, Walker N, et al. E-cigarettes versus NRT for smoking reduction or cessation in people with mental illness: secondary analysis of data from the ASCEND trial. Tob Induc Dis 2015;13(1):5.

89. Pratt SI, Sargent J, Daniels L, et al. Appeal of electronic cigarettes in smokers with serious mental illness. Addict Behav 2016;59:30–4.

90. US Department of Health and Human Services. Preventing tobacco use among youth and young adults: a report of the surgeon general. Atlanta (GA): US Department of Health and Human Services, Centers for Disease Control and Prevention, National Center for Chronic Disease Prevention and Health Promotion, Office on Smoking and Health; 2012.

91. Jamal A, Gentzke A, Hu SS, et al. Tobacco use among middle and high school students - United States, 2011-2016. MMWR Morb Mortal Wkly Rep 2017; 66(23):597–603.

92. Centers for Disease Control and Prevention (CDC). Tobacco use among middle and high school students -- United States, 2000-2009. MMWR Morb Mortal Wkly Rep 2010;59(33):1063–8.

93. Camenga DR, Kong G, Cavallo DA, et al. Current and former smokers' use of electronic cigarettes for quitting smoking: an exploratory study of adolescents and young adults. Nicotine Tob Res 2017;19(12):1531–5.

94. Dutra LM, Glantz SA. Electronic cigarettes and conventional cigarette use among U.S. adolescents: a cross-sectional study. JAMA Pediatr 2014;168(7): 610–7.

95. Gottlieb S, Zeller M. A nicotine-focused framework for public health. N Engl J Med 2017;377(12):1111–4.

96. Warner KE, Schroeder SA. FDA's innovative plan to address the enormous toll of smoking. JAMA 2017;318(18):1755–6.

97. Brown J, WR. Quit success rates in England 2007-2017. Smoking in Britian 2017;(5):5–8. Available at: http://www.smokinginbritain.co.uk/read. Accessed March 3, 2018.

98. Siu AL. Behavioral and pharmacotherapy interventions for tobacco smoking cessation in adults, including pregnant women: U.S. Preventive services task force recommendation statement. Ann Intern Med 2015;163(8):622–34.

99. Clinical practice policy to protect children from tobacco, nicotine, and tobacco smoke. Pediatrics 2015;136(8):1008–17.

100. Fiore MC, Jaen CR, Baker TB, et al. Treating tobacco use and dependence: 2008 update. Clinical practice guideline. Rockville (MD): US Department of Health and Human Services. Public Health Services; 2008.

101. Bam TS, Bellew W, Berezhnova I, et al. Position statement on electronic cigarettes or electronic nicotine delivery systems. Int J Tuberc Lung Dis 2014; 18(1):5–7.

102. Brandon TH, Goniewicz ML, Hanna NH, et al. Electronic nicotine delivery systems: a policy statement from the American Association for Cancer Research and the American Society of Clinical Oncology. Clin Cancer Res 2015;21(3): 514–25. https://doi.org/10.1158/1078-0432.ccr-14-2544.

Smoking Cessation for Those Pursuing Recovery from Substance Use Disorders

Karen J. Derefinko, PhD[a],*, Francisco I. Salgado García, PhD[a],
Daniel D. Sumrok, MD[b],[1]

KEYWORDS

- Tobacco • Cessation • Alcohol use disorder • Substance use disorder
- Concomitant treatment

KEY POINTS

- Tobacco addiction risk is profound in substance users.
- Many alcohol and substance use disorder treatment providers do not prioritize tobacco use cessation in treatment.
- Smoking cessation actually improves alcohol and substance use disorder outcomes.
- Behavioral treatment strategies are similar across substance classes.

Individuals in treatment for alcohol use disorder (AUD) or substance use disorder (SUD) face a multitude of risks that need to be addressed by their service providers. Among the many comorbid issues of AUD/SUD is concomitant tobacco use, most commonly in the form of cigarette smoking. Tobacco use, smoking, nicotine dependence, and tobacco addiction risk are terms used interchangeably in the literature. Even though dependence on nicotine is important in the area of tobacco use, there is evidence that people who smoke intermittently (ie, weekly but not daily) and consistently score low on nicotine dependence measures[1] still face the health risks associated with cigarette smoking.[2,3] As such, the aim of this article was to attend to the broadest issue by reviewing the literature on tobacco use and nicotine dependence.

According to the US Department of Health and Human Services, cigarette smoking is the leading cause of preventable death in the United States, accounting for

Conflict of Interest Statement: The authors report no commercial or financial conflicts of interest.
[a] University of Tennessee Health Science Center, 66 North Pauline Street, Suite 305, Memphis, TN 38163-2181, USA; [b] University of Tennessee Health Science Center, Department of Addiction Medicine, 6401 Popular Avenue, Suite 500, Memphis, TN 38119, USA
[1] Present address: 1894 Cedar Street, McKenzie, TN 38201.
* Corresponding author.
E-mail address: kderefin@uthsc.edu

Med Clin N Am 102 (2018) 781–796
https://doi.org/10.1016/j.mcna.2018.02.014
0025-7125/18/© 2018 Elsevier Inc. All rights reserved.

approximately 1 in 5 deaths.[4] Although the rates of smoking have been steadily declining for the past 10 years, 15.1% of those over age 18 report current cigarette use, with the highest rates among adults age 25 to 44 years (17.7%).[5] Results from the National Epidemiologic Survey on Alcohol and Related Conditions suggest that prevalence rates of nicotine dependence based on criteria in the fourth edition of the *Diagnostic and Statistical Manual of Mental Disorders* (eg, the use of nicotine to relieve withdrawal symptoms, use of nicotine more than intended) are extraordinarily high in those with an AUD (45.4%) or nonalcohol SUD (69.3%).[6] Other studies have found similar,[7,8] or even higher rates.[9] In addition to high prevalence, research has indicated that the degree of dependence using diagnostic criteria and dependence measures is stronger in those with AUD/SUD than those without,[10–13] indicating that risk for nicotine dependence is profound in substance users.

Although often overlooked, the long-term impact of tobacco use among those with AUD/SUD is undeniable. Smoking quit rates among those with AUD/SUD are significantly lower than those without comorbid substance use; Lasser and colleagues[8] found that those with a history of AUD had a quit rate of 16.9%, compared with those who have no history of AUD (42.5%). Although often treated as a secondary outcome, smoking has dire consequences among those with AUD/SUD. Results from a large study of individuals in treatment for AUD/SUD (n = 845) indicated that, among documented deaths in the sample, a significantly greater proportion were caused by tobacco use than the alcohol use that brought them into treatment (50.9% vs 34.1%, respectively).[14]

Despite known comorbidity rates and clear adverse outcomes, it is estimated that only 42% of SUD treatment centers provide tobacco cessation services.[15] With the known risk factors associated with smoking, this statistic suggests a crucial need for tobacco cessation services. This article presents a summary of the literature regarding the similar biopsychosocial mechanisms of tobacco use and AUD/SUD. This article also includes a description of the commonly held beliefs regarding smoking in those with AUD/SUD, and the argument of "harm reduction" in the broad context of addiction. Although there are clear reasons why physicians and other addiction treatment providers do not prioritize or promote smoking cessation among those with AUD/SUD, the risks to optimal outcomes should eclipse this apathy. The practicality of treatment, focusing on the methods, timing, and innovations of intervention strategies, are also presented. Finally, the common methodologies that may be used across tobacco use and AUD/SUD to prevent long-term lapse and relapse are discussed. Physicians can and should adhere to the policy that tobacco use is a common and dangerous comorbid condition that demands concomitant treatment for those with AUD/SUD and should follow the guidelines for treating tobacco use.[16]

COMMON ETIOLOGY OF TOBACCO, ALCOHOL, AND ILLICIT SUBSTANCE USE

It is critical to consider the basis for the cooccurrence of tobacco use and AUD/SUD to understand their concomitant use. Many hypotheses about the cooccurrence of these disorders exist and are generally based on biological predispositions and psychosocial/environmental factors. In addition to a possible joint genetic predisposition,[17] neurobiological models indicate that nicotine modulates neurotransmitter systems directly implicated in other SUDs, including dopamine,[18,19] serotonin,[20,21] acetylcholine,[22] endogenous opioid peptides,[23,24] gamma-aminobutyric acid, glutamate,[25–27] and norepinephrine.[28] Research has also demonstrated that nicotine increases the effects of other substances, may serve as a gateway drug, and may contribute to increased risk of drug use.[29]

Further, developmental research suggests that specific mechanisms of dysfunction underlie both tobacco and AUD/SUD, including executive cognitive function. As noted by Tarter,[30] executive cognitive function is believed to be modulated by the dorsolateral prefrontal cortex, and involves planned behavior (vs impulsivity), self-monitoring, attention, memory, and mental flexibility.[31] These mechanisms of function have been validated as reliable predictors of both tobacco and AUD/SUD in numerous empirical studies,[32–38] and cognitive tasks such as delay discounting have provided a strong link between mechanisms of dysfunction and related therapeutic techniques.[39–41]

Still other research points to the shared psychosocial or environmental mechanisms of both tobacco use and SUDs.[7] Independent but related theories[30,42,43] have been posited to explain the interactions between, and the importance of, proximal (peer and family use, access, stressors, psychopathology, novelty seeking) and distal (media and cultural influences regarding tobacco and substance use) interpersonal and environmental influences. Although each of these mechanisms have been found to be important contributors to the development of tobacco and substance use, several deserve specific mention. First, early environmental experiences have been found to have a significant effect on later substance use. The Adverse Childhood Events (ACEs) study, a collaborative effort between Kaiser and the Centers for Disease Control and Prevention, identified 10 categories of negative childhood events that predict tobacco,[44] alcohol,[45] and substance use[46] well into adulthood. These events included a household member who uses alcohol or illicit drugs. Parental substance use as a risk factor has been demonstrated repeatedly in individual studies of tobacco, alcohol, and other substance use,[47–49] as has peer substance use,[50–52] suggesting that modeling plays a large role in the etiology of all forms of substance use. Further, different forms of psychopathology have been shown to predict or cooccur with multiple forms of substance use, particularly depression,[53–55] anxiety,[55,56] posttraumatic stress disorder,[57,58] and bipolar disorder.[59,60] Results from the Epidemiologic Catchment Area study suggest that among those with a mental disorder, 29% have a lifetime prevalence of a SUD.[53]

It is clear that these multiple environmental and individual factors do not exist in isolation, and often seem to work in tandem to increase substance use risk over the life course. Numerous individual studies have contributed to emergent work on the latent factor of SUD liability,[61] which identifies the many shared genotypic and phenotypic contributors to multiple forms of substance use. In support of a common liability concept, research has documented comorbidity between substances (even among those with opposite effects),[62] cross-tolerance and cross-dependence between substances,[63,64] and consistency across individuals in "staging," or the progression from tobacco and alcohol to illicit drugs over time.[65,66]

WHY ALCOHOL USE DISORDER/SUBSTANCE USE DISORDER TREATMENT PROVIDERS TURN A BLIND EYE TO TOBACCO USE

Although the risks for tobacco use are widely known, physicians and other addiction treatment providers do not prioritize combustible (ie, cigarettes) and noncombustible (ie, e-cigarettes) tobacco cessation in treatment.[15] There are several reasons why this would be the case. First, as noted by Romberger and Grant,[67] there exists a common belief among providers that it is simply too difficult for patients to address both smoking cessation and alcohol or other substance use abstinence at the same time, leading to failures in treatment.[68] As evidence of this belief, smoking is not addressed in one of the largest attended public support groups (Alcoholics Anonymous), and a large survey conducted in 1995 that included health professionals who provide AUD/SUD treatment, suggested that two-thirds of treatment providers did not support smoking cessation during active alcohol or other substance use treatment.[69] In addition, research has found that barriers to the provision of smoking cessation interventions in substance use treatment settings include a lack of skill in the area of tobacco use treatment and few resources.[70] Also, it is possible that a number of treatment facilities may make decisions to allow smoking to engage patient populations needed to meet financial goals. Facilities with smoking bans run the risk of alienating patients who smoke, which may result in patients choosing treatment facilities that allow smoking. Although the Joint Commission on Accreditation of Health Organizations introduced indoor restrictions on smoking as a quality indicator effective December 31, 1993,[71] many health care settings continue to allow smoking outdoors in designated areas to accommodate patients and staff who continue to smoke.

Second, owing to common effects on neurotransmitters of addiction, smoking has anecdotally been considered a replacement behavior for alcohol and other drugs, with no clear associations with relapse,[72] or even concerns that smoking cessation will result in a relapse of alcohol or other substances.[73] Owing to the neurophysiological mechanisms of nicotine, it is quite possible that those in recovery for AUD/SUD do indeed experience less craving for alcohol or other substances because AUD/SUD withdrawal symptoms may, in part, be avoided by tobacco use.[74] This reliance on tobacco during substance use treatment is reflected in research on readiness to change, and concerns over smoking cessation during treatment for AUD/SUD. For instance, studies have found that methadone patients recognize the health risks of smoking, but few plan on quitting in the next 30 days.[75] Also, most patients in treatment perceive smoking cessation to be as or more difficult than quitting drugs or alcohol.[68] Similarly, patients' perceived barriers to smoking cessation include fear of relapse and lack of emotional coping.[73]

Third, tobacco use is legal and does not cause marked inebriation. Impairment in the areas of attention, impulse control, working memory, executive functioning, motor coordination, and cognitive flexibility are some of the deficits related to acute and chronic drug use.[76,77] Unlike alcohol and illicit drugs, nicotine—the common substance across tobacco products—does not produce major cognitive or behavioral impairment.[78] In fact, research has found that nicotine improves memory and attention in clinical and nonclinical populations.[78,79] Other studies have found that nicotine may increase response accuracy and speed relative to a placebo.[80] The lack of acute and visible signs of cognitive and behavioral impairment may influence the perception that tobacco products are less harmful and not a focus of substance use treatment.

Fourth, e-cigarettes and other noncombustible tobacco products have become popular,[81] are perceived to aid in cigarette smoking cessation,[82] and have received support as a harm reduction strategy for tobacco use.[83] Nevertheless, reviews on this topic[81] and a recent report of the surgeon general[84] have strongly warned against the use of e-cigarettes as a harm reduction strategy owing to the lack of evidence for its safety and efficacy in reducing or quitting smoking. Thus, physician endorsement of e-cigarettes and similar devices as a way to reduce harm is not recommended and cessation of e-cigarette should be encouraged.

There are indeed counterpoints to all of these issues, but it is important to note that these beliefs against the treatment of tobacco use exist, and are commonly held by patients and treatment providers alike. It is often the case that treatment providers are former alcohol or substance users,[85] and former (or current) tobacco users themselves.[69,86,87] These providers in recovery are likely to have personal experiences that limit their motivation to urge those in treatment for AUD/SUD to stop smoking. Owing to these arguments, it is necessary to address each of these issues, as well as others, and provide compelling evidence for the provision of tobacco cessation services to those in treatment for AUD/SUD.

WHY ALCOHOL USE DISORDER/SUBSTANCE USE DISORDER TREATMENT PROVIDERS SHOULD ENCOURAGE TOBACCO CESSATION

Although it is indeed the case that tobacco use is both legal and does not cause marked inebriation, it remains a very harmful behavior to those with AUD/SUD, especially considering that 50% of concurrent users die from tobacco use.[14] Other issues raised with evidence-based supportive research are addressed herein.

Quitting Smoking Will Not Cause a Relapse in Alcohol or Substance Use

Concerns that smoking cessation will result in a relapse of alcohol or other substances[73] have been directly challenged by research. A number of studies have found either no association between smoking cessation and alcohol or substance use relapse,[72,88,89] or that smoking cessation actually improves AUD/SUD outcomes.[90–93] For instance, Stuyt[94] reported on the 1-year outcomes of a group of alcohol or substance users that received inpatient addiction treatment. No significant effect on the duration of sobriety after treatment was observed regarding primary drug of use of participants, but the duration of sobriety between tobacco users and nontobacco users was significantly different; nontobacco users (including nonsmokers at time of entry and those who engaged in cessation during treatment) had nearly twice the duration of sobriety time compared with tobacco users (6.9 vs 3.9 months of sobriety, respectively). Prochaska[95] has provided an extensive overview of this literature, and Prochaska and colleagues[96] completed a metaanalysis of 19 randomized, controlled trials evaluating tobacco treatment interventions for individuals with substance use problems. This metaanalysis indicated that smoking cessation interventions were associated with a 25% increased likelihood of long-term abstinence from alcohol and illicit drugs. Further, other work suggests that these benefits exist for the longer term; De Soto and colleagues[97] found that 10-year abstention from alcohol and smoking are highly correlated. Taken together, these findings suggest that smoking cessation dramatically improves treatment success for AUD/SUD.

Concurrent versus Successive Treatment Could Affect Outcomes

Regarding the timing of AUD/SUD and smoking cessation, study results are mixed. Some research has demonstrated that concurrent treatment for tobacco and AUD/SUD improves the outcomes of tobacco alone (with no detriment to AUD/SUD outcomes) or of both substances,[91,96,98–100] but studies in this area suffer from notable methodologic limitations, including nonrandomized designs.[101]

In contrast, recent work has suggested that concurrent treatment may have adverse effects on the outcomes for primary drug treatment.[102] Joseph and colleagues[102] randomized 499 smokers with AUD to a concurrent (during alcohol treatment) or delayed (6 months later) smoking cessation intervention. All individuals received the same cognitive–behavioral treatment that included nicotine replacement therapy. Results indicated that, although smoking cessation rates were similar at 18 months (12.4% vs 13.7%), abstinence and prolonged abstinence rates for alcohol were significantly worse in the concurrent (vs delayed) treatment group at the 6 (41% vs 56%), 12 (33% vs 42%), and 18 month (41% vs 48%) follow-ups.[102]

As noted by others,[103] it is difficult for individuals to make multiple health behavior changes, suggesting that the timing of intervention (concurrent vs delayed tobacco cessation provision) may be best decided in the collaborative relationship between the treatment provider and patient. Work in related areas has suggested that considerable economic savings are associated with the joint behavior change,[104] indicating that, regardless of the timing, tobacco cessation services for those with AUD/SUD provide benefits to both the individual and the community.

Smoking Bans Do Not Affect Admissions

There is evidence that those in AUD/SUD treatment are interested in tobacco cessation, even among military personnel, who smoke at higher rates than the general population.[105] One may argue that expectations for smoking cessation (eg, facility-wide bans) may decrease the engagement of patients in substance use programs. Nevertheless, patients in such programs have been shown to lower resistance to such expectations over time; Brown and colleagues[106] surveyed substance use treatment facility administrators in New York before and after tobacco-free regulation implementation. These regulations increased tobacco screening and cessation services (including pharmacotherapies) among settings, and increased support for policies was demonstrated. Importantly, although patient resistance was reported, patient admissions did not decrease.[106]

Alcohol Use Disorder/Substance Use Disorder Treatment Patients Actually Want to Quit Smoking

Despite potential concerns about adverse effects on craving and sobriety, evidence suggests that those in treatment for AUD/SUD know about the harms of smoking, are interested in quitting smoking, and are willing to consider to smoking cessation during their treatment.[68,107] McClure and colleagues[107] found that 80% of individuals in opioid use disorder treatment who were receiving opioid agonist treatment would consider trying the nicotine patch to stop smoking, and more than 40% would try nicotine gum. Kozlowski and colleagues[68] surveyed clients of the Addiction Research Foundation and found that 46% indicated that they were "moderately" to "very much" interested in receiving smoking cessation services, although there was a consistent preference for receipt of services after their alcohol or drug problem was treated.

TREATMENT

Smoking cessation for those in treatment for AUD/SUD should be multifaceted, with both behavioral therapy and medication. We describe recommended smoking cessation medications and their potential positive effects on alcohol or other substance use. Then, describe traditional psychological smoking cessation techniques are described, and emergent techniques that can be used with success across different substance use treatment settings are presented.

Pharmacotherapies for Smoking Cessation

The most widely used pharmacotherapies for smoking cessation include nicotine replacement therapy and nonnicotine products such as bupropion hydrochloride (Zyban) and varenicline (Chantix). Each is approved by the Food and Drug Administration for smoking cessation,[108] and each may be used in conjunction with pharmacotherapies for other addictions. Treatment is based on the individual case.

Bupropion is an antidepressant with simulant properties that inhibits the reuptake of norepinephrine and dopamine, and has shown to be an effective pharmacologic aid in smoking cessation. Little work exists regarding the additional benefits of bupropion for alcohol or other drug craving or use. Although 1 study has indicated that bupropion may reduce the craving and effect of methamphetamine,[109] bupropion has not demonstrated efficacy for the treatment of AUD.[110] Nicotine replacement therapy is one of the most well-studied pharmacotherapies for smoking, and is available over the counter in the form of a transdermal patch, gum, or lozenge. Nicotine replacement therapy inhalers and nasal mist are available by prescription. Although there are few known benefits of nicotine replacement therapy for the reduction of alcohol or other substance use, some work has suggested that nicotine replacement therapy administration reduces positive subjective alcohol response and urges to drink.[111,112]

Varenicline is a selective α4 β2 partial nicotinic receptor agonist that diminishes nicotine's reinforcing effects. Currently, varenicline is the most effective medication for smoking cessation.[113–115] The benefits of varenicline include few side effects, and a lack of pharmacologic interaction with other medications owing to the fact that varenicline is not metabolized. Recent randomized trials with varenicline suggest that it may be effective at reducing alcohol use and craving.[116–119] However, warnings and precautions issued by the Food and Drug Administration indicate that patients may experience adverse effects when taking varenicline and drinking alcohol, including decreased tolerance to alcohol, increased drunkenness, unusual or aggressive behavior, or no memory of things that happened.[120] Thus, it is recommended that providers use varenicline with caution in patients with AUD.

Interestingly, recent work has also tested the possibility of using varenicline for opioid withdrawal. Based on work that found a relation between nicotinic acetylcholine receptor and opioid dependence, a placebo-controlled pilot study by Hooten and Warner[121] sought to test whether varenicline could decrease opioid withdrawal symptoms in patients with chronic pain during detoxification. In this small sample (only 7 patients remained in the varenicline group through completion of the study), results demonstrated that opioid withdrawal in patients receiving varenicline decreased over time whereas opioid withdrawal in patients receiving placebo increased, although results were not significant (regression coefficients were -0.116 and 0.086, respectively; $P = .26$).[121] Relatedly, in another study, varenicline was not effective for smoking cessation in smokers who were opiate dependent and undergoing methadone treatment.[122] Because this work is preliminary, further investigation of varenicline as a pharmacotherapy for concomitant smoking and AUD/SUD is warranted.

Psychological Treatments

The US Department of Health and Human Services recommended that pharmacologic treatments for smoking be accompanied by cognitive–behavioral therapy.[90] Cognitive–behavioral therapy helps individuals to learn to identify and correct maladaptive cognitions and behaviors. Accepted cognitive behavioral treatments for smoking cessation in medical settings include the "5 A's" model (ie, ask about use, advise to quit, assess willingness to make a quit attempt, assist in the quit attempt, and arrange follow-up) and motivational enhancement via discussion of the "5 R's (eg, relevance, risks, rewards, roadblocks, and repetition). These skills can be directly applied to those with AUD/SUD in the course of treatment. Other recommended cognitive–behavioral therapy skills include goal setting/making a commitment, self-monitoring of behavior, avoidance of triggers, management of cravings through alternative activities, problem-solving skills, and augmenting social support. Importantly, all of these techniques are common across treatment for different forms of substance use.[123,124]

There are also emergent areas of treatment provision that may be applicable to both tobacco use and other forms of substance use. One emergent treatment approach is behavioral economics, a model developed through psychology and economics that seeks to explain and ultimately treat the lapses in decision making commonly seen in substance users.[125] These lapses in judgment are notable in moments of extreme craving, where short-term reinforcement seems to be more valuable than the long-term goal of sobriety, thereby leading to lapse and relapse behavior.

Complementary to behavioral economics, specific forms of problem solving and mindfulness-based therapy targeting emotion regulation and the reduction of impulsive action are believed to directly address impulsivity and delay discounting deficits. Evidence demonstrates that mindfulness-based substance use treatment is effective in decreasing impulsivity, improving emotion regulation, and increasing perceived drug risk.[126,127] Moreover, a recent metaanalysis investigating the efficacy of mindfulness for smoking cessation on long-term follow-up (6 months) found that mindfulness may be as effective as other smoking cessation treatments (odds ratio, 2.52; 95% confidence interval, 0.76–8.29),[128] and individual studies have supported the efficacy of mindfulness-based approaches in relapse prevention (effect size d = 0.88, indicating a large effect size).[129] Other randomized controlled studies that have addressed potential mechanisms of mindfulness-based substance use treatment have found no significant differences with cognitive–behavioral therapy, but significant differences compared with usual care (eg, decreased anxiety, cravings, and dependence).[130]

Aside from cognitive–behavioral therapy-based methods, a related area of substance use treatment is contingency management, or reinforcing abstinence through external rewards.[131] Several clinical trials have supported the efficacy of contingency management for smoking,[92,132] alcohol,[133] cocaine,[134] and opioid use.[135] Metaanalytic reviews indicate that contingency management generates moderate effect sizes (Cohen's ds between 0.31 and 0.65, indicating small to medium effect sizes) in reducing multiple forms of substance use and other externalizing behaviors,[131,136] indicating impressive efficacy, but long-term financial feasibility has remained a significant limitation to its long-term use in most treatment settings.

Notably, combined treatment methods for smoking and AUD/SUD are lacking in this literature, despite the many common ingredients of successful treatment across these substances. Given the economic barriers to treatment (reduced duration of approved treatment and few resources available to physicians and other addiction treatment providers), the development of combined treatment methods may be of considerable individual and economic value. Although some mixed findings regarding concurrent treatment success likely dampen enthusiasm, it is clear that this work is in its infancy, and more sophisticated methods for evaluation of treatment components are becoming available. For instance, adaptive intervention methods can be developed to construct individualized treatment that varies in sequencing and intensity according to patient response, risk, burden, adherence, and preference.[137] Such modeling would be of considerable value in those with comorbid tobacco and AUD/SUD.

Relapse Prevention

It is notable that all forms of substance use come with a high risk of relapse. Smoking, for instance, is estimated to have a relapse rate of 10% per year after 1 year of abstinence.[138] Relapse prevention focuses on identifying high-risk relapse situations and problem solving possible urges to use. In addition, other skills include emotion regulation, goal adherence, and social support. Although relapse prevention is often used as a part of smoking cessation (and other substance use treatment), results from empirical work are not entirely encouraging. A metaanalysis reviewing the efficacy of 26 different relapse prevention programs for smoking, AUD, and SUD found only a small effect (r = 0.14).[139] Thus, although relapse prevention is intuitively a good practice, research does not suggest that patients are successful at using preventative skills long after treatment has ended.

It should be noted that relapse prevention in those with tobacco use and AUD/SUD may also include psychoeducation regarding the comorbidity of these behaviors, as well as the potential increases in relapse of AUD/SUD with smoking relapse. Other studies have indicated that smokers with AUD/SUD who are not ready to quit benefit from psychoeducation practices[140]; it is likely that this kind information can help former smokers with AUD/SUD to resist temptations to smoke after cessation in light of the considerable consequences to their sobriety.

SUMMARY

Many reviews of the comorbidity of smoking and AUD/SUD exist, and a number of studies have been directed at understanding concomitant risk, barriers to treatment, and the need for smoking cessation in AUD/SUD populations. These efforts have only indirectly impacted the field of practice, as evidenced by alarmingly low rates of available smoking cessation programs in AUD/SUD treatment settings, despite interest and need. Dissemination of empirically validated methods to reduce dangerous comorbid behaviors is important. It is also imperative for physicians and other addiction treatment providers to promote smoking cessation across all treatment foci to increase healthy behavior and challenge the misconception of incompatibility between smoking cessation and AUD/SUD treatment.

ACKNOWLEDGMENTS

The editors thank Hilary A. Tindle, Vanderbilt Center for Tobacco, Addiction and Lifestyle, Vanderbilt University Medical Center, for providing a critical review of this article.

REFERENCES

1. Salgado-Garcia FI, Cooper TV, Taylor T. Craving effect of smoking cues in smoking and antismoking stimuli in light smokers. Addict Behav 2013;38(10):2492–9.

2. Tverdal A, Bjartveit K. Health consequences of pipe versus cigarette smoking. Tob Control 2011;20(2):123–30.

3. Franceschini N, Deng Y, Flessner MF, et al. Smoking patterns and chronic kidney disease in US Hispanics: Hispanic Community Health Study/Study of Latinos. Nephrol Dial Transplant 2016;31(10):1670–6.

4. U.S. Department of Health and Human Services. The health consequences of smoking—50 years of progress: a report of the surgeon general. Atlanta (GA): U.S. Department of Health and Human Services; 2014.

5. Centers for Disease Control and Prevention. Cigarette smoking among adults—United States, 2005–2015. Morb Mortal Wkly Rep 2016;65(44):1205–11.

6. Grant BF, Hasin DS, Chou S, et al. Nicotine dependence and psychiatric disorders in the united states: results from the National Epidemiologic Survey on Alcohol and Related Conditions. Arch Gen Psychiatry 2004;61(11):1107–15.

7. Kalman D, Morissette SB, George TP. Co-morbidity of smoking in patients with psychiatric and substance use disorders. Am J Addict 2005;14(2):106–23.

8. Lasser K, Boyd JW, Woolhandler S, et al. Smoking and mental illness: a population-based prevalence study. Jama 2000;284(20):2606–10.

9. Gulliver SB, Kalman D, Rohsenow DJ, et al. Smoking and drinking among alcoholics in treatment: cross-sectional and longitudinal relationships. J Stud Alcohol 2000;61(1):157–63.

10. Hughes JR. Treating smokers with current or past alcohol dependence. American Journal of Health Behavior 1996;20:286–90.

11. Hughes J. Do smokers with current or past alcoholism need different or more intensive treatment? Alcohol Clin Exp Res 2002;26(12):1934–5.

12. Sobell MB. Alcohol and tobacco: clinical and treatment issues. Alcohol Clin Exp Res 2002;26(12):1954–5.

13. Marks JL, Hill EM, Pomerleau CS, et al. Nicotine dependence and withdrawal in alcoholic and nonalcoholic ever-smokers. J Subst Abuse Treat 1997;14(6): 521–7.

14. Hurt RD, Offord KP, Croghan IT, et al. Mortality following inpatient addictions treatment. Role of tobacco use in a community-based cohort. Jama 1996; 275(14):1097–103.

15. Substance Abuse and Mental Health Services Administration. Center for Behavioral Health Statistics and Quality. The N-SSATS report: tobacco cessation services. Rockville (MD): MD Substance Abuse and Mental Health Services Administration,; 2013. p. 2013.

16. 2008 PHS Guideline Update Panel, Liaisons, and Staff. Treating tobacco use and dependence: 2008 update U.S. Public health service clinical practice guideline executive summary. Respir Care 2008;53(9):1217–22.

17. Swan GE, Carmelli D, Cardon LR. The consumption of tobacco, alcohol, and coffee in Caucasian male twins: a multivariate genetic analysis. J Subst Abuse 1996;8(1):19–31.

18. Schilström B, Nomikos G, Nisell M, et al. N-methyl-D-aspartate receptor antagonism in the ventral tegmental area diminishes the systemic nicotine-induced dopamine release in the nucleus accumbens. Neuroscience 1997;82(3):781–9.

19. Clarke PB. Mesolimbic Dopamine Activation—The Key to Nicotine Reinforcement?. Bock J, Marsh J, editors. In Ciba Foundation Symposium 152- The Biology of Nicotine Dependence.

20. Awtry TL, Werling LL. Acute and chronic effects of nicotine on serotonin uptake in prefrontal cortex and hippocampus of rats. Synapse 2003;50(3):206–11.

21. Bang SJ, Commons KG. Age-dependent effects of initial exposure to nicotine on serotonin neurons. Neuroscience 2011;179:1–8.

22. Picciotto MR, Zoli M, Rimondini R, et al. Acetylcholine receptors containing the beta2 subunit are involved in the reinforcing properties of nicotine. Nature 1998; 391(6663):173.

23. Kishioka S, Kiguchi N, Kobayashi Y, et al. Nicotine effects and the endogenous opioid system. J Pharmacol Sci 2014;125(2):117–24.

24. Xue Y, Domino EF. Tobacco/nicotine and endogenous brain opioids. Prog Neuropsychopharmacol Biol Psychiatry 2008;32(5):1131–8.

25. Markou A, Paterson NE, Semenova S. Role of gamma-aminobutyric acid (GABA) and metabotropic glutamate receptors in nicotine reinforcement: potential pharmacotherapies for smoking cessation. Ann N Y Acad Sci 2004;1025: 491–503.

26. D'Souza MS, Markou A. The "Stop" and "Go" of nicotine dependence: role of GABA and glutamate. Cold Spring Harb Perspect Med 2013;3(6) [pii:a012146].

27. Perez de la Mora M, Mendez-Franco J, Salceda R, et al. Neurochemical effects of nicotine on glutamate and GABA mechanisms in the rat brain. Acta Physiol Scand 1991;141(2):241–50.

28. Picciotto M. Nicotine as a modulator of behavior: beyond the inverted U. Trends Pharmacol Sci 2003;23:494–9.

29. Kandel DB, Kandel ER. A molecular basis for nicotine as a gateway drug. N Engl J Med 2014;371(21):2038–9.

30. Tarter RE. Etiology of adolescent substance abuse: a developmental perspective. Am J Addict 2002;11(3):171–91.

31. Martin C, Earlywine M, Blackson TC, et al. Aggressivity, inattention, hyperactivity, and impulsivity in boys at high and low risk for substance abuse. J Abnorm Psychol 1994;22:177–203.

32. Doran N, Trim RS. The prospective effects of impulsivity on alcohol and tobacco use in a college sample. J Psychoactive Drugs 2013;45(5):379–85.

33. Balevich EC, Wein ND, Flory JD. Cigarette smoking and measures of impulsivity in a college sample. Subst Abuse 2013;34(3):256–62.

34. Mitchell MR, Potenza MN. Addictions and personality traits: impulsivity and related constructs. Curr Behav Neurosci Rep 2014;1(1):1–12.

35. Chase HW, Hogarth L. Impulsivity and symptoms of nicotine dependence in a young adult population. Nicotine Tob Res 2011;13(12):1321–5.

36. Holmes AJ, Hollinshead MO, Roffman JL, et al. Individual differences in cognitive control circuit anatomy link sensation seeking, impulsivity, and substance use. J Neurosci 2016;36(14):4038–49.

37. National Institute on Drug Abuse. Sensation seeking promotes initiation, impulsivity promotes escalation of substance use. 2016. Available at: https://www.drugabuse.gov/news-events/nida-notes/2016/05/sensation-seeking-promotes-initiation-impulsivity-promotes-escalation-substance-use. Accessed August 1, 2017.

38. Verdejo-García A, Lawrence AJ, Clark L. Impulsivity as a vulnerability marker for substance-use disorders: review of findings from high-risk research, problem gamblers and genetic association studies. Neurosci Biobehav Rev 2008;32(4):777–810.

39. Bickel WK, Marsch LA. Toward a behavioral economic understanding of drug dependence: delay discounting processes. Addiction 2001;96(1):73–86.

40. Sheffer C, MacKillop J, McGeary J, et al. Delay discounting, locus of control, and cognitive impulsiveness independently predict tobacco dependence treatment outcomes in a highly dependent, lower socioeconomic group of smokers. Am J Addict 2012;21(3):221–32.

41. Ashe ML, Newman MG, Wilson SJ. Delay discounting and the use of mindful attention versus distraction in the treatment of drug addiction: a conceptual review. J Exp Anal Behav 2015;103(1):234–48.

42. Bandura A. Social foundations of thought and action: a social cognitive theory. Englewood Cliffs (NJ): Prentice-Hall; 1986.

43. Petraitis J, Flay BR, Miller TQ. Reviewing theories of adolescent substance use: organizing pieces in the puzzle. Psychol Bull 1995;117(1):67–86.

44. Anda RF, Croft JB, Felitti VJ, et al. Adverse childhood experiences and smoking during adolescence and adulthood. Jama 1999;282(17):1652–8.

45. Dube SR, Anda RF, Felitti VJ, et al. Adverse childhood experiences and personal alcohol abuse as an adult. Addict behaviors 2002;27(5):713–25.

46. Dube SR, Felitti VJ, Dong M, et al. Childhood abuse, neglect, and household dysfunction and the risk of illicit drug use: the adverse childhood experiences study. Pediatrics 2003;111(3):564–72.

47. Chassin L, Curran PJ, Hussong AM, et al. The relation of parent alcoholism to adolescent substance use: a longitudinal follow-up study. J Abnorm Psychol 1996;105(1):70.

48. Patton GC, Carlin JB, Coffey C, et al. The course of early smoking: a population-based cohort study over three years. Addiction 1998;93(8):1251–60.

49. Webster RA, Hunter M, Keats JA. Peer and parental influences on adolescents' substance use: a path analysis. Int J Addict 1994;29(5):647–57.

50. West P, Sweeting H, Ecob R. Family and friends' influences on the uptake of regular smoking from mid-adolescence to early adulthood. Addiction 1999;94(9):1397–411.

51. Li C, Pentz MA, Chou C-P. Parental substance use as a modifier of adolescent substance use risk. Addiction 2002;97(12):1537–50.

52. Hu FB, Flay BR, Hedeker D, et al. The influences of friends' and parental smoking on adolescent smoking behavior: the effects of time and prior smoking1. J Appl Soc Psychol 1995;25(22):2018–47.

53. Regier DA, Farmer ME, Rae DS, et al. Comorbidity of mental disorders with alcohol and other drug abuse: results from the Epidemiologic Catchment Area (ECA) study. Jama 1990;264(19):2511–8.

54. Kessler RC, Crum RM, Warner LA, et al. Lifetime co-occurrence of DSM-III-R alcohol abuse and dependence with other psychiatric disorders in the National Comorbidity Survey. Arch Gen Psychiatry 1997;54(4):313–21.

55. Patton GC, Carlin JB, Coffey C, et al. Depression, anxiety, and smoking initiation: a prospective study over 3 years. Am J Public Health 1998;88(10):1518–22.

56. Grant BF, Stinson FS, Dawson DA, et al. Prevalence and co-occurrence of substance use disorders and independent mood and anxiety disorders: results from the national epidemiologic survey on alcohol and related conditions. Arch Gen Psychiatry 2004;61(8):807–16.

57. Acierno R, Kilpatrick DG, Resnick H, et al. Assault, PTSD, family substance use, and depression as risk factors for cigarette use in youth: findings from the National Survey of Adolescents. J Trauma Stress 2000;13(3):381–96.

58. Brown PJ, Stout RL, Mueller T. Substance use disorder and posttraumatic stress disorder comorbidity: addiction and psychiatric treatment rates. Psychol Addict Behav 1999;13(2):115.

59. Strakowski SM, DelBello MP. The co-occurrence of bipolar and substance use disorders. Clin Psychol Rev 2000;20(2):191–206.

60. Swann AC. The strong relationship between bipolar and substance-use disorder. Ann N Y Acad Sci 2010;1187(1):276–93.

61. Vanyukov MM, Tarter RE, Kirisci L, et al. Liability to substance use disorders: 1. Common mechanisms and manifestations. Neurosci Biobehavioral Rev 2003;27(6):507–15.

62. Helzer JE, Burnam A, McEvoy LT. Alcohol abuse and dependence. In: Robins LN, Regier DA, editors. Psychiatric disorders in America. The epidemiologic catchment area study. New York: The Free Press; 1991. p. 81–115.

63. Coper H. Cross-tolerance and cross-dependence between different types of addictive drugs. In: Fishman J, editor. The bases of addiction. Berlin: Abakon; 1978. p. 235–56.

64. Funk D, Marinelli PW, Le AD. Biological processes underlying co-use of alcohol and nicotine: neuronal mechanisms, cross-tolerance, and genetic factors. Alcohol Res Health 2006;29(3):186.

65. Kandel D, Yamaguchi K. From beer to crack: developmental patterns of drug involvement. Am J Public Health 1993;83(6):851–5.

66. Kirby T, Barry AE. Alcohol as a gateway drug: a study of US 12th graders. J Sch Health 2012;82(8):371–9.

67. Romberger DJ, Grant K. Alcohol consumption and smoking status: the role of smoking cessation. Biomed Pharmacother 2004;58(2):77–83.

68. Kozlowski LT, Skinner W, Kent C, et al. Prospects for smoking treatment in individuals seeking treatment for alcohol and other drug problems. Addict behaviors 1989;14(3):273–8.

69. Bobo JK, Slade J, Hoffman AL. Nicotine addiction counseling for chemically dependent patients. Psychiatr Serv 1995;46(9):945–7.

70. Daws C, Egan SJ, Allsop S. Brief intervention training for smoking cessation in substance use treatment. Aust Psychol 2013;48(5):353–9.

71. Joint Commission on the Accreditation of Healthcare Organizations. Accreditation manual for hospitals. Oakbrook Terrace (IL): Joint Commission on the Accreditation of Healthcare Organizations; 1992.

72. Hughes JR. Treatment of smoking cessation in smokers with past alcohol/drug problems. J Subst Abuse Treat 1993;10(2):181–7.

73. Asher MK, Martin RA, Rohsenow DJ, et al. Perceived barriers to quitting smoking among alcohol dependent patients in treatment. J Subst Abuse Treat 2003; 24(2):169–74.

74. Palfai TP, Monti PM, Ostafin B, et al. Effects of nicotine deprivation on alcohol-related information processing and drinking behavior. J Abnorm Psychol 2000;109:96–105.

75. Clemmey P, Brooner R, Chutuape MA, et al. Smoking habits and attitudes in a methadone maintenance treatment population. Drug Alcohol Depend 1997; 44(2–3):123–32.

76. Gould TJ. Addiction and cognition. Addict Sci Clin Pract 2010;5(2):4–14.

77. Crean RD, Crane NA, Mason BJ. An evidence based review of acute and long-term effects of cannabis use on executive cognitive functions. J Addict Med 2011;5(1):1–8.

78. Rezvani AH, Levin ED. Cognitive effects of nicotine. Biol Psychiatry 2001;49(3): 258–67.

79. Newhouse P, Kellar K, Aisen P, et al. Nicotine treatment of mild cognitive impairment: a 6-month double-blind pilot clinical trial. Neurology 2012;78(2):91–101.

80. Kumari V, Gray JA, Ffytche DH, et al. Cognitive effects of nicotine in humans: an fMRI study. Neuroimage 2003;19(3):1002–13.

81. Das S, Prochaska JJ. E-cigarettes, vaping, and other electronic nicotine products: harm reduction pathways or new avenues for addiction? Psychiatr Times 2017;34(8):24–5.

82. Sutfin EL, McCoy TP, Morrell HE, et al. Electronic cigarette use by college students. Drug Alcohol Depend 2013;131(3):214–21.

83. Nitzkin JL. The case in favor of E-cigarettes for tobacco harm reduction. Int J Environ Res Public Health 2014;11(6):6459–71.

84. U.S. Department of Health and Human Services. E-cigarette use among youth and young adults. A report of the surgeon general. Atlanta (GA): U.S. Department of Health and Human Services, Centers for Disease Control and Prevention; 2016.

85. Hecksher D. Former substance users working as counselors. A dual relationship. Subst Use Misuse 2007;42(8):1253–68.

86. Fuller BE, Guydish J, Tsoh J, et al. Attitudes toward the integration of smoking cessation treatment into drug abuse clinics. J Subst Abuse Treat 2007;32(1): 53–60.

87. Guydish J, Passalacqua E, Tajima B, et al. Staff smoking and other barriers to nicotine dependence intervention in addiction treatment settings: a review. J Psychoactive Drugs 2007;39(4):423–33.
88. Martin JE, Calfas KJ, Patten CA, et al. Prospective evaluation of three smoking interventions in 205 recovering alcoholics: one-year results of Project SCRAP-Tobacco. J Consult Clin Psychol 1997;65(1):190–4.
89. Reid MS, Fallon B, Sonne S, et al. Smoking cessation treatment in community-based substance abuse rehabilitation programs. J Subst Abuse Treat 2008; 35(1):68–77.
90. Frosch DL, Shoptaw S, Nahom D, et al. Associations between tobacco smoking and illicit drug use among methadone-maintained opiate-dependent individuals. Exp Clin Psychopharmacol 2000;8(1):97–103.
91. Bobo JK, McIlvain HE, Lando HA, et al. Effect of smoking cessation counseling on recovery from alcoholism: findings from a randomized community intervention trial. Addiction 1998;93:877–87.
92. Shoptaw S, Jarvik ME, Ling W, et al. Contingency management for tobacco smoking in methadone-maintained opiate addicts. Addict Behav 1996;21: 409–12.
93. Kohn CS, Tsoh JY, Weisner CM. Changes in smoking status among substance abusers: baseline characteristics and abstinence from alcohol and drugs at 12-month follow-up. Drug Alcohol Depend 2003;69(1):61–71.
94. Stuyt EB. Recovery rates after treatment for alcohol/drug dependence. Tobacco users vs. non-tobacco users. Am J Addict 1997;6(2):159–67.
95. Prochaska JJ. Failure to treat tobacco use in mental health and addiction treatment settings: a form of harm reduction? Drug Alcohol Depend 2010;110(3): 177–82.
96. Prochaska JJ, Delucchi K, Hall SM. A meta-analysis of smoking cessation interventions with individuals in substance abuse treatment or recovery. J Consult Clin Psychol 2004;72(6):1144–56.
97. De Soto CB, O'Donnell WE, De Soto JL. Long-term recovery in alcoholics. Alcohol Clin Exp Res 1989;13(5):693–7.
98. Cooney NL, Litt MD, Sevarino KA, et al. Concurrent alcohol and tobacco treatment: effect on daily process measures of alcohol relapse risk. J Consult Clin Psychol 2015;83(2):346–58.
99. Hurt RD, Eberman KM, Croghan IT, et al. Nicotine dependence treatment during inpatient treatment for other addictions: a prospective intervention trial. Alcohol Clin Exp Res 1994;18(4):867–72.
100. Joseph AM, Nichol KL, Anderson H. Effect of treatment for nicotine dependence on alcohol and drug treatment outcomes. Addict Behav 1993;18(6):635–44.
101. Kodl M, Fu SS, Joseph AM. Tobacco cessation treatment for alcohol-dependent smokers: when is the best time? Alcohol Res Health 2006;29(3):203–7.
102. Joseph AM, Willenbring ML, Nugent SM, et al. A randomized trial of concurrent versus delayed smoking intervention for patients in alcohol dependence treatment. J Stud Alcohol 2004;65(6):681–91.
103. Prochaska JJ, Spring B, Nigg CR. Multiple health behavior change research: an introduction and overview. Prev Med 2008;46(3):181–8.
104. Edington DW. Emerging research: a view from one research center. Am J Health Promot 2001;15(5):341–9.
105. Shealy SE, Winn JL. Integrating smoking cessation into substance use disorder treatment for military veterans: measurement and treatment engagement efforts. Addict Behav 2014;39(2):439–44.

106. Brown E, Nonnemaker J, Federman EB, et al. Implementation of a tobacco-free regulation in substance use disorder treatment facilities. J Subst Abuse Treat 2012;42(3):319–27.

107. McClure EA, Acquavita SP, Dunn KE, et al. Characterizing smoking, cessation services, and quit interest across outpatient substance abuse treatment modalities. J Subst Abuse Treat 2014;46(2):194–201.

108. U.S. Food and Drug Administration. FDA 101: smoking cessation products. 2016. Available at: https://www.fda.gov/ForConsumers/ConsumerUpdates/ucm198176.htm. Accessed August 7, 2017.

109. Newton TF, Roache JD, De La Garza R, et al. Bupropion reduces methamphetamine-induced subjective effects and cue-induced craving. Neuropsychopharmacology 2006;31(7):1537.

110. Ait-Daoud N, Lynch WJ, Penberthy JK, et al. Treating smoking dependence in depressed alcoholics. Alcohol Res Health 2007;29(3):213–20.

111. McKee SA, O'Malley SS, Shi J, et al. Effect of transdermal nicotine replacement on alcohol responses and alcohol self-administration. Psychopharmacology 2008;196(2):189–200.

112. Udo T, Harrison ELR, Shi J, et al. A preliminary study on the effect of combined nicotine replacement therapy on alcohol responses and alcohol self-administration. Am J Addict 2013;22(6):590–7.

113. Fagerström K, Hughes J. Varenicline in the treatment of tobacco dependence. Neuropsychiatr Dis Treat 2008;4(2):353–63.

114. Ebbert JO, Hughes JR, West RJ, et al. Effect of varenicline on smoking cessation through smoking reduction: a randomized clinical trial. Jama 2015;313(7):687–94.

115. Anthenelli RM, Benowitz NL, West R, et al. Neuropsychiatric safety and efficacy of varenicline, bupropion, and nicotine patch in smokers with and without psychiatric disorders (EAGLES): a double-blind, randomised, placebo-controlled clinical trial. Lancet 2016;387(10037):2507–20.

116. Mitchell JM, Teague CH, Kayser AS, et al. Varenicline decreases alcohol consumption in heavy-drinking smokers. Psychopharmacology 2012;223(3):299–306.

117. Erwin BL, Slaton RM. Varenicline in the treatment of alcohol use disorders. Ann Pharmacother 2014;48(11):1445–55.

118. Verplaetse TL, Pittman BP, Shi JM, et al. Effect of lowering the dose of varenicline on alcohol self-administration in drinkers with alcohol use disorders. J Addict Med 2016;10(3):166–73.

119. Litten RZ, Ryan ML, Fertig JB, et al. A double-blind, placebo-controlled trial assessing the efficacy of varenicline tartrate for alcohol dependence. J Addict Med 2013;7(4):277–86.

120. U.S. Food and Drug Administration. FDA drug safety communication: FDA updates label for stop smoking drug Chantix (varenicline) to include potential alcohol interaction, rare risk of seizures, and studies of side effects on mood, behavior, or thinking. 2015. Available at: https://www.fda.gov/Drugs/DrugSafety/ucm436494.htm. Accessed August 1, 2017.

121. Hooten WM, Warner DO. Varenicline for opioid withdrawal in patients with chronic pain: a randomized, single-blinded, placebo controlled pilot trial. Addict behaviors 2015;42:69–72.

122. Stein MD, Caviness CM, Kurth ME, et al. Varenicline for smoking cessation among methadone-maintained smokers: a randomized clinical trial. Drug Alcohol Depend 2013;133(2):486–93.

123. McHugh RK, Hearon BA, Otto MW. Cognitive-behavioral therapy for substance use disorders. Psychiatr Clin North Am 2010;33(3):511–25.

124. Fiore MC. US public health service clinical practice guideline: treating tobacco use and dependence. Respiratory care 2000;45(10):1200–62.

125. Bickel WK, Johnson MW, Koffarnus MN, et al. The behavioral economics of substance use disorders: reinforcement pathologies and their repair. Annu Rev Clin Psychol 2014;10:641–77.

126. Himelstein S. Mindfulness-based substance abuse treatment for incarcerated youth: a mixed method pilot study. Int J Transpers Stud 2011;30(1):3.

127. Tang YY, Tang R, Posner MI. Mindfulness meditation improves emotion regulation and reduces drug abuse. Drug Alcohol Depend 2016;163(Suppl 1):S13–8.

128. Maglione MA, Maher AR, Ewing B, et al. Efficacy of mindfulness meditation for smoking cessation: a systematic review and meta-analysis. Addict Behav 2017; 69:27–34.

129. Vidrine JI, Spears CA, Heppner WL, et al. Efficacy of Mindfulness Based Addiction Treatment (MBAT) for smoking cessation and lapse. J consulting Clin Psychol 2016;84(9):824–38.

130. Spears CA, Hedeker D, Li L, et al. Mechanisms underlying mindfulness-based addiction treatment versus cognitive behavioral therapy and usual care for smoking cessation. J Consult Clin Psychol 2017;85(11):1029–40.

131. Prendergast M, Podus D, Finney J, et al. Contingency management for treatment of substance use disorders: a meta-analysis. Addiction 2006;101(11): 1546–60.

132. Alessi SM, Petry NM, Urso J. Contingency management promotes smoking reductions in residential substance abuse patients. J Appl Behav Anal 2008;41(4): 617–22.

133. Petry NM, Martin B, Cooney JL, et al. Give them prizes, and they will come: contingency management for treatment of alcohol dependence. J consulting Clin Psychol 2000;68(2):250–7.

134. Higgins ST, Wong CJ, Badger GJ, et al. Contingent reinforcement increases cocaine abstinence during outpatient treatment and 1 year of follow-up. J consulting Clin Psychol 2000;68(1):64–72.

135. Petry NM, Martin B. Low-cost contingency management for treating cocaine- and opioid-abusing methadone patients. J consulting Clin Psychol 2002; 70(2):398–405.

136. Petry NM, Alessi SM, Olmstead TA, et al. Contingency management treatment for substance use disorders: how far has it come, and where does it need to go? Psychol Addict Behav 2017;31(8):897–906.

137. Murphy SA. An experimental design for the development of adaptive treatment strategies. Stat Med 2005;24(10):1455–81.

138. Hughes JR, Peters EN, Naud S. Relapse to smoking after 1 year of abstinence: a meta-analysis. Addict behaviors 2008;33(12):1516–20.

139. Irvin JE, Bowers CA, Dunn ME, et al. Efficacy of relapse prevention: a meta-analytic review. J consulting Clin Psychol 1999;67(4):563–70.

140. Rohsenow DJ, Monti PM, Colby SM, et al. Brief interventions for smoking cessation in alcoholic smokers. Alcohol Clin Exp Res 2002;26(12):1950–1.

Printed and bound by CPI Group (UK) Ltd, Croydon, CR0 4YY

03/10/2024

01040388-0005